**Basic Cardiac
Electrophysiology
for the Clinician**

Dedications

To Paloma, Andrea, David, Marina, Obi, Kachi, Celina, Sofía, Ilán, Sebastián, Josyane, Jean-Pierre and Late Chief C.N. Anumonwo, the Iyase of Ogwashi-Uku, Delta State, Nigeria.

Basic Cardiac Electrophysiology for the Clinician

Second Edition

José Jalife, MD
The Cyrus and Jane Farrehi Professor of Cardiovascular Research
Professor of Internal Medicine
Professor of Molecular & Integrative Physiology Co-Director
Center for Arrhythmia Research
University of Michigan
Ann Arbor, Michigan
USA

Mario Delmar, MD, PhD
Frank Norman Wilson Professor of Cardiovascular Medicine
Professor of Internal Medicine
Molecular & Integrative Physiology Co-Director, Center for Arrhythmia Research
University of Michigan
Ann Arbor, Michigan
USA

Justus Anumonwo, PhD
Assistant Professor of Internal Medicine
Cardiovascular Medicine
University of Michigan
Ann Arbor, Michigan
USA

Omer Berenfeld, PhD
Assistant Professor of Internal Medicine and Biomedical Engineering
Cardiovascular Medicine
University of Michigan
Ann Arbor, Michigan
USA

Jérôme Kalifa, MD, PhD
Assistant Professor of Internal Medicine
Cardiovascular Medicine
University of Michigan
Ann Arbor, Michigan
USA

WILEY-BLACKWELL

A John Wiley & Sons, Ltd., Publication

Library of Congress Cataloging-in-Publication Data

Basic cardiac electrophysiology for the clinician / Jose Jalife . . . [et al.]. – 2nd ed.
  p. ; cm.
Includes bibliographical references and index.
ISBN 978-1-4051-8333-8
  1. Heart–Electric properties. 2. Electrophysiology. 3. Arrhythmia. 4. Heart conduction system.
I. Jalife, Jose.
  [DNLM: 1. Heart–physiology. 2. Electrophysiology. WG 202 B3107 2009]
QP112.5.E46B37 2009
612.1'71–dc22

                                2008045638

ISBN 9781405183338

A catalogue record for this book is available from the British Library.

Set in 9.5 on 12 pt Palatino by SNP Best-set Typesetter Ltd., Hong Kong
Printed & bound in Malaysia by Vivar Printing Sdn Bhd

1 2009

Contents

Acknowledgments

Special thanks to the Jalife, Delmar, Anumonwo, Berenfeld and Kalifa families for their love, patience and unconditional support. We are also deeply indebted to all students, postdoctoral fellows, and technicians who throughout the years have contributed their work and ideas to our research program. Many of the concepts presented in this book are direct results of such contributions. We particularly thank all the current scientists, technicians, and clerical staff of the Center for Arrhythmia Research of the University of Michigan for their exceptional courage in following our lead and for sharing our vision for a bright future in the study of intercellular communication and cardiac impulse propagation. The unreserved support of our fearless administrator, Laurie Lebouef, is greatly appreciated. Thanks to Sherry Morgenstern, our in-house artist who helped with the figures. Our thanks go also to Doug Zipes, who generously took time from his busy schedule to read the manuscripts and write the forewords for the two editions of this book. We are obliged to Dr. David Pinsky, Dr. Hakan Oral, and Dr. Fred Morady and to the leadership of the University of Michigan Health System for helping make our dream for a Center for Arrhythmia Research a reality with a bright outlook. Much of the work presented was made possible by generous grants from the National Heart, Lung and Blood Institute; National Institutes of Health; the American Heart Association, Inc.; and the Heart Rhythm Society for the last 28 years.

José Jalife, MD
Mario Delmar, MD, PhD
Justus Anumonwo, PhD
Omer Berenfeld, PhD
Jérôme Kalifa, MD, PhD

Foreword to the Second Edition

A popular series of books includes the words *for dummies* in the title, to indicate the information contained has been modified so that readers—certainly not dummies, just less knowledgeable about the topic can more easily understand the subject matter presented. In fact, writing such a book requires the authors to have an even greater grasp of the material than other experts in the field because they must be able to explain complex concepts in ways the uninitiated can understand. This is accomplished by eliminating jargon and superfluous information characteristic of usual scientific writing, and explaining the "taken for granted" information in detail, i.e., focusing on the core of the topic for the less sophisticated student. Judging by the enormous success of the series, the concept is effective. In fact, Dr. Jalife and his colleagues wrote such a book about basic cardiac electrophysiology 10 years ago and have now updated and richly illustrated it with the wealth of new information attained in the last decade. As they indicate in the Introduction, the book is for all types of students of the heart—medical students, residents, fellows, postdocs, and faculty, whether basic or clinical—to educate and interest them in understanding cardiac electrophysiology and arrhythmias. It goes without saying that the basic scientist early in his or her career would be interested in such a book: I wish I had one when I started 40 years ago. But what needs to be said is that the clinician should be interested in this topic as well because acquiring this knowledge, even in its rudimentary form, will enable him or her to be more effective in critically evaluating published literature, understanding the basis of various clinical syndromes and arrhythmias, and, in the end, making more intelligent diagnostic and therapeutic decisions. From a personal perspective, I think I have been a better clinician because of my understanding of basic cardiac electrophysiology, knowledge "from cell to bedside." In the final analysis, the goal of virtually every medical scientist and physician is to provide better care for patients. This book brings the doctor closer to achieving that end and I recommend it to every student of the heart.

Douglas P. Zipes, MD
Distinguished Professor of Medicine, Pharmacology and Toxicology
Director, Division of Cardiology and Krannert Institute of Cardiology
Indiana University School of Medicine

Foreword to the First Edition

Finally a book for the clinician that explains basic cardiac electrophysiology! Pepe Jalife and his colleagues have done it at last, based on a series of lectures they presented to residents, fellows, and faculty members of the divisions of cardiology and pediatric cardiology at SLTNY Health Science Center in Syracuse, New York. Their course, "Basic Cardiac Electrophysiology for Clinical Fellows," became exceedingly popular as clinicians realized the importance of what they were learning and that this information could help them make decisions, which directly impacted on choices for patient care. This type of lecture series, with its subsequent book, could only be given by a group of scientists with feet firmly planted in the animal laboratory and at the bedside. Indeed this group of electrophysiologists represent precisely that skill set. Further, they do this in a fashion that eschews the jargon of the profession that ordinarily is certain to drive off would-be students. The importance of their teaching is underscored by the breakthrough observations over the past several years on the genetic basis for the "ionopathy" responsible for the congenital Long QT Syndrome. Knowledge of this type will increment and include more and more diseases as we hurdle toward the 21st century and the practice of genetic-based medicine. A firm grasp of the electrophysiological basis of the principles for the normal and abnormal heartbeat will be required, and *Basic Cardiac Electrophysiology for the Clinician* provides this information. Their work is very much "all you need to know, as clinicians, about basic cardiac electrophysiology but were afraid to ask." Each chapter has a similar format, beginning with an introduction and ending with a summary. I found that very helpful, and so should the clinician. Further, the figures avoid complexity and vividly make the points the authors seek to convey.

Chapter 1 deals with the bioelectricity of cardiac electrophysiology and discusses how the laws of electricity apply to movement of ions across cell membranes, using standard concepts about voltage, current, resistance, and capacitance. Basic concepts of action potentials and their differences in muscle, sinus and AV nodes, and Purkinje fibers help explain many of the clinical phenomena observed. There is a useful discussion on methodology to understand which currents flow through the various ion channels, such as use of voltage clamp method. Finally, the concept of rectification can be understood!

Chapter 2 introduces the various components responsible for the currents underlying cardiac excitation that are carried by ion channels, pumps or exchangers, and the differences between them. Gating and ion selectivity are discussed along with the various currents and the molecular structure of cardiac ion channels. The M and H gates, postulated by Hodgkin and Huxley, are explained in the light of the three confirmational states of closed, open and inactivated ion channels.

In Chapter 3 the authors present mechanisms of ion channel regulation, including enzyme systems, signaling pathways and autonomic regulation of ionic currents. Understanding control of ion channel regulation may provide insight into methods of therapeutic intervention when these systems go awry.

Chapter 4 offers a critical discussion of the concept of propagation of the cardiac impulse, explaining how the electrical signal spreads from cell to cell through the cardiac synctium to induce electrical activation of the entire heart. This chapter capitalizes on the basic information presented in the previous three chapters. A key concept, electrotonus, is clearly explained.

Intrinsic to the heartbeat is the concept of pacemaker activity, with the sinus node as the obvious prototypic example. Chapter 5 considers in-depth sinus node function, the synchronization of all of the sinus node cells to discharge in unison, phase response curves and entrainment and resetting, along with vagal modulation of sinus node activity. Many of these concepts are then applied to parasystolic foci and electrotonic modulation.

Chapter 6 focuses on rate dependent modulation of discontinuous action potential propagation, a concept underlying complex patterns of propagation such as Wenckebach and development of arrhythmias such as fibrillation. Most investigators are unaware that propagation, when viewed microscopically, is actually step wise as electrotonic currents propagate from cell to cell. Macroscopically, the action potential appears to travel uniformly and continuously. Differences in cell geometry and ionic currents, as well as non-uniform distribution of gap junctions connecting neighboring myocytes, contribute to non-uniform discontinuous propagation.

Chapter 7 is "bread and butter" for any clinical electrophysiologist and discusses clearly and at length the cellular mechanisms underlying the basic for cardiac arrhythmias. Thus, abnormal impulse formation, including normal and abnormal automaticity and triggered activity, along with alterations in conduction of the cardiac impulse that provide the basis for reentry, underlie all the therapeutic interventions used to treat patients with arrhythmias.

Chapter 8 extends these concepts by focusing in on spiral wave activity, which may be the basis for functional reentry. This chapter, to me, emphasizes a major aspect of the contributions from the Syracuse group of electrophysiologists: their insights into mechanisms of cardiac electrophysiology are rooted in "biological laws of nature," from phase response curves and resetting of parasystolic foci to spiral wave activity. One can only do this if the investigators have a clear understanding of the fundamental electrical phenomena responsible for the genesis of the heartbeat. Jalife and his group clearly demonstrate this breathtaking expanse of knowledge and it comes through vividly to the reader in chapter after chapter. This book is an exciting contribution for anyone interested in cardiac electrophysiology.

Douglas P. Zipes, MD
Distinguished Professor of Medicine, Pharmacology and Toxicology
Director, Division of Cardiology and Krannert Institute of Cardiology
Indiana University School of Medicine

Introduction

The genesis of the heartbeat is a biological process that depends on electrical phenomena that are intrinsic to the heart itself. The study of the fundamental basis of such phenomena is essential to cardiology, not only because it serves as the source from which current knowledge in clinical cardiac electrophysiology (EP) is based but, most importantly, because electrical diseases of the heart are a major health problem in society and clinical practice. In this regard, the rate of increase in our knowledge of cardiac EP has accelerated dramatically over the past 40 years. A wide variety of basic mechanisms is already well described in the experimental laboratory. Furthermore, the field has been enriched by concepts derived from other disciplines, including genetics, molecular biology, cell biology, biochemistry, biophysics, and computer modeling. Yet although several tools have been developed for the identification of the cellular mechanisms of clinical arrhythmias (mapping systems, pharmacologic agents, pacing, etc.), the understanding of the mechanisms and the appropriate treatment of such arrhythmias continue to be very difficult tasks. Nevertheless, many patients benefit annually from the use of devices or other advanced treatments aimed at diagnosis and therapy of electric diseases, and many of such advances can be traced directly to research in the basic EP laboratory.

Future progress may depend on enhanced understanding of the fundamental mechanisms underlying the heart's electrical behavior and on improved methods for detection of bioelectric phenomena and mathematical approaches to analyze more accurately the complex nonlinear processes underlying normal and abnormal cardiac rhythms. Thus, a precise quantitative understanding of electrical diseases is a major challenge faced by both basic scientists and clinicians. Achieving that understanding should have significant health benefits and should be greatly accelerated by multidisciplinary approaches that bring clinical and basic investigators to work together on

Basic Cardiac Electrophysiology for the Clinician, 2nd edition. By J. Jalife, M. Delmar, J. Anumonwo, O. Berenfeld and J. Kalifa. Published 2009 by Blackwell Publishing, ISBN: 978-1-4501-8333-8.

such a common goal. Then basic cardiac EP will play a major role in the future of clinical EP, including applications to diagnosis and therapy.

The original idea for the first edition of this book, published in 1998, materialized many years ago as a result of many informal but enlightening conversations with our dear friend and colleague, Dr. Winston Gaum, now at the University of Rochester, when he was Chief of Pediatric Cardiology at the SUNY Upstate Medical University in Syracuse, NY. This led to a series of lectures given by the authors in the 1990s to pediatric and adult cardiology residents, fellows, and faculty members at SUNY Upstate. The course, entitled "Basic Cardiac Electrophysiology for Clinical Fellows," was designed as a review of fundamental principles of EP and cellular mechanisms of arrhythmias, with the goal of refreshing our students' memories about long forgotten academic material seen during the first and second years of medical school. In addition, we had a hidden, more selfish agenda in mind. First, we wished to demonstrate to those students that such basic principles were not useless esoteric "stuff" in which only basic scientists were interested but in fact represented a solid basis for the rational management of their patients in their daily clinical practice. Second, and more important for us, we wished to spread the virus of our enthusiasm for basic cardiac EP and biophysics among those students and to entice at least a few of them to spend some time working in the basic EP laboratory. Fortunately, we succeeded on both counts. In fact, shortly after the course started, our students began to make the connection between the newly refreshed basic concepts and their knowledge of clinical electrocardiography and EP. Henceforth, the course became a series of scholarly and interesting discussions between basic scientists and clinicians. Most importantly, our success in infecting our students with the enthusiasm-for-basic-EP virus became clearly apparent shortly after completion of the course, when our clinical faculty began to encourage their fellows in cardiology and pediatric cardiology to spend 6 months to 1 year working on basic research projects under the supervision of one of us. This led to a steady flow of fellows through our laboratories, which continues to this date and is likely to continue for years to come.

This second edition of *Basic Cardiac Electrophysiology for the Clinician* represents a significant enhancement over the first edition. Outdated material has been omitted and previously existing chapters have been updated and carefully revised for errors (we thank Prof. Ketaro Hashimoto and his students for kindly pointing out some of those errors to us). In addition, three completely new chapters (Chapters 8–10) have been added.

In Chapter 1, we discuss some of the basic principles for applying concepts of basic electricity to the movement of ions across cell membranes. We start with the concept that the transmembrane flow of ions leads to electric currents and the displacement of charges across the cell membrane capacitor establishes the membrane potential. We review also some fundamental principles that determine the electric properties of the cell at rest and during activation, as well as the technology and concepts that have made it possible to unravel the ionic basis of the cardiac action potential. In the chapters that follow, we make repeated use of those concepts when discussing the properties of various membrane currents and the propagation of currents along tissues in the normal as well as the diseased heart.

In Chapter 2, we review the fundamental properties of ion channels, which, together with other protein macromolecules that include pumps and exchangers, act as "molecular machines" for the various ion translocation mechanisms across the cardiac cell membranes and that underlie cardiac excitation. A wide variety of ion channels are involved in the cardiac excitation process. These channels can be characterized by their gating mechanisms, e.g., voltage or ligand, as well as by their ion selectivity. Clearly, the determination of the molecular architecture of ion channels and the determination of structural correlates of ion channel key functions of gating and selectivity are important questions. A combination of tools of molecular and structural biology and of electrophysiology is providing important insight into ion channel function at the molecular level, and a fascinating picture is beginning to emerge. The studies implicate elements of the sequence of the ion channel protein in the two fundamental tasks of gating and ion selectivity.

Chapter 3 reviews current knowledge about how ionic currents in heart cells are regulated by several agents under physiological and pathophysiological conditions. Each regulatory agent, such as a neurotransmitter or a hormone, acts on a specific membrane receptor to affect the biophysical characteristics of several membrane currents in cardiac cells. Ion channel function is also dependent on the amount of the channel protein on the cell membrane. Overall, these changes in ion channel function will, in turn, affect the electrophysiological properties of the heart cell, with an ultimate effect on cardiac function.

In Chapter 4, we move from the ion channel and the cell to the study of intercellular communication by focusing on the role of electrical coupling on pacemaker synchronization and impulse propagation in the heart. We introduce the reader to basic concepts of electrotonic propagation and local circuit currents and their role in ensuring sinus pacemaker synchronization for the generation of the cardiac impulse as well as for successful impulse conduction. Based on those principles, the chapter discusses the concepts of phase resetting and mutual entrainment as well as the manner in which thousands of pacemaker cells in the sinus node synchronize to initiate together each cardiac impulse. In addition, the text brings attention to the fact that, although the unidimensional cable equations provide a good analytical tool to characterize the various electric elements involved in the propagation process, the heart is a highly complex 3-D structure, and its behavior commonly departs from that predicted by simple cable models. In this regard, some of the possible mechanisms by which active propagation may fail are discussed. The concept of wave front curvature, with its potential to lead to conduction slowing, the property of anisotropic propagation and the case of propagation across the Purkinje–muscle junction, as well as the presence of heterocellular interactions between myocytes and non-myocyte cells, all serve to illustrate the fact that cardiac impulse transmission does depart from simple unidimensional models.

The focus of Chapter 5 is the pathophysiology of cardiac impulse propagation, particularly in regard to the rate dependency of discontinuous action potential propagation in one-, two- and three-dimensional cardiac muscle. The chapter also discusses the dynamics and ionic mechanisms of complex patterns of propagation, such as Wenckebach periodicity and fibrillatory conduction, which provides a framework for understanding cellular and tissue behavior during high-frequency excitation and arrhythmias. Given the structural complexities of the various cardiac tissues and the complex nonlinear dynamics of cardiac cell excitation, it seems reasonable to expect that any event leading to very rapid activation of atria or ventricles may result in exceedingly complex rhythms, including fibrillation.

Chapter 6 deals with the cellular mechanisms of arrhythmias with emphasis placed on those aspects that may be relevant to the analysis of ECG manifestations. We review in detail well-established arrhythmia mechanisms and provide some insight into the appropriate tools to diagnose an arrhythmia in the clinical setting, which should reflect in our ability to provide a more rational therapeutic approach. The current focus on the development of new 3-D mapping techniques as well as the long-term recording of spontaneously occurring rhythm disturbances most likely will broaden our knowledge and offer new clues for diagnosing and managing cardiac arrhythmias.

In Chapter 7, we introduce the concept of rotors and spiral waves as a mechanism of the most complex arrhythmias. Some of the clinical manifestations of these arrhythmias are poorly explained by more conventional electrophysiological models of reentry. The theory of spiral waves, on the other hand, offers a new approach for the study of arrhythmias. Spontaneously occurring complex patterns of activation, as well as various dynamics resulting from external stimulation, are clearly predicted by theoretical and experimental studies on spiral waves. In addition, this approach offers new clues for the understanding of reentrant processes occurring in the complex three-dimensionality of the heart.

In Chapter 8, we present a brief review of contemporary ideas on atrial fibrillation (AF) mechanisms, from the bench to the bedside. We explore how studies in the isolated sheep heart enhance our understanding of AF dynamics and mechanisms by showing that high-frequency reentrant sources in the left atrium can drive the fibrillatory activity throughout both atria. Following those results and based on a large body of work investigating how measurements of AF cycle length in patients can contribute to its treatment, we focus our analysis on the organization of dominant frequency (DF) of the activity during AF in humans. We also emphasize how AF sources may be identified in human patients undergoing radio frequency ablation by the use of electroanatomic mapping and Fourier methods to generate 3-D, whole-atrial DF maps. In patients with paroxysmal AF, those sites are often localized to the posterior left atrium near the ostia of the pulmonary veins (PVs). We also contrast patients with paroxysmal vs. permanent AF by demonstrating that in the latter, high DF sites are more often localized to either atria than the posterior left atrium–PV junction. Finally, we review evidence showing how the response of the local AF frequency to adenosine tested for the mechanistic hypothesis that reentry is the mechanism that maintains human AF.

Chapter 9 reviews the most significant work demonstrating that the molecular mechanism of wave propagation dynamics during VF in the structurally and electrophysiologically normal heart may be explained in part on the basis of chamber-specific differences in the level of expression of cardiac potassium channels, particularly the inward-rectifier potassium channels responsible for I_{K1}. In addition, we review some recent experiments in 2-D rat cardiomyocyte monolayers strongly suggesting that the slow component of the delayed-rectifier current, I_{Ks}, plays an important role in the mechanism of fibrillatory conduction. We also summarize recent exciting data demonstrating that the inter-beat interval of VF scales according to a universal allometric scaling law, spanning over four orders of magnitude in body mass, from mouse to horse. Overall, a clearer picture of VF dynamics and its molecular mechanisms is emerging that might eventually lead to more effective prevention of sudden cardiac death.

Chapter 10 briefly addresses clinical manifestations, genetic bases, and cellular mechanisms of arrhythmias seen in some heritable arrhythmogenic diseases. Arguably, the intense amount of scrutiny given to these relatively rare diseases over the past 20 years has led to an explosion of new knowledge about the molecular and ionic bases of normal cardiac excitation and propagation. However, recent work has led to the conclusion that identifying a mutation in a given gene need not establish the diagnosis of a single disease and that discovering a mutation in an individual with a known disease is not enough to predict the phenotype of that individual. Therefore, important challenges remain in the understanding of the relationship between genetic defects and their clinical consequences. Nevertheless, we introduce the reader to original studies on the functional consequences of specific protein mutations in systems that approximate the physiological environment of these proteins which have been useful not only in the characterization of individual mutations, but also in the elucidation of the events underlying the initiation and maintenance of the arrhythmias in question.

In each chapter, the reader will find that most items of discussion in the text are accompanied by a substantial amount of graphic material, including simplified diagrams, color figures, and graphs, as well as schematic representations and cartoons. Whenever possible, we have intentionally avoided using original data, and, in most cases, individual concepts are explained in the simplest possible terms. Moreover, in general, we give no specific citations to original papers; rather, in the last few pages of the book, we provide a bibliography, where original articles, reviews, chapters, and monographs are presented to aid the reader interested in gaining a more in-depth knowledge of the subject matter. We are fully aware that our approach sacrifices detail and that some of our learned colleagues and critics may find such an approach offensive; we apologize for that. Yet we feel that, because our goal as educators is to spread the "gospel" of basic EP among clinicians, we needed to be didactic rather than absolutely precise.

Ten years have passed since the first edition was published and the authors of this book have moved to a new research environment with new students, fellows, and staff. Yet the same philosophy and excitement for basic and translational EP continues to drive our daily work. It is with that same excitement that we continue to teach basic cardiac electrophysiology at the University of Michigan. Thus, we have written the second edition of *Basic Cardiac Electrophysiology for the Clinician* with one major objective in mind: to give our graduate students, postdocs, and clinical EP fellows as well as clinicians everywhere a broad general outline of modern knowledge in cardiac EP from the point of view of the basic scientist. It is our hope that this edition will have a similar effect as the previous one and as that described for students who have attended our lectures. We also hope that this book will contribute somewhat to reducing the ever-expanding intellectual gap between basic and clinical electrophysiologists. Hence, the book is not written as a scholarly text and is not directed to the technically expert basic researcher. In fact, because our primary goal is to reach as broad an audience as possible, we have again written each chapter as if it were the script for one of our lectures to graduate students, postdocs, and clinical fellows.

1   Bioelectricity

The movement of selected ions across biological membranes generates changes in the intracellular environment that, either directly or indirectly, result in the contraction of the muscle cell. This passage of ions can be studied from a variety of perspectives. A practical approach is to take advantage of the fact that ions carry an electrical charge. As such, the flow of ions across cell membranes can be studied using equipment designed to measure electrical flow, and the properties of excitable membranes can be modeled after the behavior of electric devices. In fact, the subject of electrophysiology is borne out, to a certain extent, by the similarities that can be established between the flow of ions across membranes and the behavior of electrical currents moving through cables. As an introduction to the subject of cardiac electrophysiology, we will first define some basic concepts of bioelectricity to establish the fundamental principles that govern electric currents across cell membranes.

On the Electricity of Biological Membranes

Charge

Most elements in nature tend to maintain an equal number of protons and electrons. However, occasionally electrons are transferred more or less permanently from one element to another, thus creating an imbalance. For example, sodium, potassium, and chloride ions have an unequal number of protons and electrons. This imbalance turns the element into a charged particle. Particles that are charged positively are called cations. Negatively charged particles are called anions. The unit of charge is the coulomb (C). Electricity is created by the attraction of charged particles of opposite sign.

Basic Cardiac Electrophysiology for the Clinician, 2nd edition. By J. Jalife, M. Delmar, J. Anumonwo, O. Berenfeld and J. Kalifa. Published 2009 by Blackwell Publishing, ISBN: 978-1-4501-8333-8.

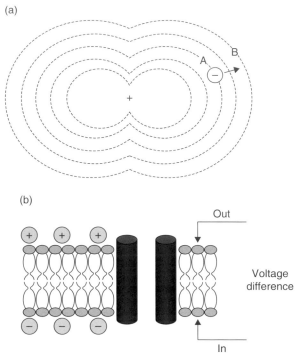

Figure 1.1 Voltage difference. (a) Dotted lines represent the distribution of an electric field around a positive charge. Voltage is the work involved in moving a charge along the electric field (e.g., from point A to point B). (b) The voltage difference across the cell membrane results from the uneven distribution of charges between the inside and the outside of the cell.

Voltage Difference

The attracting (or repelling) force generated by a charged particle in space is called the electric field. If a negative charge is free to move within a given electric field, it will be strongly attracted to a positive charge, and the field will eventually become electroneutral. There is therefore a certain amount of work involved in keeping the negative particle from rejoining its positive counterpart. More formally, we say that the work involved in moving a charge from point "A" to point "B" in an electric field (Figure 1.1a) is called potential difference (or voltage difference). In more practical terms, from the point of view of the electrophysiologist, potential differences are created when charges accumulate unequally across an insulator. For example, a potential difference is created across the membrane of cardiac myocytes because more anions are present inside than outside the cell (Figure 1.1b).

Current

As illustrated in Figure 1.2a, when the two ends of a source of voltage are separated, the potential difference is maintained. If a conductive pathway is

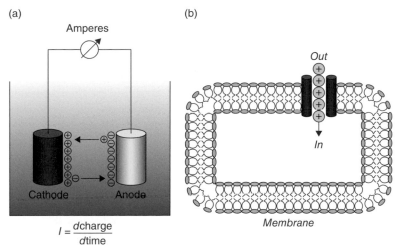

(a)

Amperes

Cathode   Anode

$$I = \frac{d\text{charge}}{d\text{time}}$$

(b)

Out

In

Membrane

Figure 1.2 Concept of electric current. (a) If a positively charged and a negatively charged electrode (anode and cathode, respectively) are placed inside a conductive medium, charge will flow from one to the other along the gradient. Current is defined as the magnitude of the charge that moves along a cross section of the conductor per unit time. (b) Hydrophilic channels allow for the flow of charge through cell membranes. The direction of the current follows the direction of the positive charges.

placed between them, charge will flow from the positive to the negative end. The negative plate will attract cations and is therefore referred to as the cathode (red). Conversely, the positively charged plate, which attracts anions, is called the anode (yellow). This movement of charges along a conductor is known as electric current. The unit of measure for electric current is the ampere (A). Current is more formally defined as the amount of charge passing through a conductor per unit time. By convention, positive current refers to the movement of cations toward the cathode.

In the cardiac cell (as in most living cells, for that matter) ions are constantly moving across the membrane, thus generating electric current. Ionic current is conceptualized as the flow of charge moving through selective hydrophilic pores or channels (Figure 1.2b). In the past, ion channels were studied only as functional entities, without any clear structural or biochemical correlate. Nowadays we know that channels are formed by integral membrane proteins that traverse the lipid bilayer and form a pathway for the transfer of selected ions between the intra- and extracellular spaces (see Chapter 2). Channels are conceptualized as electric resistors that connect the intra- and extracellular compartments. In the following section, we will describe the basic behavior of resistors in electric circuits. These concepts should be helpful in our subsequent review of the electrophysiological properties of the various ion channels in the membrane of the cardiac cell.

Resistance
Ohmic Resistors

All conductors offer a certain resistance (R) to the flow of current (if the flow of a fluid is used as an analogy, it can be said that a hose offers resistance to the flow of water). The unit of resistance is the ohm (Ω). Often, the properties of conductors are defined not by their resistance, but by their conductance. Conductance (G) is simply the inverse of resistance (i.e., $G = 1/R$) and it is expressed in siemens (S). The simplest resistors are those whose behavior is independent of time or voltage. These resistors are called "ohmic" because they follow Ohm's law:

$$I = V/R \qquad\qquad (1.1)$$

where I is current and V and R represent the magnitude of the voltage difference and the resistance, respectively. Ohm's law establishes that, given an increase in voltage across a constant resistance, there would be a linear increase in the amplitude of the current flowing through the circuit. Moreover, in an ohmic resistor, the time course of the change in current should be equal to the time course of the change in voltage. An example is illustrated in Figure 1.3. As shown by the simple circuit in panel (a), when a resistor (R) is placed between the anode and the cathode of a source of voltage (i.e., a battery), and the circuit is then closed by a switch, current flows toward the cathode. Moreover, a sudden increase in voltage induces an equivalent step in the amplitude of the current, as illustrated in panel (b). The bottom tracings represent three superimposed positive voltage steps of different magnitudes. The top tracings show recordings of the current flowing through the circuit in response to each voltage step. Thus, if current is plotted as a function of voltage (panel c), a linear function, of slope $1/R$ (or G) is obtained. This linear current–voltage ($I–V$) relation would be the same for both positive and negative voltage steps.

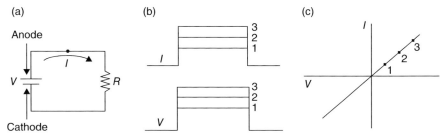

Figure 1.3 Current through an ohmic resistor. (a) An electrical circuit composed of a voltage source (V) and a resistor (R). Current (I) flows through the circuit. (b) The amplitude of the current is directly proportional to the magnitude of the voltage pulse. (c) A plot of current as a function of voltage (an IV plot) yields a straight line. Resistance is equal to the inverse of the slope of the line (slope = $1/R$).

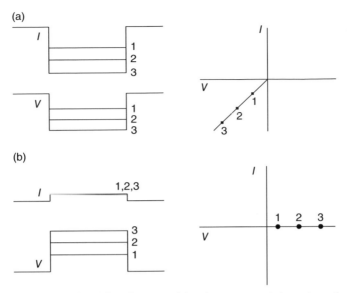

Figure 1.4 Rectification. The ability of some resistors to pass current depends on the voltage applied to the circuit. (a) In this example, current can flow in the negative direction. Negative voltage pulses 1, 2, and 3 generate progressively increasing currents of amplitudes 1, 2, and 3, respectively. (b) Positive voltage pulses do not elicit currents of increasing amplitudes. As a result, the *I–V* plot in the positive direction shows a horizontal line.

Non-ohmic Resistors: Rectification

It is common to find that the resistance of a conductor varies with the polarity of the current that flows through it. An example is illustrated in Figure 1.4. Panel (a) shows three superimposed negative tracings of current (top) obtained from our electric circuit in response to voltage steps of negative polarity (bottom). A linear relation similar to the one obtained from a purely ohmic resistor (Figure 1.3) is obtained. However, as shown in Figure 1.4b, a different behavior is observed for pulses of positive polarity. In that case, voltage steps induce only a small current step whose amplitude is essentially constant for any voltages being applied. This property of some conductors to allow the passage of current only (or largely) in one direction is called rectification. Rectification is one example of voltage dependence.

Slope Resistance and Chord Resistance

Some cardiac membrane channels rectify. In most cases, the channel allows the passage of current more effectively in the inward (i.e., from the extra- to the intracellular space) than in the outward direction. For this reason, this property is called inward-going rectification. Figure 1.5 shows the example of a current–voltage relation of an inward-rectifier cardiac membrane channel (in this case, the potassium current I_{K1}; see Chapter 2). It is clear that in this case the resistance of the channel is not constant. Indeed, the slope of the *I–V*

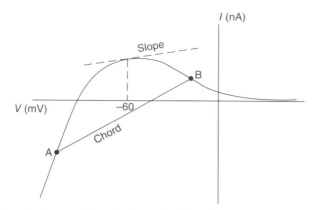

Figure 1.5 Current–voltage relation of an inward-rectifier channel. The diagram illustrates the concepts of slope resistance and chord resistance. Chord resistance is the inverse of the slope of a line joining points A and B. Slope resistance is the inverse of the slope of the line that is tangential to a specific point of the *I–V* curve. For a rectifying channel, slope and chord resistances can be different.

relation changes with the voltage. There are basically two approaches to evaluate the conductive properties of these channels. One is to determine the slope resistance. This is done by calculating the slope of a line that is tangential to the *I–V* relation at a certain point. In the case of Figure 1.5, the slope of the dashed line that touches the *I–V* function at a voltage of −60 mV is the slope conductance of that channel at that particular voltage. The inverse of the slope conductance is the slope resistance. Clearly, in a nonlinear *I–V* relation, the slope resistance varies appreciably, depending on the voltage at which it is measured. The other approach is to measure the chord resistance. In that case, two specific points (A and B) are chosen, and resistance is measured from the slope of the line (or "chord") that joins those two points. In a linear *I–V* relation, slope resistance and chord resistance are the same; however, in a nonlinear *I–V* relation, the two parameters may be different from each other, and their individual values should depend on the points chosen for measurement.

Time Dependence

Thus far, we described the properties of resistors that respond instantaneously to the changes in voltage. However, in some cases, the amplitude of the current in response to a voltage change may vary also as a function of time. An example is illustrated in Figure 1.6. In this case, a sudden change in voltage causes a progressive increase in the amplitude of the current. Because the voltage is constant, the increase in current is not due to voltage changes but rather to the intrinsic ability of the conductor to allow the passage of varying amounts of current as a function of time. Many cardiac membrane currents are time-dependent. In some cases, the current progressively increases during a voltage step, whereas, in other cases, the current decreases, and yet

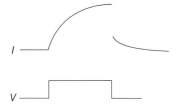

Figure 1.6 Time-dependent current. In this case, the ability of the conductor to pass current changes with time. Thus, the current amplitude increases progressively while the voltage is held constant.

(a)

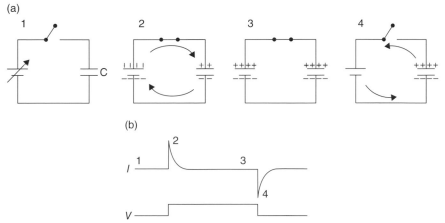

(b)

Figure 1.7 Capacitive current in an equivalent circuit consisting of a switch, a variable voltage generator, and a capacitor (C). (a) The diagrams illustrate the charge distribution along the circuit at four different times (1–4). (b) Current (*I*) generated by a voltage (*V*) square pulse. The small numbers in panel (b) correspond to the four frames in panel (a). The switch is open; no current flows across the circuit (frame 1). When the circuit is closed and a voltage step is applied from the baseline, the current surges rapidly (frame 2) (from point 1 to point 2) but then decreases to zero once the capacitor is fully charged (frame 3). An identical surge of opposite polarity is elicited when the voltage step is returned to baseline or the circuit is open (frame 4).

in other instances, completely disappears even if the voltage step is held constant for an extended period of time.

Capacitance

Capacitance is the property of an electric nonconductor that permits the storage of energy as a result of electric displacement when opposite surfaces of the nonconductor are maintained at a different potential. The measure of capacitance is the ratio of the change in the charge on either surface to the potential difference between the surfaces. Thus, a capacitor is formed when two conducting materials are separated by a thin layer of nonconducting material, an insulator (or dielectric). Cell membranes are capacitors in that the thin lipid bilayer (which is a very poor electric conductor) behaves like a dielectric interposed between the intracellular and the extracellular spaces, both of which are capable of conducting electricity. As opposed to resistors (ion channels in the case of cells), a voltage step imposed through a capacitor causes only a temporary current. This is illustrated in Figure 1.7. In panel (a), the top diagram shows an electric circuit consisting of a variable voltage generator (i.e., a battery of variable voltage), a capacitor, and a switch. Initially (step 1), the switch is off and no voltage difference is set between the anode and the cathode. When the switch is turned on, a voltage difference is established across the circuit (step 2), charge travels toward the cathode until it encounters the capacitor. Because the conductive pathway is interrupted by the dielectric that separates the two plates of the capacitor, positive charge accumulates at the plate that is closer to the anode. A steady-state condition is rapidly reached (step 3), and the flow of current stops. The tracings in panel (b) show the time course of positive capacitive current in response to voltage in this circuit. The voltage step elicits a rapid surge of current; however, the current rapidly returns to zero. When the voltage difference is switched back to zero (step 4), the capacitor is gradually discharged (i.e., charges now flow in the opposite direction) and a negative capacitive current is observed.

Capacitive current (I_C) is thus defined as

$$I_C = C \, dV/dt \tag{1.2}$$

where C is the capacitance and dV/dt represents the first derivative of voltage with respect to time. The latter can be roughly thought of as the rate at which voltage changes. When voltage is constant, dV/dt is zero (because voltage is not changing), and the amplitude of the capacitive current is also zero.

It is important to note that the capacitive properties of the cell are essential for the maintenance of a voltage difference across the membrane. Indeed, the lipid bilayer allows for the separation of charge. The voltage difference across the membrane is established by the fact that charge is unequally distributed. Therefore, the magnitude of the membrane potential reflects the extent of the disparity in charge distribution across the capacitor. Changes in membrane potential occur when ions, normally moving through the membrane channels, charge or discharge the membrane capacitance, thus changing the number of charges in the intra- and the extracellular spaces.

Parallel RC Circuits

In the previous sections, we described the behavior of the lipid bilayer of the membrane as a capacitor. We also equated membrane channels with resistors, because they allow the movement of ionic currents. Because the channels are formed by proteins that span the membrane, they are usually modeled in equivalent circuits as resistors in parallel with the membrane capacitor.

Therefore, the basic membrane circuit is that of a resistor and a capacitor in parallel (Figure 1.8a) and is usually referred to as an RC circuit. In an RC circuit, the total current flow (I_t) is equal to the sum of the current that moves through the capacitor (I_C) and the current that flows through the resistor (I_R).

$$I_t = I_C + I_R \tag{1.3}$$

Consequently, if one combines Equations 1.1, 1.2, and 1.3, then

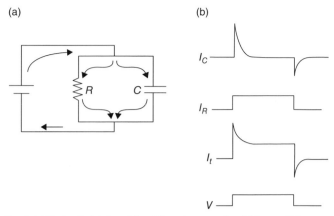

Figure 1.8 Parallel RC circuit. (a) A resistor (R) and a capacitor (C) in parallel are connected to a voltage source. (b) A voltage step (V) generates a total current (I_t), which is the sum of the current flowing through the resistor (I_R) and that flowing through the capacitor (I_C).

$$I_t = C\, dV/dt + V/R \qquad (1.4)$$

Figure 1.8b depicts the change in current in response to a voltage step in a parallel RC circuit (assuming that the resistor shows no time-dependent properties). The current flowing through the capacitor (I_C) has the properties depicted in Figure 1.7, whereas the current moving through the resistor (I_R) is directly proportional to the voltage step itself (as in Figure 1.3). Because both currents add, the total current (I_t) in Figure 1.8b shows an initial transient change, which is due to the flow of capacitive current, but rapidly reaches a steady state. The steady state corresponds to the magnitude of the current flowing through the resistor, and it is maintained for as long as the voltage step is maintained. Termination of the voltage step elicits the discharge of the capacitor, and then the current trace returns to the baseline value.

As noted earlier, cell membranes are modeled as parallel RC circuits. Accordingly, when a voltage change is imposed across the cell membrane, there is an initial transient surge of capacitive current, also called the capacitive transient. In the case of a square voltage pulse, the capacitive current rapidly drops to zero. Hence, all currents recorded after the end of the capacitive transient are currents that move through ion channels.

Origin of the Membrane Potential

Electrical current is driven by the voltage difference across a conductor. In the case of cells, this driving force is generated by the unequal distribution of electric charges and ion concentrations across the membrane. In other words, the membrane potential is electrochemical in origin. The physical basis for the establishment of electrochemical potentials is defined by the Nernst equation.

(a)

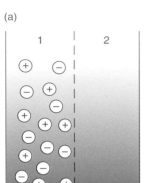

(b)

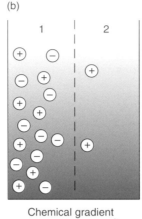

(c)

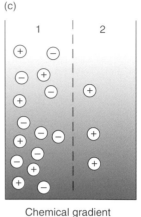

Chemical gradient →   Chemical gradient →   Chemical gradient →

← Electric gradient   ← Electric gradient

Figure 1.9 Electrochemical potential. A vessel is divided into two compartments (1 and 2) by a membrane that is permeable to positive ions but impermeable to negative ions. (a) Placing an ionizable solution into compartment 1 creates a chemical gradient for the flow of ions toward compartment 2. (b) As positive ions move across the membrane, they leave negative ions behind, generating an electric gradient whose direction is opposite to the chemical gradient. (c) Steady state is reached when the magnitude of the chemical and electric gradients are equal.

The principles of the Nernst equation can be illustrated by the example shown in Figure 1.9. A vessel is divided into two compartments (1 and 2) by a semipermeable membrane. The membrane allows for the passage of cations, but not anions. In panel (a), at the onset of the experiment, a solution of potassium chloride is placed in compartment 1. Both ions now tend to move to side 2, following the respective concentration gradients. Because the membrane is permeable to cations only, every time a potassium ion crosses to side 2 (following its concentration gradient), it leaves a negative charge (a chloride ion) behind. Two opposing forces are therefore created: (1) chemical, which pushes the potassium ions along their concentration gradient and (2) electric, which is created by the attraction that the negatively charged chloride ions exert over the cations (panel b). At steady state, a dynamic equilibrium is reached in which the magnitude of the chemical force is equal and opposite to the magnitude of the electric force (panel c). Consequently, the concentration of potassium differs in the two compartments, while at the same time a voltage difference is created. Mathematically, this equilibrium is expressed by the Nernst equation, as follows:

$$E_K = RT/F \ln [K]_2/[K]_1 \tag{1.5}$$

where T is temperature, R is a constant derived from the gas law, F is the Faraday constant, and $[K]_2$ and $[K]_1$ are the final concentrations of potassium in compartments 2 and 1, respectively. E_K is the equilibrium potential for potassium. That is, the voltage difference imposed across this semipermeable membrane is a result of the selective conductance of the membrane for potassium. If the cell membrane were exclusively permeable to potassium (and impermeable to all other ions), one could draw its equivalent circuit as a resistor in parallel with a capacitor, with the driving force (i.e., the source of membrane voltage) created by the electrochemical gradient of potassium, as predicted by the Nernst equation. In that case, the resistor represents the potassium channels in the membrane.

The concentration of potassium inside most mammalian cells is significantly larger than outside. In a cardiac ventricular myocyte, for example, the intracellular concentration of potassium is approximately 150 mM, whereas the concentration of potassium in the extracellular space is about 5 mM. Solving for the Nernst equation (Equation 1.5), one would predict a resting potential for a ventricular myocyte (kept at 37°C) of about −90 mV. The actual value, however, is slightly less negative than that. The reason is that other conductances with more positive equilibrium potentials may also contribute to the resting potential. For example, in some cells, a small permeability to sodium can be detected at rest. The concentration of sodium in the extracellular space is much larger (~140 mM) than in the inside (~10 mM); consequently, the sodium equilibrium potential is more positive than zero. A small conductivity to sodium would therefore tend to bring the resting potential to a less negative level. In the case of the ventricular myocyte, the resting potential is much closer to E_K because the membrane is much more permeable to potassium than to sodium. The final resting potential of a cell is therefore established by the balance between the equilibrium potentials for those ions to which the cell is permeable and the conductivity that the membrane may have for that ion. Mathematically, for a cell that is permeable to sodium, potassium, and chloride, the resting potential (V_m) can be predicted by the Goldman–Hodgkin–Katz (GHK) equation as follows:

$$V_m = RT/F \ln \{P_K[K]_o + P_{Na}[Na]_o + P_{Cl}[Cl]_i / P_K[K]_i + P_{Na}[Na]_i + P_{Cl}[Cl]_o\} \quad (1.6)$$

where P_{Na}, P_K, and P_{Cl} are the permeabilities of the membrane to sodium, potassium, and chloride, respectively. Hence, a complete electric diagram of the cell membrane at rest should include several sources of voltage, each providing a driving force for current across highly specific resistors. The magnitude of each source of voltage corresponds to the equilibrium potential for individual ions, and each specific resistor represents the ion channel that is specific for the ion in question. The magnitude of each resistor at rest is different. In the case illustrated in Figure 1.10, a hypothetical equivalent circuit of a cell is drawn that shows selective permeability to potassium, sodium, and chloride. In this case, the resting potential V_m, which is maintained across the cell capacitor, is established by the solution of the GHK equation (Equation 1.6) where all pertinent equilibrium potentials and conductivities are taken into account.

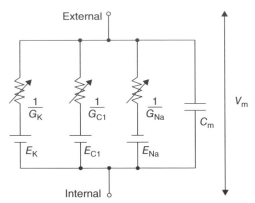

Figure 1.10 Simplified electric circuit of an excitable membrane. Three conductances in parallel are represented (G_K, G_{Cl}, and G_{Na}), each one connected to an electrochemical voltage source (E_K, E_{Cl}, and E_{Na}) created by the different concentrations of the individual ion species across the membrane. The lipid bilayer is represented by the capacitor C_m. A voltage difference (V_m) can be recorded across the membrane.

Active Currents

Most membrane conductances are not ohmic. The specific time- and voltage-dependent characteristics of various ion channels are reviewed in Chapter 2. However, it is important to note here that the conductivity of various channels changes during cardiac excitation. The action potential is therefore generated by variations in the magnitude of individual ion channel conductances, thus creating ionic currents that flow as a result of the difference between the actual membrane potential and the equilibrium potentials for the ions involved in the excitation–recovery process. As new charges enter or leave the cell, the capacitor is charged or discharged accordingly, thus displacing the resting potential. As shown in Figure 1.11a, when a positively charged ion (e.g., sodium or calcium) enters the cell, the membrane potential becomes more positive (or less negative); i.e., the cell is "depolarized." Conversely, a positive ion leaving the cell (e.g., potassium; see Figure 1.11b) increases the negativity of the cell interior. The flow of positive ions into the cell is referred to as "inward current." Inward currents are depicted as downward deflections and are represented by a negative sign. Positive ions flowing from the inside to the outside of the cell generate an "outward current." Outward currents are depicted as upward deflections and are represented by a positive sign. The amplitude and duration of the action potential results from the balance among the amplitude, time course, and direction of the specific currents involved.

Ionic currents flow through hydrophilic pores formed by membrane channel proteins. Electrically, these channels can be thought of as resistors. Thus, we can use Ohm's law to define the amplitude of the current that moves through a given channel, as follows:

$$I_x = (V_m - E_x)G_x \tag{1.7}$$

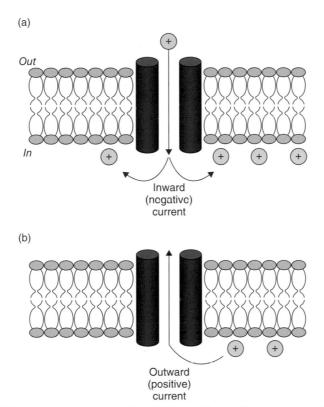

Figure 1.11 Direction of current across the membrane. (a) A positive ion entering the cell generates inward current and is represented by a negative deflection. (b) A positive charge leaving the cell creates an outward (positive) current.

Equation 1.7 indicates that the amplitude of the current flowing through "x" type of channels is a function of the channel conductance (G_x) and the driving force. The latter parameter is defined by the difference between the membrane potential (V_m) and the equilibrium potential for the ion (E_x). If the membrane potential is equal to the equilibrium potential, no current will flow (even if the channels are conductive). A current will be elicited only if the membrane potential is different from E_x and the channel is conductive. This relation also shows that, when the equilibrium potential is more negative than the membrane potential (e.g., the potassium conductance during repolarization), the current has a positive sign. Conversely, if the equilibrium potential is more positive than the membrane potential (e.g., sodium during depolarization), the current is of negative sign. Finally, it is important to note that, for time- and/or voltage-dependent channels, the value of G_x can change constantly. For example, the sodium conductance (G_{Na}) is almost zero at rest. As a result, no sodium current is present in a quiescent cell. However, if the cell reaches a critical (threshold) value, G_{Na} increases transiently, thus allowing for a large influx of sodium and consequent depolarization of the cell. On the other hand,

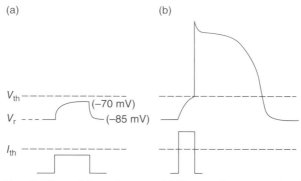

Figure 1.12 Cell excitability and the action potential. The membrane potential of a ventricular cell (top trace) stays at its resting level (V_r) if undisturbed by a current input (bottom trace). (a) A depolarizing current pulse of amplitude lower than a certain threshold value (I_{th}; bottom dotted line) will only change the membrane potential from rest (–85 mV in this example) to a constant level (–70 mV), and the membrane potential will return to rest when the current input is switched off. (b) A current pulse larger than the critical I_{th} amplitude will force the membrane potential to reach the voltage threshold (V_{th}) at which an "all-or none" action potential is elicited. In that case, the membrane potential goes through an entire cycle of changes in ionic currents that occur regardless of whether the initial input is maintained.

the amplitude of the inward-rectifier potassium current (I_{K1}) at rest is also close to zero, but in this case, the lack of measurable current is consequent to the fact that, at the level of the resting potential, there is no driving force for potassium. (Yet, the channels remain conductive.) Depolarization of the membrane elicits an outward potassium current because a driving force ($V_m - E_K$) is created for the ion. The importance of these issues will become clearer as we define the ionic bases of the action potential and discuss some of the ionic mechanisms that may be involved in cell excitability and refractoriness.

Excitability

Cardiac cells are "excitable" because they are able to generate action potentials that transfer information between cells. In Figure 1.12 we have plotted the membrane potential of a cardiac ventricular myocyte as a function of time. These types of measurements are obtained by introducing a fine-tipped glass microelectrode into the cell, and comparing the recorded potential against a reference electrode kept in the extracellular space. If no external stimulus is delivered to the cell, the membrane remains at its resting potential of about –85 mV. Panel (a) shows the changes in membrane potential that result from depolarization induced by a square electric current pulse of "subthreshold" amplitude applied through the microelectrode. In this case, the externally applied current causes the membrane potential to depolarize to a level of approximately –70 mV. After reaching that level, the membrane potential remains constant at –70 mV for the duration of the pulse. At the end of the pulse, the membrane potential returns to the resting level, and no further change is observed. However, as shown in panel (b), a stimulus of slightly larger amplitude triggers a regenerative response (an action potential) that lasts much longer than the duration of the current pulse itself. The level of voltage at which the cell needs to be depolarized to elicit the action potential is called the threshold voltage (V_{th}). Similarly, the minimum amount of current needed to trigger the active response is referred to as the threshold current (I_{th}). Threshold voltage and current are very useful variables for defining quantitatively the excitability of the cells. For instance, to measure excitability, investigators usually apply depolarizing pulses of progressively larger amplitude until threshold is reached. The larger the current needed to achieve threshold, the lower the excitability; i.e., excitability = 1/threshold current.

For the most part, excitability is determined by the availability of inwardly directed currents to depolarize the cell membrane. However, it is important to remember that outward currents are also essential determinants of excitability. Consider, for example, the case of an isolated ventricular myocyte. As noted earlier, the resting potential is established primarily by the presence of the inward-rectifier I_{K1} conductance. These highly selective potassium channels maintain the resting membrane potential close to the equilibrium potential for potassium. Figure 1.13b shows a representation of the current–voltage relation of I_{K1}, and Figure 1.13b shows the expected values of membrane

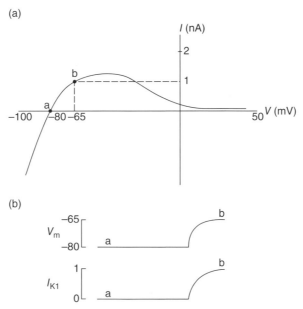

Figure 1.13 Role of the background current I_{K1} in determining the response to an externally applied subthreshold current pulse. (a) I–V relation of I_{K1}. (b) Subthreshold changes in membrane potential (V_m) and I_{K1} amplitude. Cell depolarization from point "a" (–80 mV) to point "b" (–65 mV) causes an increase in I_{K1} that is proportional to the magnitude of the depolarization, as predicted by the I–V curve. This outward current opposes the depolarizing influence of the excitatory input and, under extreme conditions, can interfere with the generation of the action potential.

potential (V_m; top) and I_{K1} amplitude (bottom) in quiescence (a) and during subsequent depolarization (b) induced by an external current source (not shown). At rest, a negligible amount of ionic current flows through these channels because the resting potential is very close to E_K. However, depolarization moves the membrane potential away from the rest and establishes the driving force ($V_m - E_K$) for the outward potassium current. This outward (i.e., repolarizing) current opposes cell depolarization; the larger the outward current, the lesser the depolarization and the more difficult it will be for the membrane to achieve threshold. In other words, excitability is determined not only by the number of sodium channels available to depolarize the cell but also by the balance between the availability of active inward currents and the amplitude of the outward conductance that opposes depolarization by the excitatory input.

Under normal conditions, I_{K1} may be a small factor in the regulation of excitability and conduction. However, conditions such as acute ischemia can induce the opening of other potassium channels (K_{ATP}) that generate large outward currents at subthreshold values of potential. Given their ability to oppose depolarization, these currents may be important in the regulation of excitability during ischemia.

Cardiac Action Potential

The action potential of a cardiac ventricular myocyte presents four distinct phases (see Figure 1.14, top panel): phase 0 corresponds to the rapid depolarization (or action potential upstroke) that ensues once the cell reaches the voltage threshold. Phase 1 corresponds to the brief, rapid repolarization that is initiated at the end of the action potential upstroke and that is interrupted when the cell reaches the "plateau level" or phase 2. During the plateau, repolarization progresses slowly; but eventually a final phase of rapid repolarization, or phase 3, ensues. Finally, phase 4 is the period between the last repolarization and the onset of the subsequent action potential. In atrial or ventricular myocytes, phase 4 corresponds to the resting membrane potential. As noted earlier, all of these changes in membrane potential are the result of the transmembrane movement of charges flowing through ion-specific, time- and voltage-dependent channels. A more detailed discussion of specific ion channel proteins is presented in Chapter 2; at this point it is appropriate to introduce some basic concepts relating the individual ionic currents to the various phases of action potential in a "generic" non-pacemaking cardiac cell.

Phase 0: Action Potential Upstroke

At rest, the dominant membrane conductance is provided by the potassium channels. However, once the cell reaches a threshold level of approximately -65 mV, membrane sodium channels suddenly open. Hence, at threshold, the membrane rapidly switches from being mostly permeable to K$^+$ to being

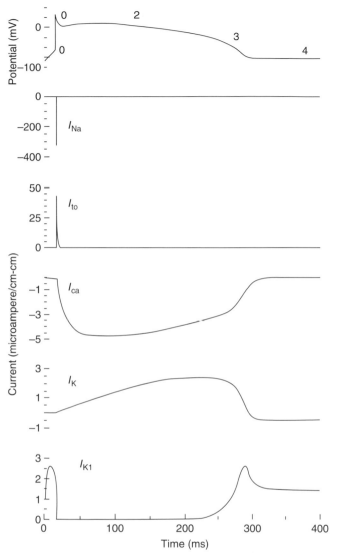

Figure 1.14 Ionic basis of the ventricular action potential. A simulated action potential (top panel) is shown in parallel with the various membrane currents that originate it (see Chapter 2 for a detailed description of ionic currents). The phases of the action potential are noted by the small numbers. I_{Na} and I_{Ca} are inward (downward deflections) sodium and calcium currents, respectively. I_{to}, I_K and I_{K1} are outwardly directed (upward deflections) potassium-dependent currents. For illustration purposes, actual magnitudes of currents shown are not scaled.

largely permeable to Na^+. The concentration of Na^+ in the extracellular space (~140 mM) is significantly larger than in the intracellular space (~4 mM). Figure 1.14 shows a computer simulation of the cardiac action potential (top) and the major ionic current components. Clearly, the sodium current (I_{Na}) represents a very large, yet rapid transition (note that each current has a different vertical scale). When the conductance to sodium suddenly increases, the large transmembrane gradient of Na$^+$ leads to a rush of ions into the cell in the form of an inwardly directed negative sodium current (I_{Na}). These ions accumulate in the intracellular side of the lipid bilayer and thus charge the membrane capacitor. Because sodium ions are positively charged, the membrane rapidly becomes less negative; i.e., it depolarizes, and results in the upstroke, or phase 0 of the action potential. In fact, given that during phase 0 the cell is mostly permeable to Na$^+$, the membrane potential becomes transiently positive as it moves toward E_{Na} (approximately +40 mV). However, the increase in sodium conductance is very brief. After a few milliseconds, the sodium channels enter a nonconductive state. The membrane potential does not quite reach the sodium equilibrium potential, but stops at approximately +20 mV and then begins to repolarize.

Phase 1: Rapid Repolarization

As shown in Figure 1.14, for the most part, the end of the action potential upstroke is brought about by the inactivation of the sodium channels. During the initial phase of repolarization of the action potential, or phase 1, potassium channels provide the dominant membrane conductance. Although there can be important differences in the ionic currents that are activated at this stage, depending on the region of the heart from which the cells originate (and also depending on the animal species studied), in most cases the so-called "transient outward current" (I_{to}) provides most of the repolarizing charge. This rapidly activating potassium conductance turns on during the action potential upstroke. When the sodium channels enter their nonconductive state, repolarization begins in earnest, with the membrane potential heading toward the reversal potential for potassium. I_{to} inactivates also very rapidly, and its contribution to the repolarizing process during phases 2 and 3 of the action potential is somewhat less than that observed during phase 1.

Phase 2: Action Potential Plateau

Other voltage-dependent membrane channels are also activated by cell depolarization, although they activate at a slower rate (Figure 1.14). Consequently, these channels provide a sizable current only several milliseconds after the end of the action potential upstroke. The two dominant currents during the plateau phase of the action potential, or phase 2, are the inward calcium current (I_{Ca}) and the delayed rectifier potassium outward current (I_K). For the sake of simplicity, we labeled as I_{Ca} all current components that are calcium-dependent (including, for example, the L-type calcium current and electrogenic sodium–calcium exchanger). As discussed in more detail in Chapter 2, the potassium current I_K includes at least two separate components: a rapid component (I_{Kr}) and a slow component (I_{Ks}). Given the concentration gradient for Ca^{2+}, opening of calcium channels leads to movement of calcium from the extracellular to the intracellular space (i.e., an inwardly directed, depolarizing current). Potassium ions, on the other hand, move in the opposite direction.

The end result is that, while the calcium channels remain open, repolarization by potassium currents is prevented by the presence of a calcium current that is moving positive charges into the cell. Thus, during the plateau, the membrane potential depends on the balance between inward I_{Ca} and outward I_K currents. Although in some cells (e.g., Purkinje fibers) outward currents dominate and the plateau tends to have a consistently negative slope, in others there may be an actual slight depolarization before repolarization continues (in a "domelike" shape).

Phase 3: Final Repolarization

Inactivation of the calcium channels leads to the end of the plateau (Figure 1.14). Only potassium conductances remain active; consequently, the membrane potential returns relatively rapidly toward E_K. The delayed rectifier currents (I_{Kr} and I_{Ks}) tend to close as the cell repolarizes, and thus the inward-rectifier current (I_{K1}) predominates.

Phase 4: Diastolic Potential

In atrial and ventricular muscle cells, the resting potential remains constant throughout the diastolic interval. In these cell types, the inward-rectifier current I_{K1} remains the dominant conductance at rest and it is largely responsible for setting the resting membrane potential. An additional small background conductance, with a more positive equilibrium potential, keeps the resting potential slightly more depolarized than the value estimated by the potassium equilibrium potential. Atrial and ventricular myocytes remain at this constant level of potential until a new excitatory stimulus brings the membrane potential to threshold, thus eliciting a new active response.

Basic Action Potential Parameters

Several parameters are commonly used by cellular electrophysiologists to quantify the time course and magnitude of changes in the action potential as a result of changes in the activation frequency, ionic concentrations, temperature, pH, or drug effects. Some such parameters are illustrated in Figure 1.15. Action potential amplitude (APA) is measured from the resting potential to the peak of action potential depolarization. Action potential overshoot refers to the magnitude of membrane potential reversal from negative to positive values. Action potential duration (APD) is usually measured between the onset of the action potential upstroke and the point at which the cell repolarizes to a certain fraction of the maximum. For example, APD_{50} refers to the APD measured at 50% repolarization and APD_{90} is the APD at 90% repolarization. In pacemaker cells, where the membrane potential is not constant during diastole, the term "maximum diastolic potential" is used to identify the most negative value of membrane potential reached after repolarization. Finally, the maximum action potential upstroke velocity (i.e., the fastest rate of depolarization measured during phase 0) is often used as a rough indicator of the

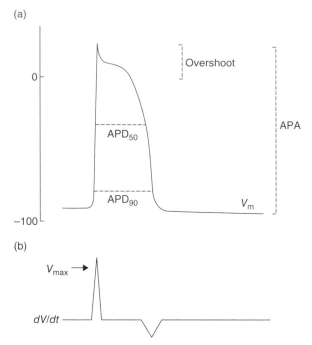

Figure 1.15 Action potential parameters. (a) A ventricular action potential. APD_{50} and APD_{90} refer to the action potential duration measured at 50% and 90% repolarization, respectively. APA stands for action potential amplitude. The overshoot refers to the segment of the action potential where the inside of the cell is positive with respect to the outside. (b) First derivative of the action potential. The maximum rate of rise of membrane potential (V_{max}) is, within certain limits, an indirect measure of the conductance of the sodium channels.

magnitude of the active inward current mediating phase 0 (see Figure 1.15b). Upstroke velocity can be estimated from the first derivative of the change in voltage as a function of time. Thus, the maximum upstroke velocity (V_{max} or dV/dt_{max}) is equal to the maximum positive value of the first derivative of the action potential.

Refractory Period

A characteristic feature of excitable cells is that, once the cell is activated, there is a period of time during which a second action potential cannot be generated. The interval of time during which the cell cannot be re-excited is called the refractory period (RP). The RP of cardiac cells is long compared with other excitable cells such as neurons and skeletal muscle cells. An important functional advantage of having a long RP is that cardiac cells cannot be activated again before enough time passed for at least partial relaxation from the previous contraction. Consequently, cardiac myocytes do not undergo tetanic contraction (i.e., tonic contraction). Although tonic contraction is indeed very important for the normal physiology of skeletal muscle, it would have fatal consequences if it were present in the heart.

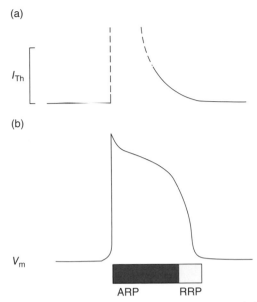

Figure 1.16 Refractory period. (a) Changes in the amplitude of the threshold current (I_{th}) during the action potential. (b) Voltage recording during the action potential. From the moment of rapid depolarization and until the end of the plateau phase (red bar), a second action potential cannot be generated regardless of the amplitude of the current input (absolute refractory period; ARP). Toward the end of phase 3 (yellow bar), an additional action potential can be elicited, but the current required is larger than during control (relative refractory period; RRP).

The recovery of excitability of a cardiac myocyte develops gradually after an action potential. Figure 1.16a shows a plot of the threshold current (I_{th}, i.e., the minimum current magnitude necessary to elicit an active response) at different times during an action potential. The membrane potential of a ventricular myocyte is shown in panel (b). An action potential is elicited after a long period of quiescence. Thus, the magnitude of current required to elicit the response reflects a baseline (or "control") level of excitability. At the onset of the action potential upstroke, there begins a period of time (marked by the solid bar at the bottom) during which I_{th} grows to infinity and a second response cannot be elicited, regardless of the magnitude of the excitatory input. This interval marked in red is known as the absolute refractory period (ARP). As the cell repolarizes, it once again becomes excitable. However, there is a period of time during which the amount of current needed to trigger the active response is much larger than the control I_{th}. This period, illustrated by the yellow bar at the bottom, is known as the relatively refractory period (RRP). As the membrane repolarizes toward resting levels, I_{th} decreases gradually, and excitability is recovered, achieving control values several milliseconds after the completion of repolarization.

The ARP occurs because, once an action potential ensues, active inward currents are no longer available to depolarize the membrane. Indeed, as discussed in Chapter 2, sodium channels become inactive (nonconductive) during depolarization. A period of recovery from inactivation (which is initiated by repolarization) is required so that these channels can become conductive once again.

The outward currents also participate in the RRP. As discussed earlier, the total membrane current results from the balance between the inward and outward currents. Outward currents oppose the depolarizing influence of inward currents. During repolarization (and briefly during diastole) the delayed rectifier channels are conductive. To re-excite the cell, the depolarizing current must overcome the repolarizing influence of the outward currents. Thus, the duration of the RRP is determined in a complex manner by the time course or reactivation of the inward currents as well as by the time course of deactivation (or "closure") of the delayed rectifier outward conductance.

Supernormal Excitability

Under normal circumstances the recovery of excitability after an action potential follows a smooth exponential time course. However, in Purkinje fibers and, under certain conditions, in working cardiac muscle as well, there is a brief period of time at the end of repolarization in which the cells are actually more excitable than at rest. This period of "supernormal excitability" (labeled "SN" in Figure 1.17) occurs at least in part because, as the membrane potential returns toward resting levels, it does so at a time when enough sodium channels are reactivated and the threshold for activation is sufficiently close to normal. As shown in Figure 1.17, as the membrane repolarizes and crosses

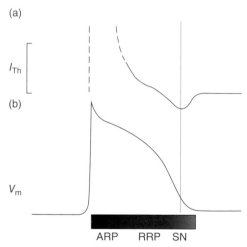

Figure 1.17 Supernormal excitability (SN). (a) Changes in the amplitude of the threshold current (I_{th}) during the action potential. (b) Voltage recording during the action potential. In some cell types, the relative refractory period (RRP) is followed by a time interval during which I_{th} is actually smaller than in the control. ARP, absolute refractory period.

the threshold for sodium channel activation (dashed vertical line), stimulation during this period requires less current than normal for a new action potential to occur. The period of supernormal excitability may be important in the generation of cardiac arrhythmias, as it allows for the new action potential to be triggered at a vulnerable time in the cardiac cycle for reentrant excitation to occur.

Action Potential Morphology in Specialized Cardiac Tissues

The preceding paragraphs describe the general concepts on the ionic currents mediating a generic cardiac action potential in the atria or ventricles. However, the magnitude and time course of action potentials vary from one cardiac region to another. In this section, we describe some of the major features in the action potentials of sinoatrial (SA) and atrioventricular (AV) nodal as well as Purkinje cells.

Sinoatrial Nodal Cells

Cardiac activation normally starts in the SA node. The specialized muscle cells in this area are capable of spontaneous (also called pacemaker) activity (see Figure 1.18), and their intrinsic frequency of discharge is, under normal conditions, faster than that of any other pacemaker in the heart. In true pacemaker cells of the SA node, the diastolic membrane potential does not remain constant. Instead, there is a spontaneous (phase 4) depolarization that brings the membrane potential slowly from the most negative value achieved at the end of the preceding repolarization (i.e., the maximum diastolic potential) to the threshold for activation, thus eliciting a new active response. It is important to note that the maximum diastolic potential of SA nodal cells is less negative (between −50 and −65 mV) than that of ventricular cells. Nodal cells have a lower permeability to potassium than ventricular cells at rest. Consequently, the repolarization process stops at less negative levels; furthermore, in nodal cells, the threshold for activation stands at approximately −35 mV because in these cells the action potential upstroke results from the inward flow of calcium through channels that are similar to those mediating the I_{Ca} current of ventricular cells. Sodium channels play a negligible role in the action potential upstroke of SA nodal cells. Therefore, the maximum rate of depolarization during the action potential upstroke is relatively slow in these cells (~1 to 10 V/s).

The slow diastolic (phase 4) depolarization that characterizes spontaneously active nodal cells results (at least in part) from activation of a hyperpolarization-activated current, commonly referred to as the "funny current" or I_f. Indeed, in the voltage range of phase 4 depolarization, the I_f channels allow for the entry of positive charges into the cell. As opposed to other channels mentioned earlier in this section, I_f channels open at voltages more negative than −60 mV (see Chapter 2). Consequently, the channels are closed during most of the action potential. Yet, when the cell repolarizes from a previous discharge, I_f channels activate. The entry of cations leads to gradual cell

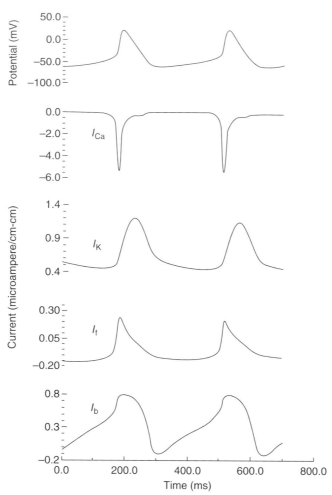

Figure 1.18 Ionic bases of the sinus nodal action potential. The simulated electric activity of the nodal cell (top) was generated by a set of differential equations describing the different relevant ionic currents. As opposed to the action potential of atrial working muscle, or ventricular tissues, in this case sodium current does not play a role. The upstroke is mediated by the calcium current (I_{Ca}). The potassium current (I_K) dominates the repolarization phase. Two additional currents are shown. The I_f current activates upon repolarization, and contributes inward current to the pacemaker potential. A time-independent background current (I_b) also changes polarity during the cardiac cycle and contributes to the different phases of the action potential.

depolarization (Figure 1.18). Depolarization progresses slowly until the membrane reaches the threshold for activation of calcium currents, at which time a sinus nodal action potential ensues. Depolarization then causes the I_f channels to close. However, during the subsequent repolarization, the I_f channels activate once again, allowing for a new entry of positive charges, thus repeating the process.

Although the presence of I_f in sinus nodal cells has been clearly documented, some authors have argued that the current provided by I_f in the voltage range of the sinus nodal pacemaker potential is not large enough to solely account for spontaneous pacemaker depolarization. An additional current during phase 4 depolarization may result from the combination of the closure of potassium channels and the activation of calcium currents. The latter hypothesis presumes the existence of a background (time-independent) current with a reversal potential near the equilibrium potential for sodium (i.e., in the positive voltage range). According to this hypothesis, the total membrane current results from the balance of currents moving through these opposing conductances. During repolarization, the outward current is larger than the background inward component. However, the progressive closure of potassium channels during repolarization is thought to unmask the depolarizing force of the background inward current. Depolarization then progresses following largely the time course of potassium current deactivation. Calcium channels are thus activated by the membrane depolarization, eventually eliciting an active response.

Of course, the mechanisms postulated here are not mutually exclusive. All individual currents (I_f, I_K, I_{Ca}, and I_b) depicted in Figure 1.18 may participate during the process of pacemaker activation. Moreover, because the SA node is a highly heterogeneous region, multiple action potential morphologies may be recorded, depending on the specific region of the node, including the center or the periphery. Thus, it is possible that pacemaking in cells with more negative diastolic potential is more dependent on I_f than in other cells where the maximum diastolic potential is never larger than −60 mV.

Atrioventricular Nodal Cells
Action potential morphology in the AV node varies widely, depending on the nodal region from which the action potentials are obtained. In the center or "N region" of the AV node, action potentials present characteristics similar to those described for the sinus nodal action potential. Briefly, as depicted in Figure 1.19, the maximum diastolic potential is more depolarized than in the ventricular or atrial cells, the action potential upstroke is slower and mostly dependent on I_{Ca}, and a pacemaker potential can be detected. The spontaneous rate of activation of the AV node is slower than that of the sinus node. Yet, in the absence of the sinus node, AV nodal cells can discharge spontaneously and act as the pacemaker for the entire heart. As illustrated in Figure 1.19, closer to the atrium, within the AN region of the AV node, the action potential morphology is somewhat intermediate between atrial and N cells, whereas in the NH region the action potential shape is intermediate between the N and His bundle cells.

Purkinje Fibers
An important characteristic of cells within the His bundle and Purkinje network is their ability to generate spontaneous action potentials. The

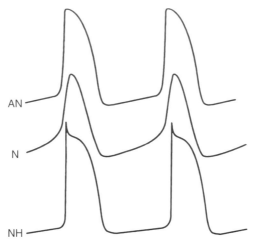

Figure 1.19 Atrioventricular (AV) nodal action potential morphology. At least three different regions of the AV node can be identified electrophysiologically: the atrio-nodal (AN), the nodal (N), and the transitional region between the node and the His (NH). Action potential morphology varies among those regions.

frequency at which His or Purkinje fibers fire their spontaneous discharges is significantly slower than in the nodes. These slow pacemaker cells can command the ventricles when activation of supraventricular origin fails. There is general agreement that the major pacemaker current of Purkinje fibers is I_f. As opposed to nodal cells, Purkinje cells are highly polarized; their action potential upstrokes are very fast and mediated by the fast sodium current.

Regional Variations in Action Potential Morphology

Differences in action potential morphology may be detected between different regions of the ventricles. In particular, ventricular subendocardial cells have longer action potentials than subepicardial cells (Figure 1.20). These and other functional differences within the heart may help to explain regional differences in the electrophysiological effects of certain antiarrhythmic drugs as well as some arrhythmic patterns that result from reentrant circuits in ventricular tissue. The implications that ventricular heterogeneities may have in the generation of cardiac rhythm disturbances are discussed in Chapter 6.

Voltage Clamp

In the preceding section, we discussed how, during the cardiac cycle, currents flow across membrane channels repeatedly changing the membrane potential. Study of the actual time and voltage dependence of individual transmembrane currents under such conditions is complicated by the dynamic nature of the voltage changes. The voltage-clamp technique allows for the control of

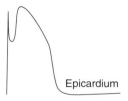

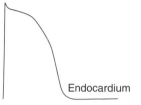

Figure 1.20 Diverse action potential morphology in the ventricles. The shape of the action potential, as well as some of its intrinsic electric properties, varies across the myocardial wall. Most noticeable, the transition between phases 1 and 2 of the action potential varies between a "spike-and-dome" morphology in the epicardium to a smooth, progressively downward deflection in the endocardium.

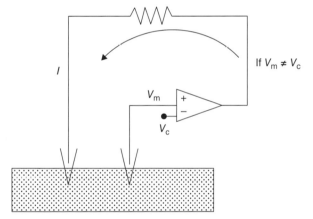

Figure 1.21 The voltage-clamp circuit. A single cell (hatched area) is impaled by two microelectrodes. One records the membrane potential (V_m); the other delivers current (I). The recorded voltage is compared against a command potential (V_c). If V_m is different from V_c, current is delivered into the cell. The current delivered by the electrode is equal and opposite to the current that moves through the cell membrane during a particular voltage pulse.

the membrane potential during specific periods of time and at preselected levels so that the biophysics of individual channels can be studied in detail.

Conceptually, the procedure is simple, and it is best explained using the configuration called "two-electrode voltage clamp" (see Figure 1.21). A fine-tipped glass microelectrode is introduced inside the cell to measure the voltage difference across the membrane (V_m). The reading of membrane potential is then compared, in an amplifier, with the value of potential chosen by the operator. This potential is usually referred to as the command voltage, or V_c. The ultimate goal is to make V_m equal to V_c. Thus, if there is a difference

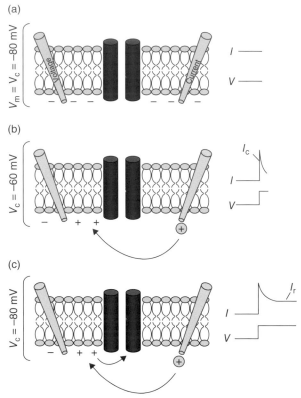

Figure 1.22 Current transitions during a voltage-clamp step. A hypothetical cell membrane, with a hydrophilic channel in the center, is illustrated in all panels. (a) The cell is impaled by two electrodes (labeled voltage and current). Magnitudes of measured voltage and delivered current are shown on the right. V_m equals the command potential, and no compensatory current is delivered by the circuit. (b) A voltage step to –60 mV requires the charge of the cell capacitor (I_c). (c) As positive charges leave the cell through the channel, they are compensated by the amplifier. Thus, the current delivered by the amplifier at this time is a reflection of the current escaping through the resistive channel (I_r).

between the two variables, the amplifier delivers current to the cell so that the membrane potential is clamped to the level of V_c. In the diagram, this current (I) is delivered by a second microelectrode placed also inside the cell.

Consider the simplest case of a cell membrane whose ion channels behave like ohmic resistors, as illustrated in Figure 1.22. Before the voltage clamp is turned on (panel a), the voltage electrode reads the membrane potential (V_m), at –80 mV. The investigator switches the voltage-clamp amplifier to exactly –80 mV. In this condition, V_m and V_c are identical, and, therefore, no current is necessary to make V_m equal to V_c. The operator now changes V_c to –60 mV (panel b). The amplifier reads the voltage difference and "injects" charge into the cell through the current electrode to force the membrane potential to

−60 mV. The current delivered by the amplifier will be used first to charge the membrane capacitance (recall that the membrane potential is the result of an electrochemical gradient across the membrane's lipid bilayer, which acts as the cell capacitor).

Most of the initial current injected by the amplifier therefore reflects the magnitude of current (I_c) needed to charge the membrane capacitance so that the voltage difference across the membrane is equal to −60 mV. In other words, the first change in the current tracing will be the capacitive transient. Current will also be moving through the ohmic resistor (the channel). The charge that moves across the channel would tend to discharge the capacitor, thus changing the membrane potential. Because the amplifier constantly compares V_m with V_c, it injects current in response to any minor deviation. Thus, the constant "leak" of charges through the resistor is immediately compensated by an injection of current by the amplifier to maintain the membrane capacitor charged to the desired voltage (panel c). The same principle applies to the case of a channel that is non-ohmic. If, for example, the channel activates slowly with time (as in Figure 1.6), progressively more charge will leave the cell through the channel, thus displacing the membrane potential. In response, the amplifier compensates by injecting more current. Again, the current injected by the amplifier is equal to the current leaving the cell through the membrane channel. In other words, once the capacitive transient is over, the current flowing through the amplifier is equal to the current flowing through the ion channels in the membrane.

A clear limitation of the voltage-clamp technique becomes apparent from the previous discussion. Indeed, most of the current injected by the amplifier at the onset of the voltage clamp is used to charge (or discharge) the cell capacitor. Therefore, ionic currents that occur during this brief interval are not properly measured. This was a major stumbling block in measuring rapid events that take place across some ion channels (see Chapter 2). Fortunately, new technology as well as the use of various alternative voltage-clamp methods helped to partially solve this important problem.

Another factor to consider when designing voltage-clamp experiments is that the entire cell membrane under study must be fixed to the desired potential. If during the voltage clamp a voltage difference exists between one region of the cell (or fiber) and another, currents will flow not only across the membrane but also between the two regions that are not isopotential. Consider the extreme example presented in Figure 1.23. A long Purkinje fiber is impaled with voltage (V) and current (I) electrodes that are relatively close to each other. During a voltage-clamp step from −80 to −60 mV, the current injected by the amplifier changes the potential of the patch of membrane surrounding the voltage electrode; however, because of the length of the fiber, the membrane potential distal to the site of impalement may be different from that near the electrode. As a consequence, current moves axially along the fiber in an effort to maintain (unsuccessfully) the entire membrane at the same level of potential. In other words, the current injected by the amplifier not only

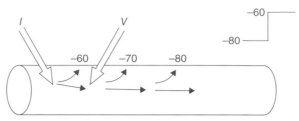

Figure 1.23 Voltage clamp requires spatial voltage control. A segment of a long fiber is voltage clamped between a voltage (V) and a current (I) electrode. The command step is from −80 to −60 mV. Although the amplifier may measure −60 mV at the site of recording, the membrane potential would not be homogeneous throughout the fiber, due to the spatial decay (see "Cable Equations" in Chapter 4). A longitudinal voltage gradient would create a longitudinal current. Accordingly, the amplifier would provide current not only to compensate for the membrane current between the electrodes but for that moving horizontally along the fiber. This condition indicates poor voltage control.

reflects the current moving through the membrane, but also the undetermined amount of current that is moving along the fiber. We shall discuss the axial flow of current in greater detail in our discussion on propagation, in Chapter 4. Suffice to say here that the lack of isopotentiality in the preparation (i.e., the lack of spatial control) is an important problem in voltage clamping. Adequate spatial control is an essential requirement of success in a voltage-clamp experiment.

In small cells, it is possible to use voltage-clamp amplifiers that both measure potential and pass current through the same electrode. This technique, called single-electrode voltage clamp, offers the great advantage of requiring only one electrode impalement. The technique is limited by the magnitude of current that can be passed across the circuit in the absence of artifacts. Large cells (e.g., *Xenopus laevis* oocytes) require large amounts of current to achieve adequate voltage control. In those cases, a two-electrode voltage clamp (Figures 1.21–1.23) is required.

Methods of Resolving Currents through Ion Channels

The ionic basis of cardiac electrical activity intrigued scientists for over a century. The initial attempts to understand the ionic bases of the cardiac impulse relied on microelectrode work carried out in isolated cardiac preparations. Although these initial studies provided important qualitative data on ionic currents, several limiting factors, for example, inadequate voltage-clamp conditions, made it difficult if not impossible to assign any meaningful functional significance to the currents measured.

Later advances, such as the development of the single-electrode voltage-clamp technique and the procedure for isolating single cardiac cells, made it possible to measure the current flowing across the membrane of an individual cardiac cell or from a single ion channel localized to a membrane patch. In the single-electrode voltage clamp, a glass capillary tube is pulled over heat to a fine tip of approximately 1–4 µm in diameter, filled with saline, and connected to a high-gain, low-noise amplifier. This recording electrode or "patch pipette," as it is often referred to, is placed on the surface of the cardiac cell and a very high-resistance (in giga-ohms, GΩ) "seal" is formed between the pipette and a patch of the cell membrane, essentially excluding ions in the extracellular space from the patch pipette contents.

Several modalities of the single-electrode voltage-clamp technique were developed through the years. The most commonly used when studying ion currents across the entire cell is the whole-cell patch-clamp technique. In this approach, after the seal is formed between the electrode and the cell membrane, a gentle suction is applied, rupturing the cell membrane in the patch and gaining access to the cytoplasm (Figure 1.24a). Consequently, the internal pipette solution enters in direct contact with the intracellular space. The membrane of the entire cell is voltage clamped, and the recorded currents are a composite of the current flowing through all the active channels. A variation of the same procedure is the perforated-patch technique (Figure 1.24b). Here, the idea is to introduce in the pipette a specific pharmacologic agent (nystatin, amphotericin B) that creates large channels in the membrane under the patch. The seal, therefore, is not broken. Instead, the electrode gains electric access to the intracellular compartment through the channels perforated by the drug. Yet, the intracellular space is not disturbed.

In another modality, a glass pipette is sealed to the membrane but, in this case, the patch is not broken (Figure 1.24c). This procedure is commonly referred to as the cell-attached patch-clamp technique. In this case, the operator controls the membrane potential only of the patch of membrane sealed inside the diameter of the microscopic glass pipette tip. The great advantage of this procedure is that the recording is obtained only from a few channels (sometimes only from a single channel). In the cell-attached configuration, the intracellular space is kept intact. Although this is ideal for studying the channel in a more "physiological" condition, it does not allow direct manipulation of the concentration of ions or other molecules that may regulate the channel under study. The latter can be done by pulling the patch of membrane out of the cell without breaking the seal (Figure 1.24d). This variant, called the cell-excised patch clamp (or inside-out patch clamp, referring to the fact that the intracellular face of the membrane is now facing the outside solution), gives the investigator direct access to the cytoplasmic side of the channel. The drawback is that the channel studied under this condition is no longer in contact with its natural intracellular environment.

Finally, yet another modality of the patch-clamp technique is called outside-out patch clamp. In this case, a pipette is sealed to the membrane, and the membrane within the patch is broken, as in the whole-cell mode. However, once the whole-cell recording is formed, the pipette is gently pulled away from the cell (Figure 1.24e). The membrane that is sealed to the glass pipette retracts, and the ends of the retracted membrane fuse. The ultimate

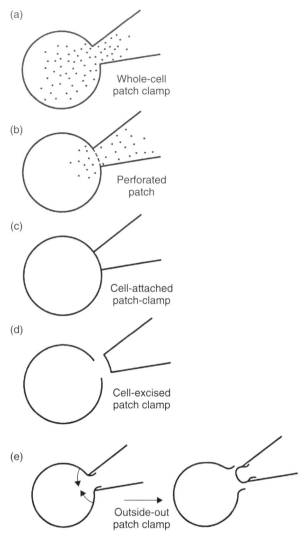

Figure 1.24 Single-electrode voltage-clamp configurations. (a) In whole-cell patch clamp, there is continuity between the intracellular space and the pipette-filling solution. (b) Dialysis of the cytoplasm is avoided when the perforated-patch technique is used. (c) When the seal between the electrode and the cell membrane is not broken, the amplifier records the electric activity of the patch of membrane within the area under the electrode; single channel recordings are thus feasible (cell-attached patch clamp). (d) The patch can also be separated from the cell (cell-excised patch clamp), thus giving access to the cytoplasmic side of the channels under recording. (e) Finally, gently pulling the pipette in a whole-cell configuration may allow for the fusion of the membrane at the edges and formation of a small patch. In this case, the "outside" phase of the membrane faces the bath (outside-out patch clamp).

consequence is that a patch of membrane is isolated from the rest of the cell and the intracellular side exposed to the pipette-filling solution.

Each of these patch-clamp configurations has specific applications in the study of ion channels. They all have advantages as well as limitations. When properly used, such techniques can provide (and have provided) highly accurate information about the physiology and pharmacology of ion channels in the cardiac cell membrane.

Some Basic Terminology

Now that we have explained the idea of the cell membrane as an RC circuit and have described some basic concepts on the study of the movement of electric currents across cell membranes, it is appropriate to define some basic terms that are used commonly in the field of cellular electrophysiology.

Direction of Current Across Cell Membranes

As noted earlier, ions move constantly across the cell membrane and generate transmembrane currents. To define whether a current is inward or outward, we use the same convention as in electricity, i.e., we follow the direction of the positive charge. Thus a positively charged sodium ion (i.e., a cation) that moves from the outside to the inside of the cell creates an inward current. Similarly, a positively charged potassium ion (also cation) that moves from the inside of the cell to the outside creates an outward current because in this case the positive charge is moving outwardly. Inward or outward currents therefore indicate whether the direction of movement of positive charges is inward or outward, respectively. The issue can be a bit confusing when discussing chloride currents. In this case, a negatively charged ion, or anion, is moving across the membrane. Because by convention we follow the direction of positive charges, in the case of a chloride ion, the direction of current is opposite to the actual direction in which the ion moves. Thus, a chloride ion that moves from the inside of the cell to the outside creates an inward current (i.e., a negative charge leaving the cell is equal to a positive charge entering the cell). When tracings of cell currents are shown, inward currents are depicted as downward deflections, whereas outward currents are conventionally depicted as upward deflections.

Components of a Voltage-Clamp Protocol

The most commonly used waveform to study ion currents is the square voltage pulse. Usually, pulses of varying amplitudes and/or durations are used to study the time and/or voltage dependence of the currents under investigation (e.g., see Figure 1.25). The membrane potential at which the cell is maintained between two consecutive pulses is referred to as the holding potential (V_h). Usually (though some exceptions apply), the cell is held at a membrane potential value at which the channel under study is closed and ready to be activated. The test potential, or command potential (V_c) is the

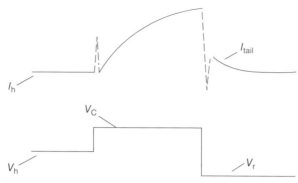

Figure 1.25 Voltage-clamp parameters. A voltage command (V_c) is applied from a holding potential (V_h). The holding current (I_h) is the current recorded while the holding potential is maintained. The voltage command may be returned to a voltage (V_r) different from the holding potential. The time-dependent current after the end of the voltage command is referred to as the tail current (I_{tail}).

voltage at which the cell is clamped during the pulse. At the end of the pulse, the cell is voltage clamped to a return potential (V_r). In many instances, the return potential is the same as the holding potential. However, in some cases, such as that illustrated in Figure 1.25, the membrane potential is clamped at an intermediate value for a certain fraction of the time before it is brought back to V_h.

The current flowing through the membrane at the level of V_h is referred to as the holding current (I_h); similarly, "pulse current" is the term used to describe the current that is activated by the test pulse. In many cases, when the membrane is switched back to the return potential, a remnant of current is observed. This remaining current is often called "tail current." Tail currents are often used to determine the conductance of the channel at the end of a specific test pulse.

What Are the Differences Among Activation, Inactivation, Reactivation, and Deactivation?

These four terms are sometimes a source of confusion. In the case of whole-cell currents, activation refers to the increase in current amplitude during a voltage-clamp pulse. It is commonly used as an indirect measure of the opening of channels following a change in membrane potential. The term "inactivation" refers to a decrease in conductance that either follows or, in some instances, occurs concomitantly with activation of the channels. Activation and inactivation are well exemplified in the case of sodium currents, as illustrated in Figure 1.26. In this hypothetical experiment, a cell is voltage clamped from a holding potential of −100 to −20 mV. The membrane current recorded shows a rapid inward deflection (activation); even though the voltage pulse is still maintained, the current spontaneously returns to the baseline. Investigators refer to that phase of current reduction as inactivation.

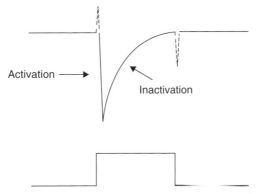

Figure 1.26 Activation and inactivation. Top trace, the membrane current; bottom trace, voltage step. The dotted lines represent the capacitive transients. The increase in current amplitude with time is referred to as "activation." A spontaneous decrease in amplitude despite the presence of the same voltage gradient is called "current inactivation."

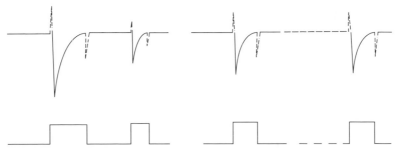

Figure 1.27 Reactivation of a membrane current. Top trace, membrane current; bottom trace, membrane potential during a voltage-clamp protocol. Left panel: two voltage steps applied with short delay. Because of its prematurity, the amplitude of the current elicited by the second step is smaller than that generated by the first one. Right panel: prolonging the delay between the two voltage commands yields two currents of equal amplitude. The process of recovery of a membrane current from inactivation is referred to as "reactivation."

On the other hand, reactivation is the repriming of the channel from its inactivated state to a state where it can be activated again. This is illustrated in Figure 1.27, where we also use the sodium current as an example. When a second pulse is applied immediately following the first one, the amplitude of the elicited current is smaller because the channels are not ready to be activated again. However, when the delay between the first and second pulses is prolonged, the amplitude of the elicited current is the same for both pulses. Once again, this process is called reactivation. Finally, some currents, such as those shown in Figure 1.25, do not seem to inactivate (at least not completely). In that case, a deactivation process is observed (I_{tail}) when the membrane voltage is returned from the pulse potential, to a voltage value in which the channel would not be activated (e.g., the holding potential).

Summary

We discussed some of the basic principles for applying electric concepts to the movement of ions across cell membranes. We established that the transmembrane flow of ions leads to electric currents and the displacement of charges across the cell membrane capacitor establishes the membrane potential. Some fundamental principles that determine the electric properties of the cell at rest, and during activation, were also reviewed. In the chapters that follow, we make repeated use of these concepts when discussing the properties of various membrane currents and the propagation of currents along tissues in the normal as well as the diseased heart.

2 | Ion Channels

Cardiac electrical excitation requires charges, primarily Na, K, Ca, and Cl ions to cross the membranes of heart cells. The task of moving charges across the lipid "hostile" environment of the cell membrane is nontrivial, and is mediated by a group of highly sophisticated, structurally complex protein molecules. As we shall see in this chapter, these protein macromolecules behave as "molecular machines" for the various ion translocation mechanisms that underlie cardiac excitation. The protein molecules are integral to the membrane (Figure 2.1), and functionally can be classified as ion channels, pumps, or exchangers. Ion channels are water-filled pores in the lipid bilayer through which ion translocation occurs in a purely passive manner. In contrast to this, ion pumps depend on metabolic energy, in the form of adenosine triphosphate (ATP) molecules, to shuttle ions across the cell membrane. Ion exchangers, on the other hand, do not depend directly on metabolic energy but use the electrochemical gradient of one ion species to translocate another ion across the lipid bilayer. Ion channels, pumps, and exchangers are important to the cardiac electrophysiologist because of their role in excitation and contraction and also because they are targets of therapeutic drugs used in the treatment of arrhythmias.

Ion channels are all characterized by two fundamental properties. First, in the face of an appropriate stimulus, ion channels open or close, a property known as gating. Second, as the channels open, there is the task of sorting out which ion species should be allowed through, a property known as ion selectivity. The cloning of the genes encoding ion channel proteins has profoundly advanced our understanding of ion channels. For example, the determination of what structural elements of the channel protein are critical to the gating and selectivity functions of ion channels has been significantly advanced for key ionic current mechanisms, e.g., Na and K ions. This chapter will provide a brief overview on the basic concepts

Basic Cardiac Electrophysiology for the Clinician, 2nd edition. By J. Jalife, M. Delmar, J. Anumonwo, O. Berenfeld and J. Kalifa. Published 2009 by Blackwell Publishing, ISBN: 978-1-4501-8333-8.

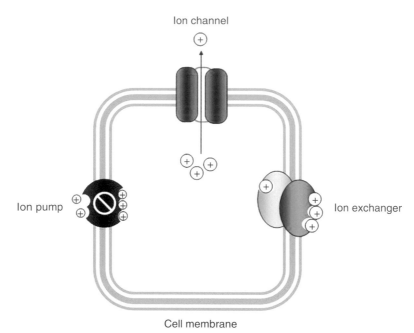

Figure 2.1 Protein macromolecules such as ion channels, ion pumps, and ion exchangers that mediate the movement of ions across the cell membrane.

of ion permeation and will rely upon a few examples of reasonably well-characterized ionic currents. Finally, a description will be given of the molecular entities putatively involved in the processes of gating and ion selectivity.

Mechanisms of Ion Permeation

Ion Channel Gating

An important feature of ion channel function is the process of gating, in which ion channels open or close to permit the movement of ions across the sarco-lemma. In fact, ion channels are usually classified based on their gating mechanisms. Channels can be gated by electrical (voltage), chemical (ligand), or mechanical (stretch) stimuli in the environment of the cell membrane. A channel is classified as voltage-gated when opening or closing of the pore is influenced by membrane voltage (Figure 2.2a). The primary Na, Ca, and several types of K currents involved in the cardiac action potential are voltage-gated.

Another group of channels, the ligand-gated ion channels, open or close in the presence of an appropriate ligand that is present in intracellular or extra-cellular spaces (Figure 2.2b). Such ligands include acetylcholine (ACh) and ATP, which gate a class of inwardly rectifying K currents, $I_{K(ACh)}$ and $I_{K(ATP)}$, respectively. Additionally, a group of channel proteins, the gap junction chan-

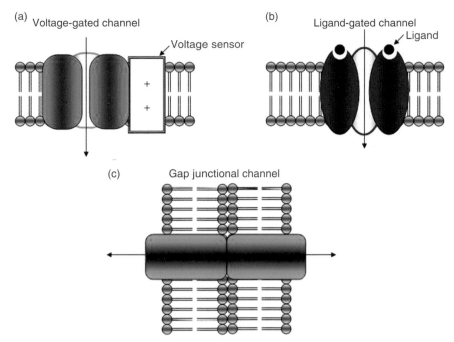

Figure 2.2 General classification of sarcolemmal ion channels. (a) Voltage-gated channels, which are open in the presence of the appropriate membrane voltage. (b) Ligand-gated channels, which are opened in the presence of the appropriate ligand molecule, such as a hormone. (c) Gap junctional channels, which permit the exchange of ions and small molecules between the neighboring cells.

nels, permit the exchange of ions and small molecules between the neighboring cells (Figure 2.2c). Evidence suggests that these channels are sensitive to changes in voltage as well as the concentration of certain molecules in the cellular environment.

The phenomenon of gating can be imagined as a change in protein conformation, i.e., a rearrangement of the channel protein molecule between forms or "states" that permit or prevent ion translocation (Figure 2.3).

A particular state is favored by changing the electric field across the membrane (for voltage-gated channels) or by the binding of the appropriate ligand (for ligand-gated channels). Ion channel gating behavior is a complex and poorly understood phenomenon. For the sake of simplicity, it can be said that ion channels can exist in one of three states: closed, open, and inactivated (Figure 2.4). For example, a channel may be closed at rest and ions do not permeate the pore. In the face of an appropriate stimulus, e.g., voltage or a ligand, the channels open and ion permeation is possible. In the inactivated state the channel is also closed, preventing any movement through the pore. Different ion channels are thought to have different numbers of states as well as different transitions between states. The complexity in ion channel gating

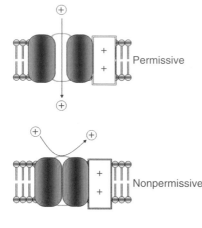

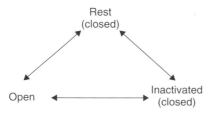

Figure 2.3 A change in channel protein conformation between permissive and nonpermissive states permits or prevents ion translocation through the channel pore.

Figure 2.4 Ion channels exist in one of three states: rest, open, and inactivated. In both rest and inactivated states, the channel pore is closed and no ion may go through the pore. Only in the open state will ion translocation occur.

is brought about partly by these differences in the transitions between states as well as in the number of states.

The pioneering work of Hodgkin and Huxely in the early 1950s on the ionic basis of the action potential of the giant axon of the squid provided a model that was used historically to explain ion channel gating mechanisms. In this model, the action potential is initiated by the activation of the Na current. The Na current rushes into the cell when the activation or "m" gates open to cause membrane depolarization. These workers postulated that the m gates are located close to the extracellular space and that three m gates interact in a cooperative manner to open the gate (Figure 2.5a). They also hypothesized that a different gate located in the cytoplasmic face of the cell membrane, the "h" gate, is responsible for terminating the influx of Na. In the model, Na influx is only possible when all three m gates and the h gate are open because the closure of either the m gates or the h gate will physically prevent ion permeation. It is easily seen how such a model may explain the existence of the three conformational states of closed, open, and inactivated.

As illustrated in Figure 2.5b, in the resting state, the channels are closed because the m gates are closed (even though the h gate is open). In the open state, both m and h gates are open. In the inactivated state, while the m gates are still open, the h gate closes the pore. How would operation of these gates lead to the transient depolarization and repolarization in the squid axon? Hodgkin and Huxely surmised that m and h gates are both increased by

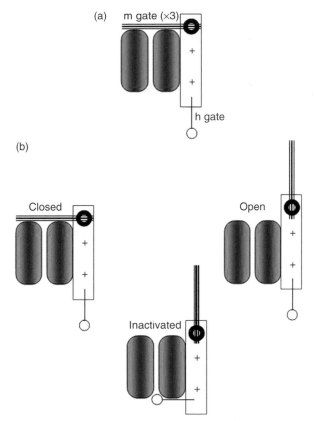

Figure 2.5 Model based on the historical work of Hodgkin and Huxely (HH) in the early 1950s and used to explain ion channel gating mechanisms in the giant squid axon. (a) The model consists of three activation or "m" gates and one inactivation or "h" gate. (b) Depiction of channel protein conformations that represent the three states of the channel, i.e., closed, open, and inactivated.

depolarization but have different time-dependent properties. Thus, with membrane depolarization the opening of the m gates is faster than the closure of the h gate (Figure 2.6).

Hodgkin and Huxely then developed a set of equations, with purely empirical bases, that describe the voltage- and time-dependent gating mechanisms responsible for the Na and K currents in the squid axon. The equation for the Na current was given as

$$I_{Na} = m^3 h G_{Na}(E_m - E_{Na}) \qquad (2.1)$$

According to this equation, the Na current (I_{Na}) is determined by the maximum Na conductance (G_{Na}, which is a function of m and h) and the difference between the Na equilibrium potential (E_{Na}) and the cell membrane potential (E_m). Similarly, the equation for the K current was given as

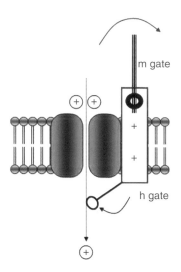

Figure 2.6 The Hodgkin and Huxely model. Because both m and h gates are activated by depolarization, their intrinsically different time-dependent properties ensure that, with membrane depolarization, the opening of the m gates is faster than the closure of the h gate to permit ion flux.

$$I_K = n^4 G_K (E_m - E_K) \qquad (2.2)$$

The activation gate for the K channel was described by n (raised to the fourth power) and, in contrast to the Na channel, there is no h gate. Hodgkin and Huxely subsequently demonstrated that these two equations well described the voltage profile of the squid axon action potential.

Although the cardiac action potential results from much more complex interaction between several ionic current types than just the Na and K currents described, and subsequent experimental investigations showed limitations of the equations, the initial work by Hodgkin and Huxely was invaluable in our understanding of the phenomenon of ion channel gating and in the development of later models, including those simulating cardiac excitation.

Ion Channel Selectivity

An equally important attribute of ion channels is their ability to discriminate among the various ion species present in the cellular environment. This sorting process is particularly challenging considering the relatively high permeation or throughput (in the order of 10^6 ions per second) of the channels. Stearic hindrance may be one method by which ion channels may achieve selectivity. For example, as depicted in Figure 2.7, it is believed that the outer mouth of a channel narrows to a very small diameter; 3.1×5.1 Å for the Na channel or 3.3×3.3 Å for the K channel, which acts as the selectivity filter. Ions with diameters larger than the opening of the narrowest region in the pore are rejected by stearic hinderance.

A closer examination of ion channel permeation will suggest that stearic considerations alone cannot explain ion selectivity, for it implies that the smallest ion will pass through all ion channels. However, this is clearly not the case because, strictly speaking, a potassium channel does not permit the

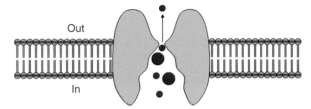

Figure 2.7 The outer mouth of an ion channel narrows to a very small diameter (~3.1 × 5.1 Å) and acts as the selectivity filter, rejecting ions with diameters larger than the opening of the narrowest region in the stearic hinderance.

passage of Na ions. Another mechanism that may be important in selectivity is the "liganding" or binding of ions to specific sites within the pore as a precondition for permeation. As will be later presented in this chapter, energy considerations favor the binding of one ion species (the permeant ion) over the other (the non-permeant ions).

Ionic Currents in Cardiac Cells

Methods of Resolving Ionic Currents

As discussed in Chapter 1, the development of the single-electrode voltage-clamp technique, together with the ability to dissociate adult ventricular myocytes using appropriate enzymatic techniques, made it possible to measure the characteristics of membrane currents of isolated cardiac cells or even those of single-ion channels in a small membrane patch. As the name of the technique implies, the same electrode is used to change the cell membrane potential and to record ionic currents, the whole cell currents, that flow across the entire cell membrane following the change in potential (Figure 2.8a). In Figure 2.8b, an idealized trace of a whole-cell rapid inward current is shown. The cell membrane potential was initially held at −100 mV and then a step depolarizing pulse was applied to −40 mV. The ionic current across the membrane rapidly increased in amplitude (activated) and then decreased (inactivated) in the face of a sustained depolarization.

Additional resolving power may be obtained in the cell-attached configuration of the single-electrode voltage-clamp technique (see Chapter 1). This approach enables the monitoring of currents through each individual ion channel (Figure 2.9a). In this example, after forming a high-resistance seal on the cell membrane, it is possible to record from a few channels or, in some instances, from a single channel in the membrane patch. If an ion channel was successfully isolated, a voltage pulse applied across the patch will cause the ion channel(s) to flicker between open and closed states (Figure 2.9b). Very clean transitions representing the opening and closing of the channel, indicative of good signal-to-noise ratio, can usually be obtained if the seal resistance is greater than 10^{10} Ω (i.e., >10 GΩ).

Although the time course of current through each channel is different from that of the whole-cell current, it is quite evident that current flowing through

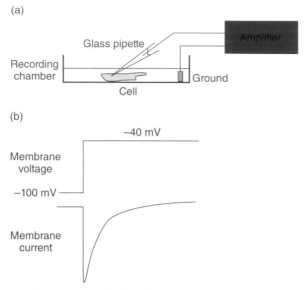

Figure 2.8 The use of the single-electrode voltage-clamp technique in recording membrane currents. (a) Single-electrode clamp recording circuitry. (b) An idealized trace of the voltage protocol (top) and whole-cell current (bottom) trace.

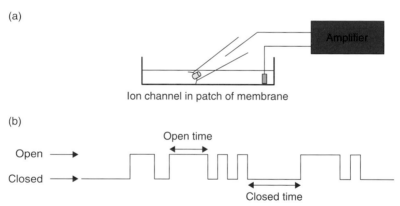

Figure 2.9 The cell-attached configuration of the single-electrode voltage-clamp technique monitors currents through individual ion channels. (a) Recording circuit in the cell-attached patch clamp. (b) Opening and closing transitions of an ion channel in a membrane patch during a cell-attached patch-clamp recording.

all the individual ion channels collectively form the basis of the whole-cell current (see Figure 2.10; compare ensemble current with membrane current in Figure 2.8). Thus, as it is often represented, the total membrane current in a cell is given by the expression:

$$I = Nip \qquad (2.3)$$

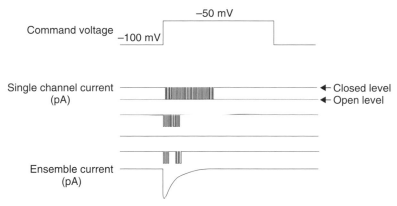

Figure 2.10 The fluctuation properties of single-channel currents are quite different from those of the ensemble current. This observation shows that current through individual ion channels collectively form the basis of the whole-cell current.

where I represents the total current, N is the number of channels on the cell membrane, i is the current flowing through a single channel, and p is the probability of each channel being open. Often, in electrophysiological analyses, this fundamentally important equation enables one to determine the mechanism by which a membrane current is modified in the face of pharmacologic agents. For example, it is clear from this relationship and from Figure 2.10 that an agent can increase a membrane current by increasing the amplitude of the current through each channel, by increasing the number of channels, or by increasing the likelihood of a channel being in the open state. With such a power of resolution, it has been possible to characterize the gating behavior of a wide variety of cardiac ion channels. It has also become possible to determine the molecular mechanism(s) responsible for abnormal cardiac excitation in inherited or acquired arrhythmias.

Functional Properties of Ionic Currents

The role of each ionic current in the different phases of the cardiac (ventricular) action potential was introduced in the preceding chapter. In this section we will examine more closely the functional properties of the major ionic currents.

Sodium Current

The major current that excites cardiac cells in the atria, the ventricles, and the Purkinje fibers is an inward current carried by Na ions (I_{Na}), which occurs during the upstroke or phase 0 (Figure 2.11a). It is believed that I_{Na} is not involved in the action potentials of the SA or AV nodal regions of the heart, either because of the absence of the Na channels or because, if at all present, the channels are inactivated by the relatively less negative membrane potential of the cells from these regions (less than -60 mV) compared with atrial, ventricular, or Purkinje cells (approximately -75 to -90 mV). As illustrated in Figure 2.11, normally closed at the resting potential (approximately -90 mV

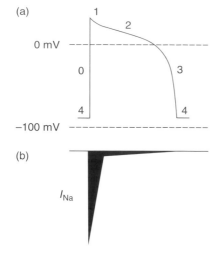

(a)

(b)

I_{Na}

Figure 2.11 A large inward Na current is responsible for depolarization in the upstroke of the action potential. (a) The five phases (0–4) of the cardiac action potential. (b) An idealized trace showing that the large activation of the Na channel current is immediately followed by a rapid channel inactivation to terminate the current.

in the working myocardium), Na channels open upon depolarization beyond threshold, allowing an influx of Na ions down their electrochemical gradient. This depolarization causes further membrane depolarization at a very rapid rate (~500 V/s in the Purkinje fibers) in a process that moves the membrane potential to positive values (Figure 2.11). The rapid voltage-dependent activation of the channel is immediately followed by an inactivation process (idealized in Figure 2.11b) that is also initiated by the depolarization. The inactivation process causes I_{Na} to be brief, resulting in the termination of the current. These properties are important for the rapid (≥1 m/s) conduction of the electric impulse in the myocardium.

Because of its extremely fast activation kinetics, as well as its very large amplitude (in nanoamps; Figure 2.12), the underlying conductance of I_{Na} is difficult to investigate electrophysiologically, and analyses are usually meaningless unless adequate precautionary measures are taken. Such measures include lowering the recording temperature, reducing the extracellular concentration of Na, and using an appropriate patch-clamp recording circuitry. Nonetheless, I_{Na} is one of the cardiac ionic currents that have been extensively investigated.

The current inactivation and reactivation are also relatively rapid processes, each with a time constant ranging from 2 to 10 milliseconds.

The influx of ions through Na channels functions as the excitatory current and as an indicator of the level of activity within the cell. For example, intracellular Na activity may rise by up to 0.3 mM following a single action potential. Therefore, during repetitive depolarization Na activity can give information on heart rate. Cardiac cells depend on the pump activity of the sarcolemmal Na-K ATPase to reestablish the gradient of Na across the cell membrane.

I_{Na} is regulated by a variety of agents, including neurotransmitters and other ions. For example, voltage-clamp studies of I_{Na} in isolated heart cells show that the current is regulated by norepinephrine at the β-adrenergic

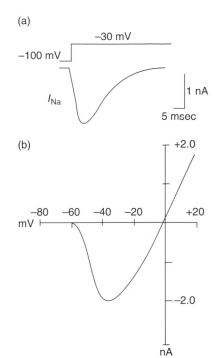

(a)

−30 mV

−100 mV

I_{Na}

1 nA

5 msec

(b)

+2.0

−80 −60 −40 −20   +20
mV

−2.0

nA

Figure 2.12 Biophysical properties of the voltage-gated Na current (I_{Na}) in a cardiac cell. (a) Idealized trace of I_{Na} showing the relatively large amplitude and very fast kinetics of activation and inactivation. (b) Idealized current–voltage (I–V) plot of I_{Na}. Because of its extremely fast activation kinetics and its very large amplitude, I_{Na} is difficult to investigate electrophysiologically unless adequate precautionary measures are taken, such as lowering the recording temperature, reducing the extracellular concentration of Na, and using an appropriate patch-clamp recording circuitry.

receptors, resulting in a shift of voltage-dependent inactivation to more negative membrane potentials (Figure 2.13a). The inhibitory effect of norepinephrine involves a cyclic adenosine monophosphate and protein kinase A (PKA)-dependent phosphorylation of the channel (Figure 2.13b, left). There is evidence also that another kinase, protein kinase C, phosphorylates the Na channel, resulting in a slowing of channel inactivation as well as a reduction in peak current (Figure 2.13b, right). The details of such regulatory pathways are discussed extensively in the following chapter. I_{Na} is also sensitive to divalent cations such as cadmium and zinc and is blocked by certain toxins such as tetrodotoxin (TTX) and saxitoxin (STX) obtained from a variety of marine animals, including newts, puffer fish, and marine snails. Because guanidinium ions can permeate Na channels and because TTX and STX contain guanidinium moieties, it is possible that these toxins inhibit I_{Na} by acting as a plug to the external mouth of the channel (Figure 2.14).

Depending on recording conditions, the single-channel conductance of the Na channel is approximately 20 pS. The behavior of individual Na channels during membrane depolarization is believed to involve stepwise transitions between conformational states of the channel, as shown in Figure 2.15. In this scheme, Na channels transit between several closed (C) states before they open (O) and then transit into the inactivated (I) state. Channels can also go into the inactivated state from the closed state without first opening. The rate constant of the transitions between states is thought to be voltage-dependent.

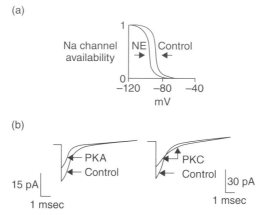

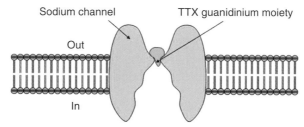

Figure 2.13 Regulation of I_{Na} in a cardiac cell. (a) Idealized plot showing the effect of norepinephrine (NE) on Na channel inactivation (a measure of Na channel availability) as a function of membrane potential. NE shifts inactivation to more negative potentials. (b) Idealized I_{Na} traces showing the effects of protein kinase A (left) and protein kinase C (right) on the amplitude and kinetics of I_{Na}.

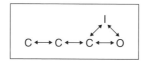

Figure 2.14 The guanidinium moiety of tetrodotoxin (and saxitoxin) inhibits I_{Na} by acting as a plug to the external mouth of the channel.

Figure 2.15 Possible transitions of Na channels during membrane depolarization. Na channels may transit between several closed (C) states before they open (O) and then transit into the inactivated (I) state. Channels can also go into the inactivated state from the closed state without first opening. The rate constant of the transitions between states is thought to be voltage-dependent.

The effects of the different class I antiarrhythmic agents (e.g., quinidine and flecainide) have been investigated at the single-channel level, and these studies revealed important drug mechanisms. The effects of the class I antiarrhythmic agents known to depend on whether the channel is in the resting, the activated, or the inactivated condition, imply that the agents have preferred binding with some of these states. This so-called modulated receptor concept can be used to explain certain properties of antiarrhythmic agents on

Table 2.1 Biophysical and pharmacological profiles of cardiac T- and L-type Ca currents

	T-type	L-type
Activation threshold	Positive to –60 mV	Positive to –30 mV
Inactivation threshold	–90 to –60 mV	Positive to –40 mV
Conductance (unitary) ($[Ca^{2+}]_o$ = 5 mM)	8.5 pS	16 pS
Pharmacological sensitivity		
Dihydropyridines	No	Yes
Nickel	High	Low
Cadmium	Low	High

the heart. For example, Na channel blocking antiarrhythmic agents that combine avidly and preferentially with channels in depolarized cells will be expected to selectively depress conduction in the depolarized tissue. Similarly, in the case of ectopic foci, the depolarization-induced activity can be suppressed by the blocking drugs preferentially combining with the Na channels in the depolarized cells. These concepts were used to explain, specifically, the selective effects of drugs such as lidocaine and phenytoin on ventricular and Purkinje cells compared with atrial cells. It is argued that atrial cells, with their characteristic short action potential duration, are depolarized for a significantly shorter duration, and hence drug binding (and effect) is much reduced, compared with the effect in the ventricular or Purkinje cells.

Calcium Current

Cardiac cells also have another transient inward current that is activated by membrane depolarization but lacks sensitivity to TTX. This current is carried by Ca ions flowing through two types (L and T) of channels, which mediate, respectively, long-lasting and transient currents. As shown in Table 2.1, the T-type Ca current [I_{Ca-T}] is activated by weak depolarizations and it inactivates rapidly. In addition, I_{Ca-T} is relatively insensitive to dihydropyridines or cadmium but is blocked by nickel. On the other hand, the L-type current (I_{Ca-L}) is activated by strong depolarizations and is slowly inactivating (Table 2.1). Under similar ionic conditions, the conductance of the L-type channels is about twice that of the T-type channel (16.0 pS vs. 8.5 pS). Compared with I_{Na}, I_{Ca-L} is activated at more depolarized membrane potential and has relatively slower activation properties: threshold of activation is –35 mV, with a time constant of 5–20 milliseconds. Inactivation and reactivation time constants are also slow, ranging from 30 to 300 milliseconds.

Similar to I_{Na}, the analyses of the activation of I_{Ca-L} show that channel behavior can be modeled using the state diagram and involves two closed states and one open state, with each step being voltage-dependent.

In general, I_{Ca-L} plays two important roles in cardiac cells (Figure 2.16a). First, it provides a sustained inward current that produces longer depolarization that is partly responsible for the plateau phase (phase 2) of the cardiac action potential. Second, it couples the electric phenomenon of cell

(a)

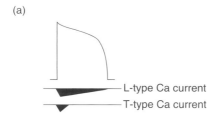

(b)

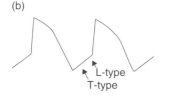

Figure 2.16 Functional roles of cardiac T- and L-type Ca currents. (a) Relative roles of T- and L-type Ca currents in ventricular action potential. (b) Roles of T- and L-type Ca currents in pacemaker potential and in the action potential upstroke.

depolarization to other cell functions such as contraction. Also, in pacemaker cells (Figure 2.16b), I_{Ca-L} is involved in generating the action potential upstroke. On the other hand, I_{Ca-T} is putatively involved in the generation of the pacemaker potential (Figure 2.16b).

Calcium channels are regulated by a wide variety of agents, and several studies showed that I_{Ca-L} is a major target for β-adrenergic agonists. I_{Ca-L} is increased by β-adrenergic agonists through a mechanism involving changes in the opening probability of the ion channel without an effect on the single-channel conductance.

Potassium Current
Delayed Rectifier Potassium Currents (I_{Kr}, I_{Ks} and I_{Kur})
The delayed rectifier currents were originally described as a single conductance mechanism and termed I_K. Important in the repolarization phase of the cardiac action potential (Figure 2.17a), the potassium currents are activated as the membrane potential becomes more positive than −40 mV, producing outward currents that repolarize the cell. Studies in cardiac single-cell preparations show that I_K is composed of two conductances that can be distinguished based on their biophysical, pharmacologic, and regulatory properties (Table 2.2): I_{Kr}, a rapidly activating and inwardly rectifying current with a sensitivity to the class III antiarrhythmic agent sotalol and its analogue, E-4031, and I_{Ks}, a slowly activating, non-rectifying current, which has no sensitivity to these class III antiarrhythmic agents. There is evidence that I_{Ks} but not I_{Kr}, is regulated by adrenergic stimulation. Which of these two conductances plays a greater role in cardiac repolarization? Under voltage-clamp conditions the amplitude of recorded I_{Ks} is over 10 times in magnitude greater than I_{Kr}. However, during an action potential, given differences in kinetics and voltage dependence of activation, it is believed that both conductances contribute equally to the process of repolarization. In a variety of species including humans, another very rapid delayed rectifier has been described. The

(a)

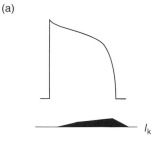

I_k

(b)

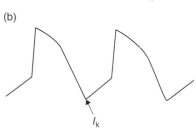

I_k

Figure 2.17 The role of the cardiac delayed rectifier K current, I_K. (a) In the working myocardium, I_K is activated as the membrane potential becomes more positive than –40 mV, producing an outward current that repolarizes the cell. (b) Also, I_K is one of the ionic mechanisms believed to be responsible for diastolic depolarization.

Table 2.2 Properties of the two components of cardiac delayed rectifier current, I_K

	I_{Ks}	I_{Kr}
Activation time constants (0 mV)	400, 2500 ms	50 ms
Rectification	Slight	Marked
Conductance (unitary) ([K⁺]ₒ = 150 mM)	1–3 pS	10 pS
Block by class III antiarrhythmic agent, E-4031	No	Yes
Activation by isoproterenol	Yes	No

ultrarapid delayed rectifier current (I_{Kur}) is present preferentially in human atria myocardium but has been demonstrated in the murine myocardium. I_{Kur} has outward rectification properties, slow inactivation, and is blocked by quinidine.

Subsequent to action potential repolarization, the activated potassium currents decay during diastole, and in the original description of the current, it was suggested that the decay of I_K during diastole, in the presence of a background current, leads to membrane depolarization in pacemaking cells (Figure 2.17b). Consistent with K channels being the most diverse group of ion channels, several other potassium currents have been described in isolated heart cells. These currents, some of which are shown in Table 2.3, have a wide variety of biophysical and regulatory properties and perhaps the only common feature being that they are permeated by K ions.

Inward-Rectifier Potassium Currents
The inward-rectifier current (I_{K1}) is responsible for the relatively high resting permeability of cardiac cells to potassium ions and is involved in setting the resting membrane potential. Inward-rectifier channels are abundant in atrial,

Table 2.3 Functional roles of other major cardiac potassium currents

K channel type	Functional role in the cardiac cell
Inward rectifier	Opens with hyperpolarization; establishes the cardiac cell resting potential
Transient outward	Opens transiently after initial depolarization; involved in phase 1 repolarization
ATP-sensitive	Opens at low ATP levels in cardiac cells, such as in metabolically compromised myocardium
Acetylcholine-sensitive	Opens in the presence of ACh, such as with vagal stimulation; efflux of K causes hyperpolarization, which shortens the action potential
Calcium-activated	Opens in the presence of high levels of intracellular Ca

ventricular, and Purkinje cells but relatively scanty in nodal cells. The relative distribution of I_{K1} channels in the cell types may therefore explain differences in resting potentials in the cells. Outward current through this classical inward-rectifier current plays a role in phase 3 repolarization of the action potential.

$I_{K(ATP)}$ is another inward-rectifier channel that is sensitive to cytosolic levels of ATP. The channels are closed at normal levels of cytosolic ATP. In the presence of low (<0.5 mM) ATP levels, such as during ischemia, $I_{K(ATP)}$ channels are activated, resulting in K efflux and hyperpolarization of the cell. The channels are therefore thought to play an important role under ischemic conditions.

$I_{K(ACh)}$ is inwardly rectifying similar to I_{K1} and is activated by the binding of acetylcholine to the muscarinic receptor on the sarcolemmal membrane. As discussed in more detail in the following chapter, the muscarinic receptor is coupled to this K channel via a membrane-bound, guanine triphosphate-binding (G) protein. It is an important ionic mechanism that underlies the modulation of heart electric properties under vagal stimulation. The binding of acetylcholine of the muscarinic receptor opens this class of K channels and results in K efflux and in the hyperpolarization of the cell.

Transient Outward Currents

The transient outward current (I_{TO}) is voltage-gated and is activated without a delay such as is seen for the activation of I_K. I_{TO} amplitude depends on membrane potential; the current is inactivated by partial membrane depolarization. In human atrial cells, I_{TO} is activated by depolarizations in the plateau range of membrane potential and is responsible for the transient repolarization in phase 1. I_{TO} amplitude also depends on frequency of stimulation. Because recovery from inactivation is slow, at fast rates I_{TO} amplitude is smaller, resulting in action potential prolongation. Similar to the delayed rectifier currents, I_{TO} has more than one ionic conductance mechanisms, a fast component, $I_{TO(f)}$, and a slow component, $I_{TO(s)}$.

Finally, a class of K channels is termed Ca-activated [$I_{K(Ca)}$] because they open in the presence of elevated levels of cytosolic Ca ions, which initiates

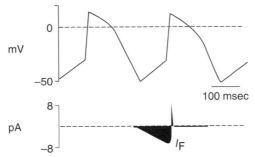

Figure 2.18 A hyperpolarization-activated current (I_f) is activated in the range of diastolic depolarization in cardiac pacemaker cells. Because I_f is an inward and depolarizing current, it is presumably important in generating pacemaker activity.

contraction. $I_{K(Ca)}$ will help terminate the action potential by providing an outward K current for repolarization. Additionally, the activity of $I_{K(Ca)}$ may protect the heart from Ca overload.

Pacemaker ("Funny") Current

The hyperpolarization-activated current (I_f) is one of the current systems putatively involved in generating pacemaker activity (Figure 2.18). The subscript "f" stands for "funny," because of the unusual properties of the current. Although usually referred to as the "pacemaker current," I_f is present in several cardiac and noncardiac cells, including non-pacemaking cells. In several cardiac preparations, I_f is nonspecific because its activation depends on both Na and K. Na ions are the charge carriers through the channel and current activation starts at approximately −40 to −50 mV, providing an inward current that depolarizes the cell. I_f is blocked by low concentrations (1–2 mM) of cesium ions. The limited single-channel study on I_f estimates the unitary conductance as 1 pS, which is a rather small value for a nonselective channel. I_f activation properties are regulated by cholinergic and adrenergic stimulation.

Background, Pump, and Exchanger Currents

Electrophysiological studies have suggested the presence of a background current in cardiac cells (Figure 2.19). With Na, Ca, and K as charge carriers, the net current is inward and time-independent, and is particularly important in pacemaker cells where its elimination arrests pacemaker activity. A Na-dependent background current in the pacemaker potential range of the SA node was identified, which has a density of approximately 0.7 pA/pF (by normalizing ionic current in this manner, one normalizes for cell size) at −50 mV and a reversal potential of approximately −20 mV. A current with such properties is a good candidate to provide membrane depolarization in the pacemaker potential range.

Cardiac cells have pumps and exchanger current mechanisms that are important for reestablishing ion gradients following activity. The Na-K pump,

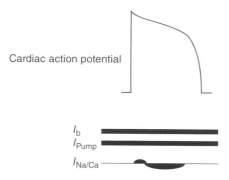

Cardiac action potential

I_b

I_{Pump}

$I_{Na/Ca}$

Figure 2.19 Background (I_b), Na-K pump (I_{pump}), and exchanger (I_{Na-Ca}) currents in the heart. Na, Ca, and K are the charge carriers for I_b, and the net current is inward and time-independent. The Na-K pump, with a coupling ratio (Na:K) of 3:2, generates an outward current. I_{Na-Ca} exchanger current depends on electric activity and the cell membrane potential. I_{Na-Ca} is an inward current throughout the range of diastolic depolarization in pacemaker cells, providing a background, depolarizing current during diastole.

with a coupling ratio (Na:K) of 3:2, will tend to cause an outward current because of the extra positive Na^+ that is moved out of the cell. Estimates of pump current amplitude in the guinea pig ventricular cell averaged 160 pA at 0 mV, with an intracellular Na concentration of 34–41 mM. It is believed that the Na-K pump will not have significant effects on the electric activity of pacemaker cells because the physiological changes in intracellular Na or extracellular K are small. In pacemaker cells, the Na-Ca exchanger current is an inward current throughout the range of diastolic depolarization; therefore, the Na-Ca exchanger will provide a background current that, in association with the decay of the delayed rectifier K current, will result in depolarization during diastole.

Gap Junctional Current

Evidently, the sarcolemmal voltage-gated Na, Ca, and K channels are critical for determining cardiac cell excitability in the heart. However, to ensure an effective contractile function, the spread of excitation from one heart cell to its neighbor must be through a rapid and efficient process, and it is generally believed that gap junctional channels provide the necessary low-resistance pathways for the intercellular propagation of the impulse. Gap junctional channels, unlike these other channels, are located in the intercalated disk, a membrane separating the interiors of two adjacent myocardial cells (Figure 2.20). Gap junction nomenclature and ultrastructure will be discussed in detail later.

Permeation studies on the gap junctional channel indicate that they are aqueous pores with large diameters (approximate channel diameter = 16 Å) and relatively low ionic selectivity. Unitary channel currents show widely varying unitary conductance values, ranging from 20 to as high as 360 pS from various channel protein (connexin) types and from different experimental conditions. Some cardiac connexins appear to be regulated by transjunctional voltage, i.e., gap junctional currents show time- and voltage-dependent activation properties. It is possible that a voltage-dependent decline in channel open probability is responsible for the time-dependent properties of the channels. Gap junctional channels are blocked by lipophiles such as heptanol and

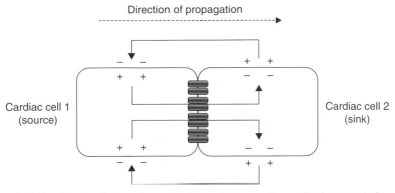

Figure 2.20 Gap junctional channels provide low-resistance pathways for the spread of excitation from one heart cell (source) to its neighbor (sink). Gap junctional channels are located in the intercalated disk, a membrane separating the interiors of two adjacent myocardial cells.

octanol, decreases in intracellular pH, and elevations in levels of cytosolic Ca, as further discussed in Chapter 3. There is evidence that low levels of intracellular ATP increase intercellular resistance, presumably by intercellular uncoupling at the gap junctions. Like other ion channels, gap junctional channels are also under regulation by neurotransmitters; however, the regulatory properties are less well understood.

Molecular Structure of Cardiac Ion Channels

Families of Glycoproteins Mediate Ion Flux

For many years, electrophysiologists have studied currents through ion channels, with only imaginary ideas as to the molecular architecture of the channel. The first insight into the structure of a voltage-gated ion channel came with the revolutions in the areas of electrophysiology and recombinant DNA technology. With the development and advances in DNA technology, it became possible to make millions of copies or "clones" of the gene of a protein, and to manipulate (genetically engineer) the DNA sequences in the clones. These molecular biological approaches require large quantities of highly purified protein as starting material and once the complementary copy of a DNA (cDNA) is obtained, it is used for heterologous expression and the electrophysiological and/or biochemical characterization of the protein. The usual expression system is the egg of the frog, *Xenopus*, or mammalian cell lines. The cells used for heterologous expression will usually not endogenously express the channel protein under study.

Such studies provided the first insights into the molecular picture of an ion channel. Experimental evidence shows that ion channel proteins are embedded in the cell membrane (Figure 2.21). Investigations on the molecular prop-

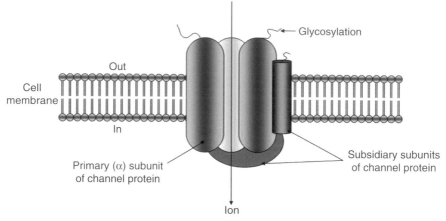

Figure 2.21 The molecular picture of an ion channel. Ion channel proteins are embedded in the cell membrane and provide a hydrophilic path in the interior of the channel for ion translocation across the cell membrane. Frequently, ion channels have multiple subunits.

erties of ion channels revealed that several of these pore-forming protein macromolecules are products of closely related genes and imply closeness in ancestral origin. It is believed, for example, that ion channels belong to one large superfamily that would have evolved by the gene duplication, mutation, and selection processes.

Once synthesized, channel proteins are inserted into specialized microdomains (channelosomes) in the membrane where they interact with several other proteins. The processes involved in channel assembly into microdomains (i.e., from channel protein trafficking to channel protein insertion into the membrane) are not understood. There is evidence, nonetheless, that normal functioning of the channel depends on its interactions with other proteins within the microdomain.

Subunit Structure of Ion Channels
Sodium Channel

First insight into the structure of a voltage-gated ion channel came in 1984, when the primary sequence and the putative membrane topology of the voltage-gated Na channel were described. The source of starting material for the cloning was the electric organ (electroplax) of the eel *Electrophorus electricus*. In the experiments, oligonucleotides and antibodies that were directed against small segments of the Na channel enabled the cloning of the primary (alpha), pore-forming subunit of the channel (Figure 2.22a). Depending on the tissue source for the isolation, the Na channel protein was composed of an α subunit of 260–280 kilodaltons (kD) that associates with from 0 to 4 auxilliary beta subunits. The α and β subunits are glycosylated in a variety of Na channels, e.g., nerve and muscle, and involve long chains of polylinked sialic acid groups. These side chains con-

(a)

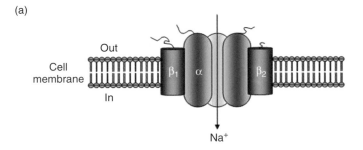

(b)

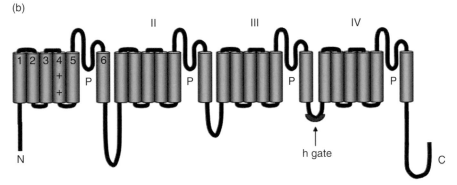

Figure 2.22 Subunit composition and membrane topology of the voltage-gated Na channel. (a) Primary (α) and ancillary (β_1, β_2) subunits of the Na channel. The Na channel α and β subunits are glycosylated in a variety of tissue types, e.g., nerve and muscle. The ion permeation path is formed by the α subunit. (b) The α subunit has four homologous, covalently linked domains (I–IV), and each domain consists of six α-helical transmembrane segments (S1–S6). The region between S5 and S6 (known as the P region) from each domain come together to form the pore. The S4 segment of each domain has a unique structure that consists of repeats of positively charged and hydrophobic residues and is a good candidate for the "voltage sensor" or the m gate. The short segment linking S6 of domain III and S1 of domain IV was identified as a possible candidate for the h gate, involved in channel inactivation by a proposed "hinged lid" mechanism.

tribute significantly to the overall weight of the protein and serve to stabilize the channel protein. Removal of the sialic acid residues in some Na channels results in dramatic reductions (to as low as one-fourth of normal) in unitary conductance as well as in a shift in the voltage dependence of activation. This latter effect may arise from the removal of negative surface charges (of the sialic acid) on the extracellular surface of the channel.

The α subunit has four homologous, covalently linked regions (I–IV, Figure 2.22b), known as domains, which are arranged such that an ion pathway is formed in the middle of the protein. Putatively, each domain consists of six α-helical transmembrane segments (S1-S6), and the region between S5 and S6 (known as the P region) from each domain come together to form the pore. Each domain of the α subunit presumably contributes to one-quarter of the wall of the channel pore. From each of these domains, segments S1 and S3, which contain negatively charged residues, and segment S2, which has both positive and negative charges, are thought to surround the ion permeation path. The hydrophobic S5 and S6 segments surround the inner walls of the pore and form part of the intracellular and extracellular vestibules of the channel while interacting with hydrophobic core of the lipid bilayer.

The S4 segment of each domain has a unique structure and consists of repeats of positively charged and hydrophobic residues (Figure 2.22), which form a spiral ribbon around the segment. The positive charges of the S4 pair up with the negative charges on segments S1, S2, and S3, thereby forming a structure that is a good candidate for the "voltage sensor" or the m gate. The short segment linking S6 of domain III and S1 of domain IV was identified as a possible candidate for the h gate that is involved in inactivation. Regions around this segment may cause channel inactivation by providing a "hinged lid" that occludes the channel pore. The α subunit has sites for binding TTX and STX and is also a substrate for PKA.

What is the role of the β subunit in the Na channel? Although the expression of the α subunit alone is enough for the formation of the ion permeation pathway, the β subunit(s) influence channel function by modulating the gating behavior of the α subunit. Co-expression of the α and β subunits accelerates activation and inactivation as well as influences the voltage dependence of inactivation of the channel.

Compared with the brain and skeletal muscle Na channel, properties of the cardiac Na channel have been less studied. Recently, it was shown that SCN5A, a gene located on chromosome 3, encodes a cardiac Na channel and that mutations in the SCN5A gene are responsible for one type of the inherited form of long QT syndrome, LQT3 (see Chapter 10). How would a defect in the Na channel affect cardiac repolarization? Evidently, the mutant SCN5A channels, because of their incomplete channel inactivation, provide persistent depolarizing current in affected individuals. In the case of LQT3, therefore, it is the gain in channel function that is responsible for the electrophysiologic abnormality.

Calcium Channel

The initial molecular characterization of the Ca channel was carried out using purified preparations from the skeletal muscle. Advantage was taken of the high density of the channels in the transverse tubule of the skeletal muscle as well as the specific binding of the dihydropyridine antagonist to this channel. The Ca channel consists of two α subunits (α_1 and α_2), and one each of β, γ, and δ subunits (Figure 2.23). The α_1 subunit has an apparent mass of 212 kD, and α_2 has an apparent mass of 140 kD. Similar to the Na channel, the α_1 subunit of the Ca channel forms the pore and is a substrate for phosphorylation by PKA. The hydrophobic δ subunit has an apparent mass of 27 kD and is linked by a disulfide bond to the α_2 subunit. The intracellularly located β subunit (Figure 2.23) is a 54-kD peptide that is not glycosylated and is a substrate for multiple protein kinases. The γ subunit has an apparent mass of

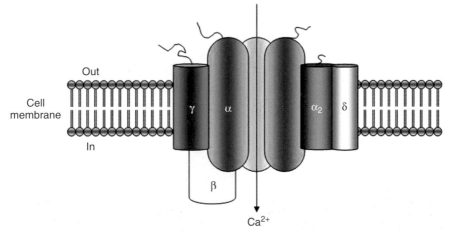

Figure 2.23 Subunit composition and membrane topology of the voltage-gated Ca channel. The Ca channel consists of two α subunits (α_1, α_2), one each with β, γ, and δ subunits. The α_1, α_2, γ, and δ subunits are hydrophobic, and δ subunit is linked by a disulfide bond to the α_2 subunit. The ion permeation path is formed by the α_1 subunit, and the β subunit is located on the cytoplasmic phase of the cell membrane.

30 kD, is hydrophobic, and has several N-linked glycosylation sites. The precise roles of these ancillary subunits are still unclear and are currently under investigation.

Potassium Channels

The structure of any K channel protein was unknown for many years because, unlike Na and Ca channels, high-affinity ligands for isolating and purifying K channels were not available. Fortuitously, a behavioral mutant of the fruit fly *Drosophila melanogaster* (called "shaker" because of the abnormal shaking of the fly's legs when exposed to ether) was discovered that had abnormalities in action potential properties and in neuromuscular transmitter release. The electrophysiological properties of the mutant were indicative of an abnormality in a K channel gene, which was later identified in the shaker locus. Subsequently, the cloning of the shaker locus and the study of the gene products revealed that the main gene product from this locus was a protein with remarkable structural similarities with the main subunit of the Na or the Ca channel protein (Figure 2.24). Furthermore, injection of cRNA from the shaker locus gene products resulted in the expression of K^+-selective channels. Using the shaker gene for sequence homology, a wide variety of K channels was now cloned, including several classes of delayed rectifier and the transient inward currents.

Currently, it is believed that shaker-related K channels belong to the superfamily of cation channels with a primary α subunit, a group that includes other voltage-gated channels such as the Na and the Ca channels. There is, however, one major difference between the K and the Na or Ca channels in

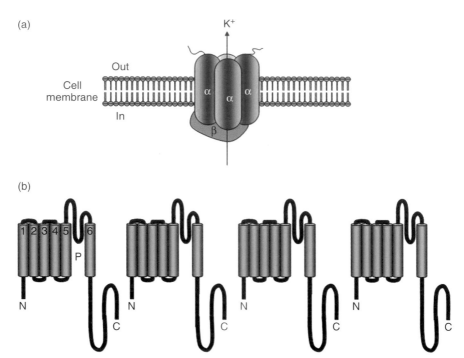

Figure 2.24 Subunit composition and membrane topology of the shaker-related K channels. (a) Membrane topology of the primary and ancillary K channel subunits. (b) In shaker-type K channels, the primary subunit responsible for ion permeation pathway is formed by a tetrameric non-covalent association between four α subunits. Thus, each primary unit of the K channel tetramer is presumably equivalent to one domain of the Na or Ca channel α subunit. The α subunit S4 segment and the P regions in K channels have similar structural designs as those in the Na and Ca channel α subunits and probably play similar roles of voltage sensing and ion permeation, respectively.

relation to their α subunits. In Na and Ca channels (Figures 2.22 and 2.23), the four homologous domains (I–IV) are covalently linked, unlike in the K channel (Figure 2.24b), where the α subunit is presumably formed by a tetra-meric non-covalent association between different units or peptides. Each unit of the K channel tetramer is equivalent to one domain of the Na or Ca channel α subunit, and the tetrameric assembly of K channels can be homo- or het-eromultimeric. It has been suggested that this is one mechanism by which K channels achieve their very diverse nature. The α subunit S4 segment and the P regions in K channels, which have similar structural designs as those in the Na and Ca channel α subunits, probably play similar roles of voltage sensing and ion permeation, respectively. In contrast to Na and Ca channels, voltage-gated K channels undergo inactivation in a process involving the physical plugging of the intracellular mouth of the channel by a particle formed by the N-terminal by what is termed the "ball and chain" mechanism (Figure 2.25). K channels can also inactivate by a different method, termed "C-type

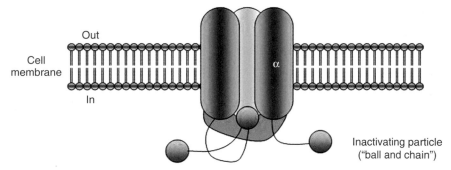

Figure 2.25 The N-terminal or "ball and chain" mechanism of K channel inactivation. A particle (ball) formed by a few N-terminal residues physically plugs the open, intracellular mouth of the K channel, preventing ion translocation.

inactivation," which involves the occlusion of the external mouth of the K channel pore. There is experimental evidence suggesting that some cardiac K channels use both N-type and C-type inactivation mechanisms to regulate ion permeation through the pore.

Molecular and electrophysiological studies shed some light on the molecular nature of two important cardiac delayed rectifier channels, I_{Kr} and I_{Ks}. I_{Kr} is encoded by the product of a recently cloned gene, HERG, for human ether-a-go-go-related gene and is localized to chromosome 7. The HERG protein is similar to the shaker channel protein in terms of the number of putative membrane topology. As discussed in more detail in Chapter 10, HERG mutations were shown to be responsible for another type of the inherited long QT syndrome, LQT2, in which the affected K channels have primarily a loss in channel function. The channel protein underlying I_{Ks} is thought to be formed by the co-assembly of the KvLQT1 gene product (another shaker-type channel protein) and the minK protein, a relatively small (~120 amino acid) and promiscuous protein. Mutations in the KvLQT1 gene result in defective K channels and in abnormal repolarization. The ensuing arrhythmia has the assignation of LQTI (see Chapter 10).

Compared with the voltage-gated K channels such as the delayed rectifiers and the transient inward currents, available information on the molecular properties of the inward-rectifier K channels is less extensive but suggests a different molecular plan. Expression cloning was used to identify the first inward-rectifier channel protein and it was shown that, unlike the shaker K channels, these channels have only two transmembrane segments (M1 and M2), which are similar to the S5 and S6 of the shaker channels (Figure 2.26). Interestingly, the M1 and M2 segments flank a region that is reminiscent of the P region of the shaker channels (see Figure 2.24), and it is believed that this region also is involved in the formation of the ion permeation pathway. Similar to the shaker K channels, the inward rectifiers also form a pore by a tetrameric assembly of the channel protein. Recent investigations have shown that multiple isoforms of the channel can heteromerize as tetramers to provide

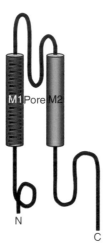

Figure 2.26 Subunit structure of the inward-rectifier K channel. The channels have only two transmembrane segments (M1 and M2), which flank a putative pore (P) region. The inward rectifiers may also form a pore by a tetrameric assembly of the channel protein.

channels with unexpected biophysical and regulatory properties. Differential tissue expression of the isoforms may explain regional and tissue-dependent differences in the inward-rectifier current. As we shall see later, a closely related family member of inward rectifiers from bacteria was recently used to carry out X-ray crystallography and to breathtaking view of the ion permeation pathway of a potassium channel.

Gap Junction Channel

Structurally, gap junctional channels are different from voltage-gated ion channels of the non-junctional membrane (Figure 2.27). Gap junction channels are made up of two connexons, one from each of the adjacent cells. A connexon is composed of six subunits known as connexins, which entails that each gap junctional channel has a dodecameric structure.

Several homologous connexins were obtained by cloning and are usually identified by their respective molecular weights. The major cardiac connexin has a molecular weight of 43000 and is usually referred to as connexin43. Each connexin characterized so far, irrespective of molecular weight, has four putative transmembrane domains, and sequence analyses show no apparent relationship to other ion channels. The N- and C-termini of connexins are cytoplasmic and two extracellular loops are important in determining "docking" of one connexon to another of the neighboring cell. The other connexins that were identified in the heart include connexin40, connexin45, and connexin30.2, and there is evidence that there may be tissue-dependent expressions of these different connexins. For example, while connexin43 is the most abundant protein in mammalian ventricular muscle, connexin40 is primarily expressed in the atria and the subendocardial Purkinje fibers, whereas connexin30.2 was shown to be expressed in the cardiac conduction system, predominantly in SA and AV nodes. Precise tissue localization, biophysical properties, and the regulation by cytosolic agents, including

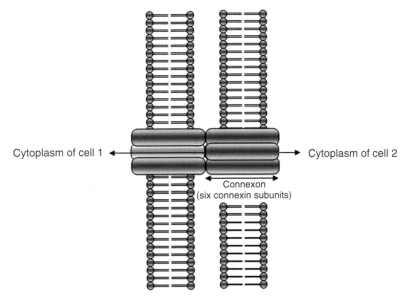

Cytoplasm of cell 1 ← → Cytoplasm of cell 2

Connexon
(six connexin subunits)

Figure 2.27 A gap junctional channel connects the interiors of two adjacent cardiac cells. Gap junction channels are made up of two connexons, one from each of the adjacent cells, and a connexon is composed of six connexins subunits. The N- and C-termini of connexins are cytoplasmic and two extracellular loops are important in determining "docking" of one connexon to another of the adjacent cell.

kinases, Ca, and pH, are currently an area of intense research in cardiac electrophysiology.

Structural Requirements for Gating and Selectivity in Ion Channels

Recent advances in several areas of science have begun to shed some light on the molecular entities responsible for gating and selectivity in ion channels. The emerging picture is that of regions of the ion channel protein, in a cooperative manner, function to gate the channel pore and to select for the appropriate ion. As can be imagined, these "modules" and the way they work in the key ion channel proteins are under investigation in several laboratories. The discussion below summarizes the postulated gating and selectivity mechanisms as mediated by these modules.

Selectivity and Gating Modules

The work in the laboratory of MacKinnon and his colleagues has been key in our understanding of permeation through ion channels. In the studies, a bacterial (*Streptomyces lividans*) inward-rectifier channel protein was overexpressed in *Escherichia coli* to produce large quantities of the protein suitable for X-ray crystallography. The crystallographic analysis of the K channel (dubbed "KcsA") provided the first detailed picture of the selectivity module (Figure 2.28a). As shown, the pore region of an ion channel is a very

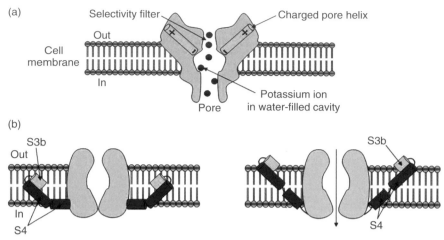

Figure 2.28 Modules for ion selectivity and gating in a potassium channel. (a) Ion selectivity module showing an aqueous cavity, negatively charges helices, and a selectivity filter. (b) Gating module in a potassium channel. The module assumes a "paddle" model of voltage gating in which the S4 acts as a sensor close to the cytoplasmic surface. Modules are based on results from X-ray crystallographic studies of a bacterial (*Streptomyces lividans*) inward-rectifier channel protein (KcsA).

specialized structure; the permeation pathway has three important structures: (1) aqueous cavity, (2) negatively charges helices, and (3) a selectivity filter. The four subunits of the channel contribute to the formation of the module. The aqueous cavity reduces the energy barrier in the otherwise hostile hydrophobic environment of the lipid bilayer. Four pore helices (only two are shown) stabilize an ion in the cavity just before it transits into the selectivity filter. Note that the selectivity filter allows multiple ion occupancy. Repulsion forces among adjacent ions within the filter are thought to enable final exit into the extracellular space. A number of models have been proposed for voltage-dependent gating, all of which have the positively charged S4 segment as central. Again, a similar cooperative action of the different subunits is thought to be involved in gating. In the relatively recent "paddle" model of voltage gating from the MacKinnon laboratory (Figure 2.28b), the S4 acts as a sensor, which is close to the cytoplasmic surface. The investigators suggest that paddle-like motion of the sensor (in contrast to an originally proposed rotating helix) gates the pore. Their crystallographic data from open and closed channels suggest that the formation of a "kink" in transmembrane helix is key to the opening of the pore.

In Figure 2.29 we reproduce a molecular ribbon model based on the original work of MacKinnon of the transmembrane and cytoplasmic domains of a putative inward-rectifier potassium channel (Kir2.1). The model highlights amino acids that are critical for inward going rectification by polyamine block; D172 (blue), E224 (red), E299 (yellow), and D259 (orange). A D172N mutation was demonstrated in a family with short QT syndrome (see Chapter 10).

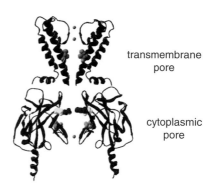

transmembrane
pore

cytoplasmic
pore

Figure 2.29 Molecular ribbon model of the transmembrane (KirBac1.1) and cytoplasmic domain (Kir2.1) highlighting positions in Kir2.1 critical for inward-going rectification by polyamine block: D172 (blue), E224 (red), E299 (yellow), and D259 (orange). (Adapted from Rodríguez-Menchaca *et al.*, *Proc Natl Acad Sci U S A* 2008; 105:1364–8 with permission.)

Summary

A wide variety of ion channels is involved in the cardiac excitation process. These channels can be characterized by their gating mechanisms, e.g., voltage or ligand, as well as by their ion selectivity. Clearly, the determination of the molecular architecture of ion channels and the determination of structural correlates of ion channel key functions of gating and selectivity are important questions. A combination of tools of molecular and structural biology and of electrophysiology is providing important insight into ion channel function at the molecular level, and a fascinating picture is beginning to emerge. The studies implicate elements of the sequence of the ion channel protein in the two fundamental tasks of gating and ion selectivity.

3   Ion Channel Regulation

The autonomic nervous system has profound effects on all cardiac functions, including chronotropy in pacemaker cells, conduction through the atria, AV conducting system, and ventricles, and in myocardial contractility. Stimulation of sympathetic or parasympathetic nerve fibers results in the release of neurotransmitters, respectively, norepinephrine (NE) and acetylcholine (ACh) from the nerve button or terminal. The neurotransmitter molecules diffuse and then combine with a specific receptor on the extracellular face of the cell membrane. A chain of events triggered by the receptor–ligand complex alters the gating properties of a variety of ion channels and pump mechanisms and consequently influences the electric and mechanical functions of the heart.

In addition to ACh and NE, other agents and factors such as neuropeptides, other hormones, monovalent and divalent cations, and temperature also influence permeation through ion channels and thus influence cardiac electric activity. Divalent cations (e.g., Ca^{2+}), as well as monovalent ions such as H^+, were shown to have very important regulatory effects on the properties of the different cardiac ion channels and pumps. Because the literature on this subject is extensive, this chapter will focus on the basic regulatory mechanisms of ion channels, including the role of the enzyme cascades and cations in the cellular environment. This will be followed by a discussion on properties of autonomic regulation in reasonably well-described ionic currents.

Mechanisms of Ion Channel Regulation

The Second Messenger Signaling Concept

The concept of second messenger signaling is key to understanding regulation of ion channels by neurotransmitters and hormones. The regulatory pathway involves a cascade of events from the receptor–ligand interaction on the cell surface to the alteration in ion channel function by phosphorylation

Basic Cardiac Electrophysiology for the Clinician, 2nd edition. By J. Jalife, M. Delmar, J. Anumonwo, O. Berenfeld and J. Kalifa. Published 2009 by Blackwell Publishing, ISBN: 978-1-4501-8333-8.

of the channel protein. The various steps in the cascade have some important historical aspects and stem from the pioneering work of Earl Sutherland and his associates while studying hormone-induced breakdown of glycogen in the supernatant fraction from liver extracts. Sutherland and colleagues discovered an important heat-stable molecule now known as cyclic 3′,5′-adenosine monophosphate (cAMP). This molecule turned out to be a key regulatory element, a "second messenger" in the entire cascade. Subsequently, investigations by this and several other groups identified crucial elements of the signaling pathway. It has been since shown that a variety of membrane-bound and cytosolic enzymes, including cyclases and kinases, are involved in a coordinated chain of events that eventually results in the phosphorylation of a target protein. Support for the importance of these pathways was obtained over the years in various experiments using synthetic analogues that specifically activate individual steps in the cascade. For example, forskolin, which stimulates the enzyme known as adenylate cyclase (ADC), is often used to demonstrate the involvement of the cyclase in a given pathway. Also, the extracellular application of membrane-permeable phorbol esters (e.g., phorbol 12-myristate 13-acetate [PMA]), which activate a membrane-bound protein kinase C (PKC), was used to establish the involvement of the enzyme in a regulatory pathway.

Figure 3.1 is a simplified schematic illustrating the major steps in a typical second messenger signaling pathway. The coupling of the agonist or ligand to a receptor on the extracellular surface of the membrane is the initial step in the cascade. The ligand–receptor interaction triggers a chain of events involving a membrane-bound, guanosine triphosphate-binding and hydrolyzing protein (G-protein) and a membrane-bound enzyme that generates a second messenger in the cytosol. The second messenger subsequently acts on a protein kinase, usually located at an intracellular site, which in turn acts on the target or effector proteins, such as the ion channels.

These kinases act by catalyzing the transfer of the terminal phosphate group from an adenosine triphosphate molecule to specific residues, such as serine,

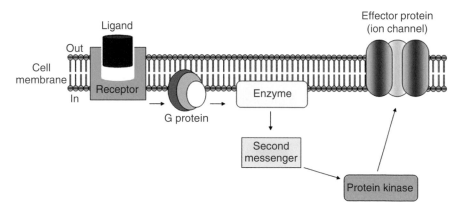

Figure 3.1 A simplified schematic illustration of the major steps in a typical second messenger signaling pathway.

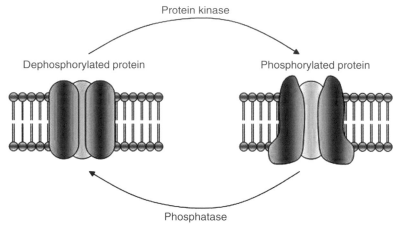

Figure 3.2 Protein kinases, by phosphorylating specific residues, such as serine, tyrosine, or threonine, located on the target protein, cause a change in the conformation of the ion channel protein and result in the modulation of function such as conductance. The modulatory effect on the target protein is terminated by the removal of the phosphate molecule by another group of enzymes known as phosphatases.

tyrosine, or threonine, located on the target protein. It is believed that in the phosphorylation process, the transfer of the phosphate molecule, a highly charged moiety, causes a change in the conformation of the ion channel protein (Figure 3.2), resulting in the modulation of function such as conductance. The modulatory effect on the target protein is terminated by the removal of the phosphate molecule by another group of enzymes known as phosphatases. Thus, in this model, the membrane-impermeable neurotransmitters or hormones are regarded as the "first" messengers which translate their message to an increase in cytosolic agents (the "second messengers") with an ultimate effect on a wide variety of the cell proteins, including ion channels.

Over the decades, it was demonstrated that several enzyme cascades involving a variety of membrane receptors and second messengers mediate neurotransmitter/hormonal signaling in different cells. For a complete description and to fully understand ion channel regulation as a topic, it is necessary to consider a few of these pathways. The cascade involving the β-adrenergic receptor stimulation and the second messenger cAMP is a classic for demonstrating second messenger signaling, and we will begin by examining in some detail this pathway for transmembrane signaling.

The Classical Signaling Cascade: The Adenylate Cyclase Enzyme System

The ADC enzyme cascade is initiated by the coupling of the ligand (e.g., NE) to a β-adrenergic receptor on the extracellular surface of the cell (Figure 3.3). How does this coupling lead to the production of the second messenger cAMP and finally to the production of the protein kinase? Interestingly,

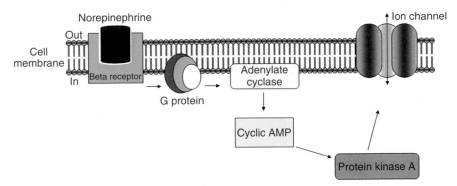

Figure 3.3 The adenylate cyclase (ADC) signaling cascade. This classical cascade is initiated by the coupling of the ligand (e.g., norepinephrine) to a β-adrenergic receptor on the extracellular surface of the cell. The G-protein involved in this cascade is of the G_s subtype. The subsequent ADC-induced production of cyclic 3′,5′-adenosine monophosphate (cAMP) leads to the production of protein kinase A (PKA), which then phosphorylates the effector (e.g., ion channel) protein.

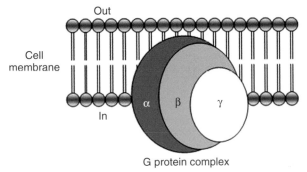

G protein complex

Figure 3.4 Guanine nucleotide-binding and -hydrolyzing (G) proteins are heterotrimeric, and consist of α (39–46 kD), β (37 kD), and γ (8 kD) subunits.

this second step was actually the final step of the cascade to be understood chronologically.

In the 1970s, G-proteins were recognized as involved in coupling agonist–receptor interaction to cAMP production. G-proteins (Figure 3.4) are a family of heterotrimeric guanine nucleotide-binding and -hydrolyzing proteins, which, for simplicity, can be classified as G_s (stimulatory), G_i (inhibitory), and G_o (also termed G_p). As illustrated in Figure 3.4, each protein consists of three separate subunits: α (39–46 kD), β (37 kD), and γ (8 kD). The G_s is the subtype involved in the ADC cascade. One important property of this subtype is that its α subunit has an arginine residue that is involved in adenosine diphosphate ribosylation by cholera toxin. G-protein α subunit binds the guanine nucleotides guanosine diphosphate (GDP) or guanosine triphosphate (GTP). At rest, each G-protein binds a GDP molecule and moves freely in the lipid membrane, and, if it recognizes an agonist–receptor complex in the membrane, the G-protein substitutes the GDP for a GTP molecule from the cytosol. The G-protein is then split into α-GTP and βγ, both of which are mobile in the membrane.

As the α-GTP moves freely in the membrane, it encounters and interacts with the ADC and initiates the synthesis of cAMP (see Figure 3.3). This synthesis continues for as long as there is an interaction between the two molecules. However, the inherent GTPase activity of the G-protein hydrolyzes the bound GTP to GDP, finally terminating cAMP production. The synthesized cAMP activates the catalytic subunit of protein kinase A (PKA, also termed A-kinase) present ubiquitously in the cell, which then phosphorylates serine and threonine residues of the target proteins, the ion channels, and pumps.

Two important features of enzymatic cascades in general are signal amplification and signal termination. In the case of amplification, for example, each agonist–receptor complex can interact with and activate several G-proteins, with each G-protein activating an ADC (see Figure 3.3). A single ADC can synthesize several cAMP molecules, each activating a PKA. Furthermore, each PKA can phosphorylate residues on several target proteins. Signal termination is achieved by several mechanisms such as by the hydrolytic action of the G-protein, the conversion of cAMP to AMP by phosphodiesterase (PDE), and by the dephosphorylation of target proteins by phosphatases (e.g., Figure 3.2). In some channels, such as in the ligand-gated ion channels, the process of receptor desensitization, in which the channel is inactivated in the presence of the agonist, prevents uninhibited ion flux through the channel.

Phospholipase C Enzyme System

The phospholipase C enzyme system involves α-adrenergic receptors. The functional existence of α-adrenoceptors in the heart has been recognized for some time, and several studies demonstrated that α-adrenergic stimulation modulates normal electrical activity in a wide variety of cardiac tissues. However, in comparison with β-adrenoceptors, α-adrenoceptor-mediated effects are not fully understood mechanistically. This is so, perhaps, because the α-adrenoceptors are linked to the relatively more complex phospholipase C enzyme cascades, which involve two second messengers and a host of other membrane and cytosolic agents (Figure 3.5). In this enzyme system, α-adrenoceptor stimulation by NE initiates the metabolism of a membrane lipid, phosphatidylinositol 4,5-bisphosphate (PIP_2). The G-protein involved in this cascade is of the G_o subtype and couples the α-receptor stimulation to PIP_2 metabolism. The enzyme phospholipase C (PLC), a membrane-bound, Ca-sensitive phosphoinositidase, splits PIP_2, resulting in the production of two second messengers, soluble inositol 1,4,5-triphosphate (IP_3) and membrane-bound diacylglycerol (DAG). Subsequently, the IP_3 diffuses into the cytosol and causes the release of Ca from intracellular stores, e.g., the sarcoplasmic reticulum. Ca ions have second-messenger functions; the ions can directly activate a protein kinase known as type II Ca-CaM-dependent kinase. DAG, the other second messenger, remains in the membrane and activates a

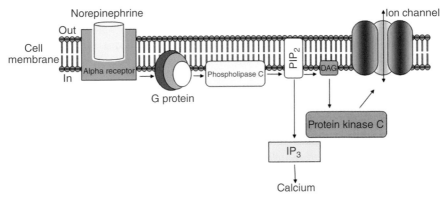

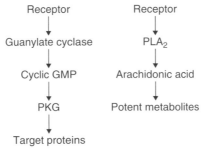

Figure 3.5 The phospholipase C enzyme signaling cascade. This classical cascade is initiated by the coupling of the ligand (e.g., norepinephrine) to the α-adrenergic receptor on the extracellular surface of the cell. The G-protein involved in this cascade is of the G_o subtype and couples the α-receptor stimulation to phosphatidylinositol 4,5-bisphosphate (PIP_2) metabolism. The subsequent production of the second messengers inositol 1,4,5-triphosphate (IP_3) and diacylglycerol (DAG) leads to the release of Ca from intracellular deposits, and protein kinase C (PKC), respectively. The effector protein, e.g., an ion channel, is then phosphorylated by the kinase. The ion channel may also be regulated by the IP_3-induced release of Ca.

Receptor	Receptor
↓	↓
Guanylate cyclase	PLA_2
↓	↓
Cyclic GMP	Arachidonic acid
↓	↓
PKG	Potent metabolites
↓	
Target proteins	

Figure 3.6 Other second messenger systems putatively involved in the regulation of electrical activity in the heart. The guanylate cyclase enzyme system is present either in the membrane or in the cytosol and synthesizes guanosine 3′,5′-cyclic monophosphate (cGMP) from guanosine triphosphate, which activates a specific protein kinase (protein kinase G, PKG). Also, phospholipase A_2 (PLA_2) acts on membrane phospholipids to release fatty acids such as arachidonic acid, which in turn are acted upon by lipooxygenase and cyclooxygenase to produce potent metabolites such as leukotrienes and prostaglandins.

membrane-associated protein kinase, PKC. Alternatively, as discussed in the following section, DAG may be broken down to arachidonic acid. Finally, the PKC phosphorylates its target proteins, including ion channels, pumps, and other kinases.

Other Enzyme Systems

The two enzyme systems described involve α- and β-adrenoceptor-mediated responses. In relative terms, these two enzyme systems are reasonably well studied. Other second messenger systems, some yet to be elucidated, are also intimately involved in the regulation of electrical activity in the heart. One example (Figure 3.6) is the guanylate cyclase enzyme system, which is present either in the membrane or in the cytosol and synthesizes guanosine 3′,5′-cyclic monophosphate (cGMP) from GTP. The synthesized cGMP then activates a specific protein kinase (protein kinase G, PKG), resulting in the phosphorylation of the target proteins.

Other examples are the fatty acids and their metabolites as second messengers. These systems deserve consideration, given that fatty acids and their metabolites are released as a result of hormonal action or during ischemia. In this pathway (Figure 3.6), phospholipases, e.g., phospholipase C and A_2, act on membrane phospholipids to release fatty acids such as arachidonic acid, which are then acted upon by agents including lipooxygenase and cyclooxygenase, with the resultant production of a host of short-lived and very potent molecules, e.g., leukotrienes and prostaglandins. Arachidonic acid is also generated from the metabolism of DAG from the phospholipase C system. The fatty acids and their metabolites, by activating protein kinase C, can indirectly (and perhaps also directly) affect ion channel properties.

Enzyme Cascade Shortcut
Direct G-Protein Regulation of Ion Channels

It is abundantly clear that the electric properties of a cell are modulated by a process in which G-proteins couple membrane receptors to a system of cytosolic enzymes. However, evidence is mounting for the presence of a shortcut of this signaling cascade in several ion channels. In a shortcut, several elements of the cascade are bypassed, and the G-protein, acting within the membrane, regulates the ion channel directly by interacting with it or through a yet-to-be-determined intermediary, which is also present in the membrane (Figure 3.7). This pathway is said to be membrane delimited because all the elements are membrane bound. It is thought that this pathway may be a possible mechanism for rapid (in milliseconds) regulation of ion channels. Although direct G-protein modulation has been described in quite a few ion channels such as the Ca and the Na channels, the most extensively studied was the modulation by the atrial muscarinic receptor of the ACh activated K ($K_{(ACh)}$) channel and will be used as an example.

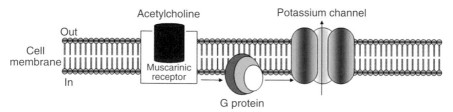

Figure 3.7 Direct (membrane-delimited) G-protein regulation of ion channels. In this shortcut, several elements of the classical cascade are bypassed, and the G-protein directly regulates the ion channel.

In the 1980s, in a set of insightful experiments from different laboratories, Pfaffinger and coworkers, Breithwieser and Szabo, and Yatani and coworkers provided independent demonstration of direct G-protein regulation of the $K_{(ACh)}$ channel. First it was shown that channel activation required a G-protein: the opening of the K channel required intracellular GTP and was blocked by the pertussis toxin (PTX) (G-protein is a substrate for PTX). Also, it was demonstrated that the $K_{(ACh)}$ channels activated by a non-hydrolyzable analogue of GTP were persistently activated. Very importantly, in cell-excised patch experiments, K channels could be activated by washing in previously activated G_i proteins into the intracellular face of the patch. These experiments therefore clearly showed that the $K_{(ACh)}$ channels are coupled to the muscarinic receptors without the involvement of cytoplasmic factors as demonstrated for the enzymatic cascades involving second messengers.

A dual pathway is also believed to exist for the regulation of the Ca current. During β-adrenergic stimulation, in addition to the indirect pathway involving ADC and cAMP, Ca channels can be regulated directly and rapidly with a time constant of less than 400 milliseconds (compared with over 30 seconds for the indirect pathway).

What could be the possible role of the direct G-protein regulation of ion channels? It was suggested that such a rapid effect may be important in the control of heart rate on a beat-by-beat basis. In the case of the Ca channel, for example, it is possible that this regulatory pathway may play an important role during increased vagal tone. Under such conditions, in which there is a block of the ADC system, the direct G-protein activation channels can provide a shortcut to override the system.

Cross Talking in Signaling Pathways

The description of the different enzyme systems may give the impression that the regulation via a pathway operates independently of the other. This, however, is not the case. Actually, there is a very complex interaction among the various pathways at every imaginable step. The result of this is that, in the presence of a neurotransmitter or hormone, for example, not one but several ion channel types are modulated, such that, depending on the path, the effects are additive or antagonistic. The overall effect is that there is an effective transmission of the message to the cell. This concept is further developed later in this chapter, where it will be shown that the coupling of a specific ligand to one receptor type has disparate effects on different ion channels.

Regulation by Protons
Sensitivity of Heart Cells to pH Changes

An understanding of proton-dependent effects on ion channels is important, considering that acidification of the cellular environment is a major factor in both myocardial ischemia and myocardial infarction. Acid loading a cell, in general, will result in membrane hyperpolarization due to the activation of the Na-K pump. Increases in intracellular protons following acid loading will stimulate the extrusion of protons and the accumulation of Na ions

(Na-H exchanger). The accumulation of Na ions in the cell then stimulates the Na-K pump.

Importantly, acidification of the cellular environment alters electric activity of cardiac myocytes, mediated through changes in normal ion channel function. For example, changes in the pH alter the properties of K, Ca, and Na channels and cause the disruption of cell-to-cell communication in the heart. Specifically, protons inhibit currents through channels and cause a shift in the voltage dependence of channel gating. Although still poorly understood, the following section describes possible molecular mechanisms underlying this regulation.

Mechanisms of pH-Dependent Effects of Ion Channels

Changes in intra- and extracellular pH can regulate ion channel function by one or more mechanisms. These possible mechanisms of regulation include effects on gating, surface potential, and acid groups.

The gating theory proposes that low pH affects gating kinetics and has no effect on the channel conductance. This proposal is the least attractive of all. The surface potential theory proposes that, by titrating surface negative charges around the pore of the channel, low pH causes a reduction in the single-channel conductance. Evidence for this was provided for several cardiac ion channels and is consistent with available evidence demonstrating the presence of negatively charged residues on channel proteins as well as on the surrounding sarcolemma. The acid group theory proposes that an acid group within the pore of the channel is titrated, with the result that the channel conductance is reduced. Although the latter two theories are more favored, frequently, from an experimental point of view, the surface potential and the acid group theories cannot be separated.

For the cardiac ion channels, including the Na, Ca, and K channels, extracellular protons reduce single-channel current amplitude in a dose-dependent manner. Also, extracellular protons shift the voltage-dependent activation

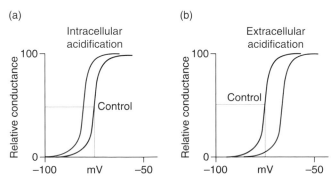

Figure 3.8 Comparative effects of intracellular (a) vs. extracellular acidification (b) on Na channel conductance. The shift in the voltage-dependent activation in each case is thought to reflect proton interaction with intracellularly or extracellularly located negative charges.

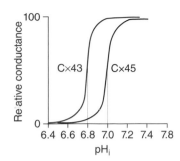

Figure 3.9 Some connexins have distinct pH sensitivities. Relative junctional conductance plotted against intracellular pH (pH$_i$) indicates that connexin45 (Cx45) is relatively more pH-sensitive than connexin43 (Cx43) (cf. pKa = 7.0 vs. 6.8).

properties to more positive potentials (Figure 3.8), which is in contrast to the effect of intracellular acidification, in which activation is shifted in the negative direction, presumably reflecting proton interaction with intracellularly located negative charges. The explanations based on the acid group theories are consistent with evidence that shows that pore region acidic residue (Glu) in the Ca and the cyclic gated nucleotide channels are the molecular mechanism of channel block by cations in these channels. However, in a cloned inward-rectifier K channel, one of two pore region cysteines was implicated, which act allosterically by stabilizing a channel conformation that exposes a titrable acid residue.

The mechanism by which gap junctional channels are regulated by protons is less understood; however, experimental studies showed that different connexins have different pH sensitivities (Figure 3.9). Available evidence suggests that connexin45 is very pH-sensitive. It is generally known that gap junctions close following increases in intracellular proton concentration, but it is not clear whether protons interact at sites within the pore, directly bind to the channel protein causing conformational changes that lead to closure, or whether protons interact with cytoplasmic factors to close the pore. There is evidence, however, that the intracellularly located, C terminal domain of connexin43 plays a critical role in the pH regulation of the channel protein. It is thought that this domain may act in a manner similar to the "ball and chain" mechanism of inactivation of voltage-gated potassium channels (see Chapter 2).

Regulation by Temperature

Changes in temperature influence permeation through ion channels, and evidence for this regulatory effect was already available in the early studies on membrane currents. The temperature-dependent effects are indicative of ion permeation as an aqueous diffusion process as well as reflective of conformational changes associated with channel gating. For example, in the case of the Na current, a 10°C change in temperature enhances the current amplitude by 1.3- to 1.6-fold and causes approximately a three-fold increase in the current time course (Figure 3.10). The higher temperature dependence of the effect on channel kinetics may reflect an effect on conformational changes associated with channel gating.

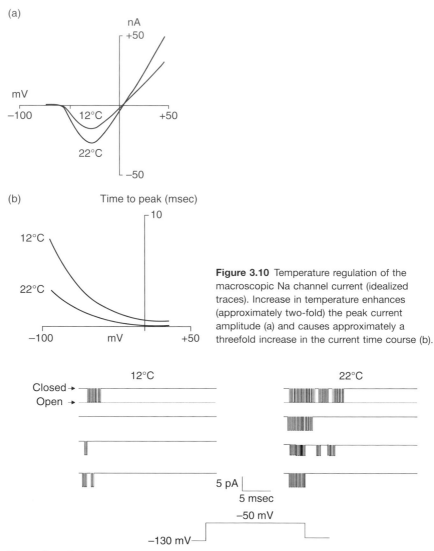

Figure 3.10 Temperature regulation of the macroscopic Na channel current (idealized traces). Increase in temperature enhances (approximately two-fold) the peak current amplitude (a) and causes approximately a threefold increase in the current time course (b).

Figure 3.11 Temperature regulation of unitary Na channel current (idealized traces). A rise in temperature increases the frequency of channel opening. The Na current was activated by membrane depolarization to −50 mV from a holding potential of −130 mV.

In more recent studies, experiments analyzing single-channel current properties in heart cells indeed show that unitary currents through the Na channel have relatively mild dependence on temperature (~1.3-fold change per temperature decade). Also, in these experiments, the important temperature effects are on the channel gating behavior because raising the temperature increases the frequency of channel opening (Figure 3.11), consistent with an effect on changes in channel conformations.

Regulation of Ion Channel Expression

An examination of Equation 2.3 in Chapter 2 shows that total current through a cardiac cell membrane also depends on the number of channels in the membrane. Normally as well as in pathophysiology, the number of channel protein molecules on a cell membrane for any given ion channel can be altered. The phenomenon of up- or down-regulation of ion channels as a mechanism underlying and/or exacerbating certain arrhythmias is increasingly drawing some attention. In a number of cardiac arrhythmias, especially for the inherited diseases, electrophysiologists are interested in understanding the underlying mechanisms for the changes in amount of a channel protein on the cardiac cell membrane. Atrial fibrillation and heart failure are known to result in, respectively, up-regulation and down-regulation of the inward-rectifier current. The question therefore arises whether the changes are due to alterations at the transcriptional or translational levels, or due to abnormalities of trafficking the synthesized channel protein to the appropriate cellular microdomains.

Autonomic Regulation of Ionic Currents in Cardiac Cells

Autonomic regulation results in profound changes in the properties of membrane currents in cardiac cells and consequently the action potential characteristics, with the ultimate effect on cardiac performance. Sympathetic stimulation via the release of NE has positive chronotropic effects on the pacemaker cell (Figure 3.12a), shortens conduction time through the AV node,

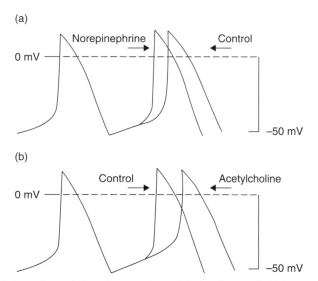

Figure 3.12 Autonomic regulation of pacemaker activity in a heart cell. (a) Sympathetic stimulation, via the release of NE, increases pacemaker frequency. (b) Vagal stimulation, via the release of acetylcholine, inhibits pacemaker activity.

and augments myocardial contractility. On the other hand, the release of ACh following vagal stimulation inhibits pacemaker activity (Figure 3.12b), prolongs conduction time through the AV node, and weakens contraction of the working myocardium, in particular, the atrial myocardium.

As discussed previously, modulators of ion channel properties, such as neurotransmitters, do not have effects that are limited to only one ion channel type; on the contrary, and as shown in Figures 3.3 and 3.5, the coupling of a ligand to a receptor, e.g., the β-adrenergic receptor, through the cascade of events involving the second messengers, will modulate several ion channels on the membrane. This modulation may be direct or indirect, involving membrane-bound and cytosolic enzymes as well as G-proteins. The resultant effects may therefore be enhancement or inhibition, depending on the ion channel. In the remainder of this section, we will examine the manner in which individual ionic currents are regulated primarily by neurohormonal agents. This will provide a basis for understanding the link between autonomic input and the electric activity of the heart.

Sodium Current (I_{Na})

The Na current is important in determining the threshold of activation in cardiac cells, and, because its very large amplitude and extremely fast kinetics ensure that action potentials are faithfully transmitted, the expectation was that the Na current was not regulated. Accordingly, few data are available on the regulation of the current in cardiac myocytes. With the cloning of the channel, it became clear that the α subunit has at least three phosphorylatable sites (Figure 3.13). In vitro experiments demonstrate that these sites are

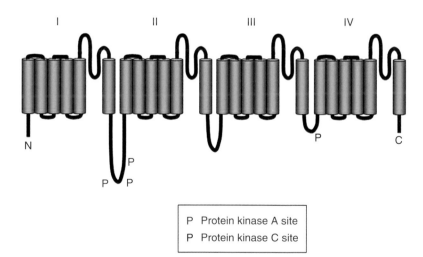

P Protein kinase A site

P Protein kinase C site

Figure 3.13 Phosphorylation sites for the regulation of I_{Na} in a cardiac cell. The cAMP-dependent protein kinase sites (red) are located in the intracellular loop connecting domains I and II of the α subunit. The phosphorylation site for PKC involves a serine residue (blue) in the intracellular loop connecting domains III and IV of the α subunit.

located in the intracellular loop connecting domains I and II of the α subunit. Indeed, experiments showed that the α subunit from different tissues is rapidly phosphorylated by cAMP-dependent protein kinase. Under experimental conditions, phosphorylation inhibits the peak Na current by 50%, without affecting the time course or the voltage dependence of the kinetics of the current. A similar inhibition of the current was demonstrated in isolated heart cells following adrenergic receptor stimulation by NE. The regulation involves two mechanisms: a direct path involving the G_s protein and an indirect path involving the activation of ADC by the G-protein. Both pathways reduce peak current by causing a negative shift in the voltage dependence of current activation.

The Na channel may also be regulated by other enzyme systems, e.g., the enzyme cascade involving DAG and Ca. Evidence for this derives from the observation that the α subunit is phosphorylated by PKC activation using DAG analogues. As illustrated in Figure 3.13, the phosphorylation site on the Na channel involves a serine residue in the intracellular loop connecting domains III and IV of the α subunit. Unlike the regulation by the ADC system, PKC has effects on both inactivation and current amplitude, resulting in the slowing of inactivation and inhibition of peak current amplitude.

L-type Calcium Current (I_{Ca-L})

Regulation of the L-type Ca current is believed to play a major role in positive chronotropic and inotropic effects of sympathetic stimulation on the heart. In ventricular cells, catecholamines were shown to shift the plateau of the action potential to more positive values (Figure 3.14), and, in pacemaker cells, adrenaline causes a more rapid phase 4 depolarization and upstroke; both effects were attributed to the enhancement of current through the Ca channel. The effect of the β-adrenergic agonist isoproterenol on the two types of Ca current studied at both the macroscopic and single-channel current level demonstrated that the effect of isoproterenol was on the L-type, not the T-type, Ca current.

It is widely accepted that responses to adrenergic stimulation are mediated by the binding of the agonist to the adrenergic receptor and may act, directly,

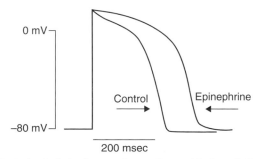

Figure 3.14 The effect of catecholamines on the cardiac ventricular cell. Compared with control, catecholamines (e.g., adrenaline) shift the plateau of the action potential to more positive values.

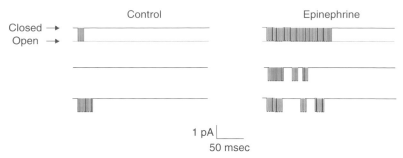

Figure 3.15 Ca channel activity (idealized) during depolarization to +10 mV from a holding potential of –70 mV, in control and in the presence of epinephrine. Because there are fewer blanks in the presence of the drug, and because the unitary current amplitude is unchanged from control value, epinephrine probably enhances the macroscopic Ca current amplitude by altering (increasing) the channel open probability.

through the G-protein in the membrane-delimited pathway (see Figure 3.7) or indirectly through the activation of the ADC system (Figure 3.3). Although evidence is limited for the direct pathway, a large body of evidence shows that phosphorylation results in the enhancement of current through the Ca channel, suggesting the significance of the indirect pathway. What mechanisms could underlie this increase in current at the single-channel level? As discussed in the previous chapter, the whole-cell (macroscopic) current is determined by three parameters: the number of channels in the cell membrane that are available for opening (N), the probability that any one of these channels will open (P_O), and the amplitude of current through an individual ion channel (I). As illustrated in Figure 3.15, it seems clear that the number of openings is augmented by adrenergic stimulation.

It is clear also that muscarinic receptor stimulation has effects on I_{Ca}; however, mechanistically these effects are less understood when compared with the effects of stimulating the β-adrenergic receptors. Consistent with this is the observation that the final phase of the action potential upstroke in nodal cells is sensitive to ACh. However, results from other cardiac cell types are not as clear-cut and are controversial.

An important effect of ACh on I_{Ca} in isolated cardiac cells is that the muscarinic agent has little or no effect on basal I_{Ca} levels. However, ACh antagonism of β-adrenergic stimulated I_{Ca} is a widely observed phenomenon in heart cells, and the site of this inhibition is presumably at a step preceding the synthesis of cAMP and involves G_i protein (Figure 3.16). Evidence for this locus includes the observation that the inhibition is prevented if I_{Ca} is stimulated by dialysis of cAMP or its analogue.

Delayed Rectifier Potassium Currents (I_{Kr}, I_{Ks})
The delayed rectifier current as originally described (I_K), is regulated by the stimulation of sympathetic nerves (Figure 3.17). Following the delineation of I_K into the two components, I_{Kr} and I_{Ks}, it was shown that the effect on I_{Ks} alone

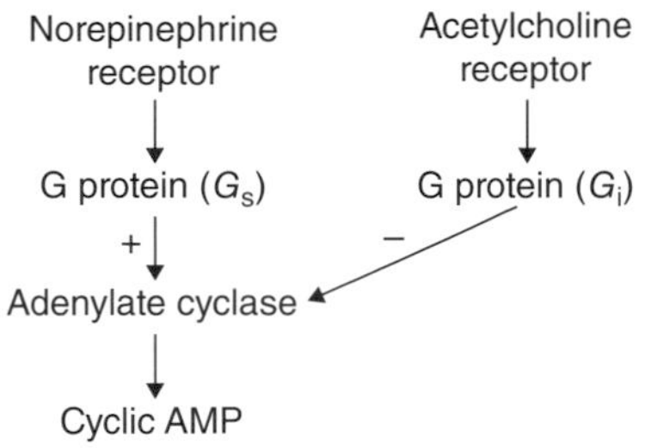

Figure 3.16 The site of acetylcholine antagonism of β-adrenergic stimulated I_{Ca}. The site of this inhibition is a step preceding the synthesis of cyclic 3′,5′-adenosine monophosphate (cAMP) by adenylate cyclase.

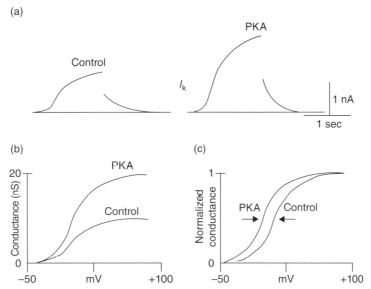

(a)

(b)   (c)

Figure 3.17 Regulation of the delayed rectifier current I_K by sympathetic (protein kinase A, PKA) stimulation. (a) Idealized traces showing that PKA increases I_K amplitude. (b) The effect of PKA on the I_K conductance. (c) PKA shifts the voltage-dependent activation negatively on the voltage axis. Experimental results depicted here represent the delayed rectifier as a mixed (I_{Kr}, I_{Ks}) or lumped conductance as originally described.

underlies the increase in current seen with β-adrenergic stimulation. The effect may involve PKA stimulation, and, in voltage-clamp experiments, the voltage-dependent activation of I_{Ks} is shifted negatively on the voltage axis (Figure 3.17b,c).

At the single-channel level, the mechanism responsible for the regulation of I_K by β-adrenergic stimulation is not very well understood because there is a paucity of data on the single-channel properties of the delayed rectifier current. However, using noise analysis, a technique that studies channel gating behavior by investigating fluctuations (noise) associated with the openings and closings of membrane channels, it was suggested that adrenergic stimulation has no effect on single-channel current but that it increases the number of functional channels or open probability of the channels.

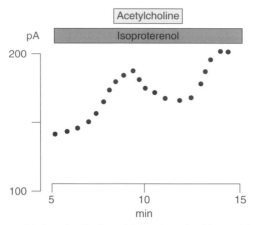

Figure 3.18 Isoproterenol-induced activation of I_K is antagonized by acetylcholine. The antagonistic effect is probably a step preceding the activation of protein kinase A by cyclic 3′,5′-adenosine monophosphate. The delayed rectifier is represented as a lumped (I_{Kr}, I_{Ks}) conductance as originally described.

I_K is also regulated by muscarinic receptor stimulation. In isolated ventricular cells, muscarinic receptor stimulation has an antagonistic effect on forskolin- and isoproterenol-induced activation of I_K (Figure 3.18). Studies also indicated that the site of the antagonism is a step preceding the activation of PKA by cAMP. Given that properties of delayed rectification may depend on cell type, e.g., sinus nodal vs. ventricular, it is conceivable that there may be differences in regulatory mechanisms of I_K in different parts of the heart.

There is evidence that I_K is also regulated by PKC. Indeed, stimulation by phorbol esters was shown to enhance the current in isolated ventricular cells. Presumably, this stimulation does not depend on the activity of the Ca channel. PKC and PKA may phosphorylate the channel at different sites based on differences in the regulatory properties of the channel by these agents (Figure 3.19). For example, unlike PKA, PKC stimulation does not cause a shift in the voltage-dependent activation but affects the slope of the activation curve. Experiments also showed that the PKA and PKC effects are additive: following maximal stimulation by PKA, PKC stimulation causes a further enhancement of the current.

Hyperpolarization-Activated Current (I_f)
Adrenergic stimulation causes an increase in I_f associated with a positive shift in the activation curve of the current (Figure 3.20a). Macroscopic currents at −100 mV (i.e., with full current activation) show that the current kinetics were accelerated without any effect on the current amplitude (Figure 3.20b). Consistent with this was the observation that single-channel current data in the presence of adrenaline show an increased probability of channel opening with no change in conductance.

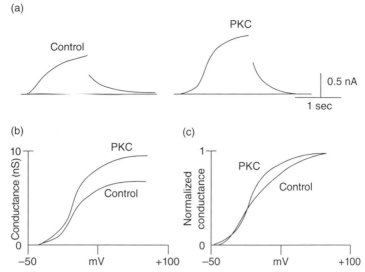

Figure 3.19 Regulation of the delayed rectifier current I_K by protein kinase C (PKC) stimulation. (a) Idealized traces showing that PKC increases I_K amplitude. (b) The effect of PKC on the I_K conductance. (c) PKC does not shift the voltage-dependent activation but alters the slope (cf. Figure 3.17).

Evidence suggests that some pacemaker cells are more sensitive to catecholamines than others; a shift in pacemaker site from primary to subsidiary pacemaker cells can be observed in the presence of catecholamines. It is thus possible that, in the presence of a catecholamine, the increase in I_f in the subsidiary pacemaker cells will cause these cells to become the dominant pacemakers. Given these observations, it is conceivable that the main role of I_f in pacemaking might be to serve as the means by which pacemaker rate is modulated by catecholamines.

As illustrated in Figure 3.21, low concentrations of ACh (0.03–1 µM) inhibit I_f. In voltage-clamp experiments, ACh shifts the activation to more negative voltages (Figure 3.21a). The current inhibition appears to involve the muscarinic receptor because the ACh-induced inhibition can be antagonized by atropine. Also, the ACh-induced inhibition of current (Figure 3.21b, left) can be abolished in the presence of pertussis toxin, suggesting the involvement of a G-protein (Figure 3.21b, right). Experimental evidence suggests that the ACh-induced modulation of the I_f channel involves a second messenger. Thus, in pacemaker cells preloaded with cAMP or with the PDE inhibitor isobutylmethylxanthine, ACh-induced current inhibition was abolished, suggesting the involvement of a second messenger. It was then concluded that the inhibition occurred via a decrease in cAMP, resulting from inhibition of the high ADC activity normally present at rest in the cells.

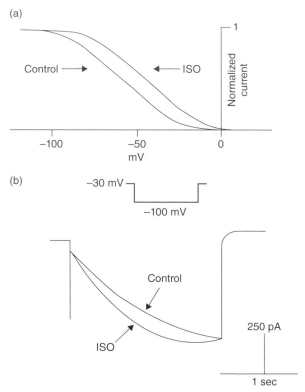

Figure 3.20 Adrenergic stimulation enhances I_f in cardiac cells. (a) Idealized plot showing that I_f activation curve is shifted positively by isoproterenol (ISO). (b) I_f recorded at –100 mV (Holding Potential = –30 mV) in control and in the presence of ISO. The traces show that the current kinetics are accelerated without any effect on the current amplitude.

Gap Junctional Currents

Junctional conductance in mammalian tissue is sensitive to neurotransmitters and second messengers; stimulation of β-adrenergic receptors or the use of cAMP or its analogues results in an increase in junctional conductance. Perhaps this increase in junctional conductance may be important in ensuring adequate electrical coupling in the face of decreases in refractoriness associated with the catecholamine-induced increase in heart rate. These regulatory processes are poorly understood and controversial. For example, in isolated cell pair experiments, evidence for increases in junctional conductance using cAMP or the catalytic subunit of PKA was difficult to obtain. The effect of muscarinic stimulation on gap junctional channels is also poorly understood and controversial. Some available data show that junctional conductance is decreased by carbachol, an analogue of ACh, and that the regulation may involve a cGMP-dependent protein kinase. However, it was also reported that PKC augments junctional conductance in the mammalian heart. Other

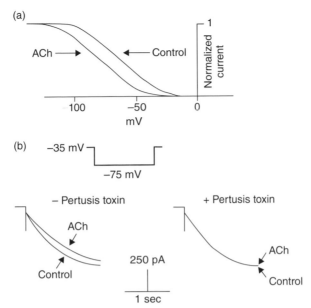

Figure 3.21 Cholinergic stimulation depresses I_f in cardiac cells. (a) Idealized plot showing that I_f activation curve is shifted negatively by acetylcholine (Ach). (b) I_f recorded at −75 mV (Holding Potential = −35 mV) is inhibited by Ach (left panel). The ACh-induced inhibition of current can be abolished in the presence of pertussis toxin (right panel).

experiments suggest that the mechanism underlying these effects may involve phosphorylation of serine residues on the channel protein.

Summary

Ionic currents in heart cells are regulated by several agents under physiological and pathophysiological conditions. Each regulatory agent, such as a neurotransmitter or a hormone, acts on a specific membrane receptor to affect the biophysical characteristics of several membrane currents in cardiac cells. Ion channel function is also dependent on the amount of the channel protein on the cell membrane. Overall, these changes in ion channel function will in turn affect the electrophysiological properties of the heart cell, with an ultimate effect on cardiac function.

CHAPTER 4

Impulse Initiation and Propagation in Cardiac Muscle

Cell-to-cell communication is essential for electrical impulse generation and propagation in the heart. In previous chapters, we discussed the electro-physiological properties of individual cardiac cells and considered the behavior of the excitable cell membrane as an equivalent circuit consisting of a resistor (the ion channel) in parallel with the membrane capacitor (the lipid bilayer). In addition, we established that the transmembrane flow of current through the ion channels leads to the charge or discharge of the membrane capacitor and thus to a change in membrane potential. In this chapter, we explore the manner in which cardiac cells communicate electrically with each other to maintain two essential aspects of cardiac function: the manner in which cardiac pacemaker cells in the sinus node synchronize to initiate together each heartbeat, and the mechanisms by which that impulse propagates throughout the cardiac tissues. The overall discussion centers on how the ionic currents that move across the cell membrane and from one cell to its neighbors lead to both pacemaking coordination of thousands of cells in the SA node and to the organized electrical activation of the entire heart.

Electrotonic Propagation

As discussed in Chapter 1, an excitable ventricular cell can be modeled by a set of resistors, each one connected to a specific voltage source, and in parallel to a capacitor (Figure 4.1). Current moving through any of the resistors (the resistances are different in case of nodal cells) charges or discharges a single capacitor, thus modifying membrane potential. In this model, however, an electric charge entering the cell has only one possible return path to complete the circuit, i.e., through the cell capacitor. In other words, according to the model depicted in Figure 4.1, all currents are moving across the membrane.

Basic Cardiac Electrophysiology for the Clinician, 2nd edition. By J. Jalife, M. Delmar, J. Anumonwo, O. Berenfeld and J. Kalifa. Published 2009 by Blackwell Publishing, ISBN: 978-1-4501-8333-8.

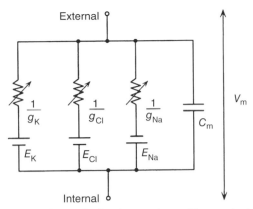

Figure 4.1 Equivalent circuit of a patch of active membrane. Three major ion channels are represented (Na, K, and Cl), each with its respective driving force (equilibrium potential, E) and variable conductance $g = 1/r$; C_m = membrane capacitance; V_m = membrane potential.

This condition is valid only for the case of an isolated single cell. Yet, cardiac tissue is a conglomerate of millions of cells, all of which are connected to each other through low-resistance intercellular channels (the gap junctions). As such, ions entering the cytoplasm of a given cell not only charge the capacitor of that individual myocyte but also move through gap junctions, thus depolarizing the neighboring cells. This "electrotonic" passage of electrical charge enables neighboring pacemaker cells to coordinate their intrinsic activity and underlies the propagation of the generated impulse throughout the heart.

Pacemaker Synchronization in the Sinus Node

The rhythmic contraction of the heart is initiated by the periodic electric discharges of its natural pacemaker, the SA node. The SA node is a somewhat diffuse and ill-defined conglomerate of thousands of specialized cells located on the roof of the right atrium, between the crista terminalis and the junction of the right atrium with the superior vena cava. In the 1970s and '80s, microelectrode studies in isolated tissue preparations from rabbits and other mammals revealed that the largest proportion of cells in the SA region of the heart shows the characteristic oscillatory transmembrane potential changes associated with pacemaker activity, including unstable diastolic potential and gradual depolarization toward threshold for an action potential (see Figure 4.2a), after which a new cycle ensues. This autonomous self-sustaining activity is apparent even in the absence of any form of neural or hormonal control because it can be demonstrated also in single SA node cells after enzymatic dispersion. Moreover, although normally the SA node contains the fastest discharging pacemaker cells, pacemaker activity is a ubiquitous property and occurs in other cardiac cells as well. Indeed, cardiac excitation can result also from impulses generated by groups of subsidiary pacemaker cells in the atria, the AV node, or the Purkinje fibers. Under normal conditions, pacemaker

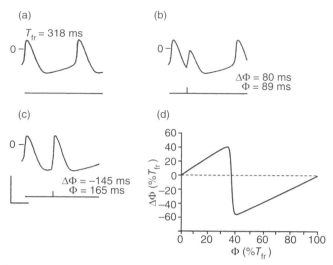

Figure 4.2 Phasic effects of brief depolarizing pulses on pacemaker activity of a single, enzymatically dissociated pacemaker cell from the sinoatrial region of the rabbit. In all panels, top trace is transmembrane potential; bottom trace is membrane current. (a) Control free-running period (T_{fr}) is 318 ms. (b) A brief (30 ms, 0.5 nA) depolarizing current pulse applied at a phase (φ) of 89 ms prolonged the pacemaker period by 80 ms. This prolongation is expressed as a phase shift ($\Delta\varphi$). (c) A similar stimulus applied at a later phase abbreviated the pacemaker period (i.e., $\Delta\varphi$ is negative). (d) Phase–response curve; ordinates $\Delta\varphi$ as percent of T_{fr}; abscissa, φ, also expressed as percent of T_{fr}. (Modified from Anumonwo et al., Circ Res 1991; 68:1138–53, with permission from the American Heart Association, Inc.)

activity does not originate in the contractile atrial or ventricular muscle but can be demonstrated as a result of membrane depolarization, ischemia, or certain drug effects.

As already discussed in Chapter 2, the precise subcellular basis of pacemaker activity in the SA node, while not fully elucidated to this day, has been explained in terms of the properties of ionic channels and exchangers on the cell membrane. On the other hand, the dynamic mechanisms involved in the communication and rhythm coordination of large numbers of spontaneously active pacemaker cells were the subject of intense controversy and, at times, wild speculation for many years. In the 1980s, a number of theoretical and experimental studies provided strong evidence in support of the hypothesis that the initiation and maintenance of the mammalian heartbeat by its natural pacemaker is a dynamic process whereby thousands of sinus node cells communicate electrically with each other and reach a consensus as to when to discharge and initiate together each beat. Furthermore, it was shown that the rules that determine the coordination of the electric activity of neighboring pacemaker cells apply also to the mechanisms by which cardiac pacemaker rhythms originated in the SA node and elsewhere synchronize to external periodicities, including nerve activity and cardiac impulses initiated in neighboring sites. Indeed, the analysis of the dynamic behavior of cardiac pacemaker rhythms led to the demonstration that, like other biological oscillatory systems, cardiac pacemakers show a phasic sensitivity to discrete perturbing stimuli. Whether the stimulus is a subthreshold depolarization or a brief vagal discharge, it can alter the periodicity of a pacemaker by an amount that depends on the timing, amplitude, and duration of the stimulus. Under these conditions, repetitive stimuli can entrain the pacemaker and force it to discharge at rates that may be faster or slower than its own rate.

Resistive Coupling and Mutual Entrainment

Many studies in the sinus node support the idea that cell-to-cell communication and pacemaker coordination are based in part on a resistive type of electric coupling. Indeed, although for many years electrophysiological studies consistently indicated that electrical coupling was present in the sinus node, early investigations failed to demonstrate the existence of direct cell-to-cell connections in the region. Such connections would act as low-resistance pathways to allow the free exchange of charge-bearing ions between the interiors of two neighboring pacemaker cells. In the late 1970s, the elegant studies by Bouman's group in Amsterdam provided direct morphological evidence that sinus node cells are indeed connected through gap junction channels, which correlates quite well with measurements of passive electric properties of tissue preparations from this region. As discussed in previous chapters, gap junctions are found joining cells in a wide variety of tissues, including cardiac muscle, and are known to permit the flow of ions and small molecules. Although in the sinus node, gap junctions are probably smaller and sparser than those found in other types of cardiac tissue, investigators found at least one gap junction per cell-to-cell contact when exploring systematically the entire SA region.

Recent studies using immunofluorescence localization techniques in various species, including human, have shown that in the center of the sinus node there is expression of Cx45 and Cx30.2, whereas in the periphery of the sinoatrial node, Cx43 and Cx45 are expressed.

Regardless of its specific molecular nature, the general consensus is that the gap junction permits electrotonic coupling between cardiac cells and allows them to function as an electric syncytium. This accounts for action potential propagation throughout the entire heart. In the case of the sinus node, it was assumed that the electrical currents generated by the fastest firing cell propagate electrotonically through the gap junction and force its neighbors to fire prematurely. The problem with this idea is that electrotonic current propagation is not unidirectional. In fact, electrotonic currents generated by the belated discharge of the subsidiary pacemaker cells would be expected to propagate to the dominant cell and somehow force it to change its rhythm. Accordingly, electrotonically mediated pacemaker coordination must be a bidirectional process in which the dynamic beat-to-beat interaction of neighboring pacemaker cells forces them to achieve a consensus as to when to fire. Thus, synchronization requires that the fastest cell must slow down and the slowest cell must accelerate. These changes may be explained on the basis of the process known as "mutual entrainment," which was defined as the condition of dynamic interaction between two or more pacemaker cells, with the result that either all cells discharge at the same frequency (i.e., 1:1 entrainment) or their frequencies become related in some harmonic fashion (e.g., 3:2, 2:1, and 3:1).

The Phase–Response Curve Predicts Entrainment

Output Phase Shift as a Function of Input Phase

The mechanisms by which cardiac pacemakers coordinate their activity to external periodicities in their surroundings were extensively studied in isolated tissue preparations and computer simulations as well as in the human. The use of programmed stimulation techniques in the analysis of the dynamic behavior of pacemaker rhythms led to the conclusion that, just as in other biological oscillatory systems, the sensitivity of the pacemaker rhythm to the external perturbation is phasic in the sense that it depends on the timing of the perturbation: the change in the period of the pacemaker is a function of the phase of the input with respect to the pacemaker period. Moreover, as a result of this phasic sensitivity, such repetitive perturbations are capable of phase locking the pacemaker, thus forcing it to discharge at frequencies that may be faster or slower than its intrinsic frequency.

In 1951, Silvio Weidmann, at the University of Berne, pioneered the use of microelectrode recording and stimulation techniques in isolated Purkinje fiber pacemakers. He demonstrated that depolarizing current pulses of relatively brief duration and subthreshold magnitude, applied early in diastole, can produce a slowing of diastolic depolarization, thus delaying the approach to threshold for a subsequent discharge. Hyperpolarizing pulses had the opposite effect. Jalife and Moe used the Purkinje fiber sucrose gap preparation to study the changes in pacemaker activity induced by subthreshold currents propagating across an area of depressed conduction. The results of that study demonstrated that subthreshold depolarizations applied early in the cycle delayed the subsequent pacemaker discharge, whereas those applied at later phases captured the pacemaker discharge and abbreviated the pacemaker period. This biphasic influence had the same qualitative characteristics whether it was the result of transmembrane current from an external stimulator or the electronically mediated effect of action potentials blocked across an area of reduced conductivity.

Additional studies were carried out in small strips of rabbit sinus node and in computer simulations of cardiac pacemaker activity based on ionic models. Subsequently, phasic effects of brief subthreshold depolarizing and hyperpolarizing current pulses on the spontaneous pacemaker cycle were demonstrated in single, enzymatically dispersed SA nodal cells. The common denominator in all examples is the fact that the sensitivity of the pacemaker is phase-related. This is illustrated by the results presented in Figure 4.2.

Panels (a) through (c) show the transmembrane potentials recorded from a single SA node cell using a patch pipette. Transmembrane potential is shown in the top traces; input current is shown in the bottom traces. In panel (a), the control spontaneous pacemaker period is 318 milliseconds. In panel (b), a 30-millisecond depolarizing current pulse applied at a phase (Φ) of 89 milliseconds, corresponding to approximately 28% of the pacemaker period (T), delays the subsequent discharge. In panel (c), a similar pulse applied at a later phase advances the subsequent discharge. These changes are short-lived, and, after the perturbation, the pacemaker rapidly returns to its original rhythm. Accordingly, the delaying or advancing effects can be described as phase shifts ($\Delta\Phi$) of the new discharge with respect to the old rhythm. In panel (d), we present the "phase–response" curve (PRC) obtained for a complete scan of the pacemaker period of the sinus node cell with single depolarizing current pulses of the same duration and magnitude as for the examples in panels (b) and (c). The horizontal broken line represents the intrinsic period in the absence of perturbation. The effects are expressed as percent of this period. Upward changes represent prolongation; downward changes represent abbreviation. It is clear that stimuli applied in the first half of the cycle delay the subsequent discharge and, consequently, prolong the cycle. Perturbations occurring during the second half abbreviate that cycle. Hyperpolarizing pulses result in a quantitatively different PRC.

Pacemaker Entrainment by Repetitive Input

The PRC is an accurate representation of the dynamics of the cardiac pacemaker to a given perturbation and can be used to predict the behavior of the pacemaker in response to that perturbation when it occurs repetitively. Figure 4.3 was taken from an experiment in which a single sinus nodal cell was subjected to the application of repetitive subthreshold depolarizing pulses (0.7 nA, 20 milliseconds). The intrinsic period of the pacemaker was 280 milliseconds (not shown). Panels (a–d) show the beat-to-beat responses to repetitive stimulation at fixed frequencies. In panel (a), stimulation at a basic cycle length (BCL) of 200 milliseconds resulted in $1:1$ $n:m$ entrainment, where n is the number of stimuli and m is the number of sinus cell responses. In panel (b), changing the BCL to 180 milliseconds resulted in an $n:m$ ratio of $5:4$. In panel (c), at a BCL of 160 milliseconds, $n:m$ was $3:2$. Finally, in panel (d), subthreshold stimuli applied at a BCL of 120 milliseconds yielded an $n:m$ pattern of $2:1$. The overall entrainment behavior is illustrated in panel (e), in which the ratio of m/n is plotted against the stimulus BCL. At BCL values around the spontaneous cycle length, $1:1$ entrainment was always obtained. Progressive reductions of driving BCL down to ~185 milliseconds did not change the m/n pattern, as seen by the large plateau at BCLs between 185 and 240 milliseconds. On the opposite side, at a BCL of approximately half the spontaneous cycle, a $2:1$ entrainment ratio was maintained between BCLs of 90 and 120 milliseconds. Between these two large entrainment plateaus, Wenckebach-like patterns were seen (i.e., $5:4$, $3:2$, and $4:3$). Presenting the

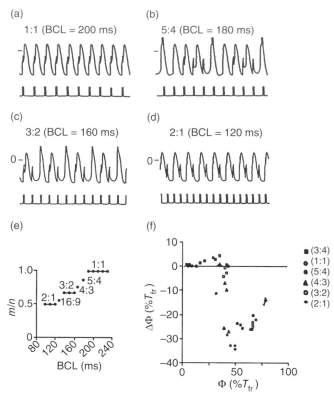

Figure 4.3 Entrainment behavior of a single pacemaker cell isolated from the sinoatrial region of a rabbit heart. The free-running pacemaker period (T_{fr}, not shown) was 280 ms. (a) 1:1 entrainment at a basic cycle length (BCL) of 200 ms. (b) Stimulation at BCL = 180 ms resulted in 5:4 entrainment. (c) BCL = 160 ms yielded 3:2 entrainment. (d) At BCL = 120 ms, 2:1 entrainment was established. (e) Plot of m/n where m is the number of responses and n is the number of stimuli, as a function of BCL. (f) Phase–response curve obtained as an inverse solution from data in panels (a) to (d), as well as other data not shown. Symbols correspond to steady-state entrainment rates indicated. (Modified from Anumonwo *et al.*, *Circ Res* 1991; 68:1138–53, with permission from the American Heart Association, Inc.)

data in this manner shows some important attributes of the behavior of pacemakers. Any m/n region in the m/n vs. BCL plot can be predicted using the following simple rule: the largest region between m/n and M/N will typically be $(m + M)/(n + N)$, where n and N are numbers of pulses and m and M are numbers of pacemaker discharges. For example, the 5:4 pattern ($m/n = 0.8$) occurred between the 1:1 ($m/n = 1$) and 4:3 ($m/n = 75$) patterns, and the 3:2 pattern ($m/n = 0.66$) occurred between 2:1 and 4:3.

Note in Figure 4.3 that, at each BCL, not only the $n:m$ pattern is different but also the phasic relationship between the stimulus and the pacemaker discharge. At some BCLs (e.g., panels a and d) phase relations are fixed, whereas at others (panels b and c) phase relations change on a beat-to-beat basis. The derived PRC presented in panel (f) of Figure 4.3 was obtained from the same data by measuring the change in phase ($\Delta\Phi$) of the pacemaker discharge, as a function of the phase (Φ) of the stimulus within the pacemaker cycle, both expressed as percent of the free-running pacemaker period (T_{fr}). The different symbols represent data obtained at the various entrainment ratios indicated on the right. These data provide direct confirmation of the relationship between the PRC and the entrainment behavior of the pacemaker. Similarly, the PRC may be used to predict the dynamic interactions of two or more cardiac pacemakers connected electrically through low-resistance junctions and forms the basis of the mutual entrainment hypothesis for coordination in the sinus node.

Interaction of Two Pacemakers (Mutual Entrainment)

In all experimental and theoretical models used thus far to study the interaction between coupled cardiac pacemakers, the reciprocal influence of the firing of one pacemaker on the periodicity of another is phase-dependent. In addition, the magnitude of this influence is a function of the degree of electrical coupling between cells. The example presented in Figure 4.4 illustrates the

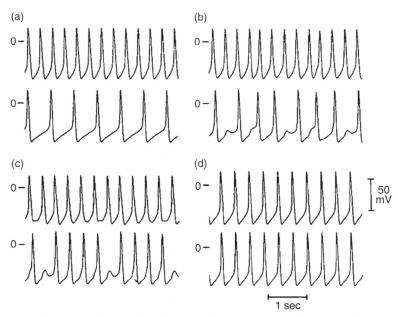

Figure 4.4 Mutual entrainment of two simulated sinus pacemaker cells connected by varying coupling resistances (R_{coup}). (a) $R_{coup} = \infty$, each cell fires at its intrinsic period undisturbed by the rhythm of the other cell. (b) $R_{coup} = 300$ kΩ. A 5:3 mutual entrainment pattern is established in the steady state. Note beat-to-beat changes in phasic relations that are accompanied by changes in the respective interbeat intervals. (c) $R_{coup} = 200$ kΩ, the pattern is now 5:4. (d) $R_{coup} = 10$ kΩ. A steady-state pattern of 1:1 mutual entrainment is established. Note that the two pacemakers now beat at a common constant period that is different from the respective intrinsic periods. (Modified with permission from Michaels *et al.*, *Circ Res* 1986; 58:706–20).

behavior expected from two sinus pacemaker cells with different harmonic frequencies when they are connected electrically and allowed to interact and phase lock at simple harmonic or more complex ratios. Panel (a) shows transmembrane potentials of the two cells in the absence of electric coupling. Cell 1 (top trace) discharges at the intrinsic cycle length of 300 milliseconds. The intrinsic cycle length of cell 2 is slower (600 milliseconds). Panels (b) through (d) show the interactions at various degrees of electrical coupling. Because of resistive coupling, the current from cell 1 to cell 2 (and vice versa) is derived from Ohm's law as the difference in their potential divided by the "intercellular" coupling resistance (R_{coup}). This current is thus supposed to add algebraically to the ionic currents flowing in each cell at each individual time step. In panel (b), R_{coup} is relatively high. The two pacemakers continued to beat at different rates. However, a 5:3 phase-locking pattern of mutual entrainment is established, with individual periods varying predictably in a manner that depends on the phasic relations between cells 1 and 2. When R_{coup} is decreased slightly (panel c), the degree of communication is increased and the locking pattern changes to 5:4. Finally, in panel (d), setting R_{coup} to a still lower value yielded a 1:1 pattern with cells 1 and 2 discharging at fixed phase relations and mutually entraining to a common period of 395 milliseconds. This period, which is different from the intrinsic period of either cell, can be accurately predicted by the PRCs of the individual pacemakers (see Figure 4.2) in response to perturbations generated by the discharge of their counterparts.

Mutual Entrainment and the Generation of the Heartbeat

The mammalian SA region is a heterogeneous multicellular structure composed of many thousands of cells forming small bundles that intertwine in all directions and give rise to very complex geometric patterns of arrangement. In addition, electrophysiological mapping studies identified several cell types within this region, including "true" and "subsidiary" pacemaker cells, as well as non-pacemaker cells, which add to the complexities one can face when attempting to determine the mechanisms of initiation and maintenance of the heartbeat. Moreover, there is enough interspecies variability in the morphology, ultrastructure, and patterns of electric activation in the node to make any consensus about mechanisms difficult to achieve. Nevertheless, on the basis of recent electrophysiological studies in isolated heart tissue preparations from rabbits and other species, some authors contend that the heartbeat is generated by the rhythmic electric discharges of a small group of cells located within the center of the SA node and that the majority of cells in that region serve only to conduct the electric impulse to the neighboring atrial tissue. However, as discussed earlier, computer simulations using large arrays of cells and more recent experimental studies in the sinus node lend support to the idea that the origin of the heartbeat may be more widespread in the SA region than previously thought. In the 1980s, we simulated the complex

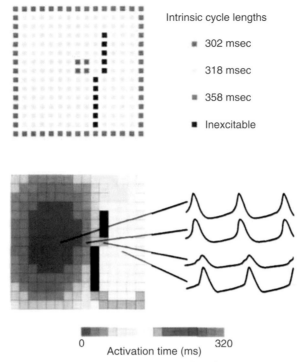

Intrinsic cycle lengths

■ 302 msec

318 msec

■ 358 msec

■ Inexcitable

0   Activation time (ms)   320

Figure 4.5 A model of the rabbit sinoatrial node consisting of 15 × 15 array pacemaker cells. Cell dimensions are 50 × 50 × 50 µm; specific resistivity is 2000 Ω·cm; surface-to-volume ratio is 8000 cm⁻¹. Location of cells with different intrinsic frequencies (top panel). Unexcitable cells (black) have no active inward membrane currents. Activation map after 10 beats of mutual 1:1 entrainment at an axial resistance of 40 kΩ (bottom left panel). Tracings show distinct action potential morphologies depending on cell location. Color bar shows times of firing of each cell. (Reproduced with permission from Michaels *et al.*, *Circ Res* 1987; 61:704–14).

activation pattern of the rabbit SA region in activation maps of a bidimensional array of 225 electrically coupled sinus node cells. By appropriately selecting a hierarchy of pacemaker cycle lengths and allowing for electric coupling and interactions among all pacemakers in the array, we were able to provide a faithful macroscopic representation of the "propagation" wave front of the rabbit SA node, as previously recorded experimentally. As illustrated in the top panel of Figure 4.5, in this version of the model, four cells in the center (red) were programmed to discharge at a relatively brief cycle length (302 milliseconds). Most other cells in the matrix (yellow) had an intrinsic period of 318 milliseconds, but the pacemakers in all four borders of the sheet (blue) had a slightly longer intrinsic period (358 milliseconds). In addition, in an attempt to simulate the conditions of low excitability in a narrow region, the band of 11 black cells was made completely unexcitable by deleting all inward excitatory currents from each of these cells. Thus, in the absence of coupling, these cells were quiescent at a resting potential of

−40 mV (not shown) and were incapable of generating action potentials. However, they could be depolarized passively by their immediate neighbors when the conditions of electric coupling were allowed.

The simulation results are shown in the bottom panel of Figure 4.5. Clearly, at the appropriate value of coupling resistance (20 kΩ), the model was able to mimic very accurately the activation sequence of the isolated rabbit SA node. Again, as a result of the dynamic interactions among all cells, there is a pattern of apparent conduction from a leading pacemaker region to the periphery. Note, however, that such a leading pacemaker region in the simulation does not correspond to that of the intrinsically fastest cells (black squares in the top panel) but is displaced toward the left border of the matrix. This occurs because the unexcitable zone exerts a constant slowing influence on these four cells. In addition, the activation sequence is such that, similar to what is seen in experiments, all cells at the left of the unexcitable zone activate within the first 40 milliseconds (bottom panel). Further, because the unexcitable cells form an additional resistive barrier to the mutual interactions between the faster cells and the right side of the sheet, the activation front appears to circumnavigate over the superior margin of the black zone, reaching the inferior border with an apparent delay of 70–80 milliseconds. Finally, as shown by the transmembrane potential tracings in the bottom right panel of Figure 4.5, the unexcitable cells (third trace) appeared to give rise to notched action potentials. These responses are very similar to those recorded experimentally at an equivalent site of the rabbit SA node. In the model, the notches resulted from summation of purely passive depolarizations originating in neighboring pacemakers at opposite sides of the unexcitable band.

More recent computer simulations using a parallel processing machine to simulate very large arrays of electrically coupled cardiac pacemaker cells provided qualitative confirmation to the initial predictions described earlier. Moreover, very recent studies in other species using high-resolution optical mapping techniques confirm the validity of the mutual entrainment hypothesis and the applicability of the aforementioned model to explain the coordinated activation of thousands of cells in the SA node. This is illustrated in Figure 4.6, obtained from one such experiment in the isolated sinus node from a normal mouse. On the left is a real image of the endocardial SA preparation showing the typical landmarks of the right atrium including the crista terminalis (CT), the superior vena cava (SVC), the inferior vena cava (IVC), the right atrial appendage (RA), and the border of the interatrial septum (IAS). On the right is a color isochrone map demonstrating that the impulse is initiated in a coordinated manner by a conglomerate of pacemaker cells in the so-called "compact region" located in the center of the node (Figure 4.6). From this region, an excitation wave appears to propagate rapidly toward the CT activating it in its entirety in less than 5 milliseconds. On the other hand, in the opposite direction the atrial free wall and IAS activate with a delay as long as 10 milliseconds. These results provide strong support to the idea that pacemaking in the sinus node is a "democratic" process whereby all its

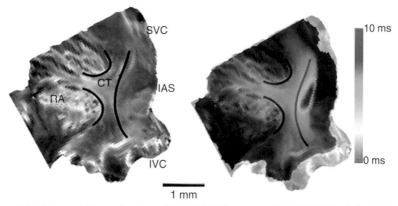

Figure 4.6 High-resolution optical map (Redshirt CCD camera, Di-4-ANEPPS) of sinoatrial activation in the isolated sinus node of a normal mouse. Real image of the right atrial endocardium (left). Landmarks include the crista terminalis (CT), superior vena cava (SVC), inferior vena cava (IVC), right atrial appendage (RA), and border of the interatrial septum (IAS). Color isochrone map showing site of impulse initiation in the center of the SA node (right).

component cells communicate with each other electrotonically and contribute together to the initiation of each cardiac impulse.

Propagation of the Cardiac Impulse

Let us now think about what happens to the cardiac impulse after it moves beyond the SA node boundaries. To address this issue mechanistically, we consider first the propagation of current in a passive linear array of parallel RC circuits (a cable) depicted in Figure 4.7, where all resistors are ohmic, i.e., there are no "active currents." As shown in Figure 4.7a, there are three different types of resistors in this model: r_m is the membrane resistance; r_i is the "intercellular resistance," equivalent to the lump sum of the resistance of the cytoplasm (r_c) and the resistance of the gap junctions (r_j); the cytoplasmic resistance is considered to be much lower than the gap junctional resistance. The term r_o represents the resistance of the extracellular space and is provided by the relatively low resistance of the extracellular solution bathing the cable. As shown in Figure 4.7b, the electrical charge associated with a brief depolarizing pulse applied across the membrane of cell 1 will divide to propagate simultaneously (1) across the capacitor of the injected cell to depolarize the membrane of that cell and (2) across the intercellular resistances to depolarize neighboring cells. At cell 2, the charges will once again divide; some of them will move across the RC circuit of that cell to induce membrane depolarization, while some others will continue across r_i and into cell 3, and so on. The same process repeats at that site; yet, as the current moves farther along the fiber, less charge is available to depolarize the next cell, in such a way that no current reaches site labeled n. Notice also that all of the current that moves

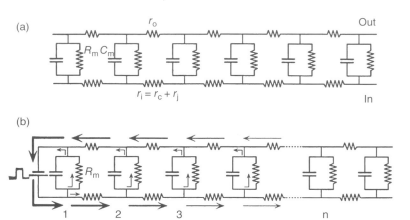

Figure 4.7 Decay of voltage along a passive cable of infinite length. (a) Equivalent circuit of cable; r_o, extracellular resistance; r_m, membrane resistance; r_i, intercellular resistance; r_c, cytoplasmic resistance; r_j, gap junction resistance; C_m, membrane capacitance. (b) When a transient potential difference (square pulse) is established at one end of the cable, local circuit currents move along the cable but decay very rapidly with distance.

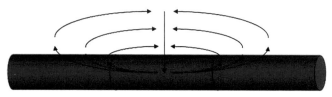

Figure 4.8 Local circuit currents at the moment of current injection at the center of an idealized cable composed of cardiac cells connected electrically through gap junctions.

across the membrane returns, through r_o, to the site of injection, so that the circuit can be completed (Figure 4.8). This is called the "local circuit" or "electrotonic" current and describes the way in which currents travel along linear arrays of cells.

As the current spreads laterally from the site of injection, it discharges the capacitors of the neighboring cells, with a consequent change in membrane potential. The circuit illustrated would be more or less equivalent to the case of a thin, unbranched Purkinje fiber to which subthreshold current pulses are applied. (A different situation arises when the current pulse elicits an action potential, as will be discussed later.) Figure 4.9 depicts the changes in membrane potential that would be observed in a similar passive cable when a square hyperpolarizing current pulse is applied at the site labeled "0." Clearly, the largest voltage deflection is observed at the site of injection (I_o). As current density decreases with distance, so does the change in membrane potential ($V_{1..3}$); at a very large distance, membrane potential is unchanged by the current pulse. The manner in which voltage changes along this circuit is predicted by the cable equations.

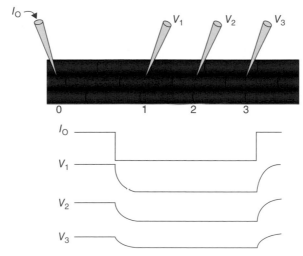

Figure 4.9 Decay of voltage along an infinitely long and homogeneous fiber of electrically connected cardiac cells during application of hyperpolarizing current (I_o) at the left end of the cable. The tracings show the rapid decay of ΔV with distance from injection site.

Cable Equations

The cable equations were developed by Lord Kelvin in 1855 to characterize the changes in current and voltage observed along the transatlantic telegraphic cable. The actual mathematical treatment of this problem goes beyond the scope of this volume. Details can be found in numerous texts that are written on the issue. Here, we will limit ourselves to the presentation of the basic concepts that are essential for the general understanding of cardiac impulse propagation.

In the simplest case, the cable equations predict the distribution of voltage along a continuous, passive, unidimensional fiber of infinite length (as already seen in Figure 4.7). The cable is continuous in the sense that individual resistors of a given type (r_m, r_i, r_o) have a constant magnitude along the fiber and the resistive elements are homogeneously distributed. The properties of all capacitors are also assumed to be constant along the cable. Thus, no abrupt discontinuities (i.e., decreases or enhancements) in the flow of current are present. The cable is passive because all resistors involved behave ohmically. Thus, these equations describe the behavior of the membrane below the threshold level. The cable is unidimensional in that current can flow only across the membrane and along the length of the fiber. The cable is of infinite length in that electrotonic propagation does not face boundary conditions imposed by the abrupt end of the fiber.

As shown in Figure 4.10, when a current pulse injected at point 0 in the fiber, the amplitude of the elicited electrotonic potential decays exponentially with distance. Experimentally, a plot correlating amplitude of the electrotonic potential vs. distance yields an exponential function of the form

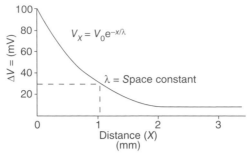

Figure 4.10 Plot of voltage change (ΔV) as a function of distance (x). V_o, voltage at $x = 0$; λ, space constant.

$$V_x = V_o e^{-x/\lambda} \tag{4.1}$$

where λ is the space constant (see Figure 4.5). Practically, λ corresponds to the distance at which the amplitude of the voltage drop decreased to 63% of maximum. λ is defined also as

$$\lambda = \sqrt{\frac{r_m}{r_i + r_o}} \tag{4.2}$$

If we assume r_o to be much smaller than r_i, then Equation 4.2 can be simplified to

$$\lambda = \sqrt{\frac{r_m}{r_i}} \tag{4.3}$$

Another experimental parameter that can be measured from the changes in voltage brought about by current injection is the so-called time constant (τ), which describes the time taken for the voltage deflection, recorded at the site of current injection, to reach 84% of maximum. The time constant is defined also as

$$\tau = r_m C_m \tag{4.4}$$

Finally, the input resistance (r_{in}), that is, the total resistance that the current faces as it enters the fiber from its site of injection, can be estimated from the ohmic relation between the applied current pulse amplitude (I_{in}) and the amplitude of the voltage step at the site of injection as

$$R_{in} = \frac{V}{I_{in}} \tag{4.5}$$

Input resistance can also be expressed as

$$R_{in} = \sqrt{\frac{(r_m r_i)}{2}} \tag{4.6}$$

Thus, using Equations 4.1–4.6, the three cable parameters, r_m, r_i, and C_m can be calculated.

It is also worth noting that the cable equations predict an inverse relation between r_m (or r_i) and the fiber diameter in such a way that

$$r_m = \frac{R_m}{2\pi a} \tag{4.7}$$

and

$$r_i = \frac{R_i}{\pi a^2}, \tag{4.8}$$

where a is the radius of the fiber (in centimeters) and r_m and r_i are, respectively, the specific membrane and intracellular resistivities (i.e., resistance corrected for surface area or cross-sectional area). Cell capacitance is also corrected for surface area by the following relation:

$$c_m = 2\pi a C_m, \tag{4.9}$$

where C_m is the specific cell capacitance. This value is approximately 1 $\mu F/cm^2$ in cardiac cells.

In summary, the diameter of the fiber has a major influence on its cable properties. Both membrane and intracellular resistances increase as the fiber diameter is reduced. Combining Equations 4.3, 4.7, and 4.8, we obtain

$$\lambda^2 = \frac{R_m a}{2R_i} \tag{4.10}$$

which shows that the space constant is directly related to fiber diameter. In other words, the length of fiber influenced by a given current pulse from a point source is greater in a thick than in a thin fiber.

The use of the cable equations provided crucial information about the passive electrical properties of the cardiac fibers. For example, it was through the use of these equations that Silvio Weidmann reached the conclusion that communication between cardiac cells is electric in nature and that these cells behave as a functional syncytium. Weidmann's demonstration of the existence of low-resistance pathways between cardiac cells long preceded the morphological or biochemical demonstration of cardiac gap junction channels. In addition, the use of cable equations was instrumental in the demonstration of the effects of certain antiarrhythmic agents on the passive properties of cardiac cells. Finally, a more elaborate treatment of the cable equations has allowed some authors to determine the roles of intercellular communication and cell excitability on action potential propagation failure during ischemic conditions (see, e.g., work by the group of André Kléber).

It is important to note that there are significant limitations to the use of cable equations. First, propagation along cardiac tissues is not perfectly uniform or continuous. Indeed, the sole existence of the gap junction between cells constitutes a microscopic discontinuity because the gap junctional resistance is appreciably larger than the cytoplasmic resistance. Yet, under normal circumstances, when propagation is analyzed along the whole fiber, the small delays imposed by these microscopic obstacles are unnoticed. However, if a localized area of higher resistance is established between cells (e.g., by the presence of blood vessels separating cardiac cell bundles, or by deposits of fibroid tissue between bundles), propagation becomes discontinuous and the cable equations no longer apply.

Second, the condition of unidimensionality is difficult to fulfill for cardiac tissue. This is easily understood after comparing the case of a Purkinje fiber (the closest to a unidimensional cable in the heart) with that of an axon. Although in axons there is only one cell membrane dividing the intra- and the extracellular space, in the Purkinje fiber there are many rodlike cells that are stacked together (see Figure 4.9), forming bundles that are oriented parallel to the long axis of the cells. Yet, because the cells are electrically well connected, we assume that no voltage drop occurs inside the fiber, transverse to the orientation of the bundle. The assumption is that current decreases either along the fiber or homogeneously across all membranes so that current is the same throughout the cross-sectional area. This condition, however, may fail if the fiber is too thick in relation to the size of the current source or if the cells are not properly connected in the side-to-side direction.

This assumption, of course, is untenable if instead of a Purkinje fiber we consider the case of a sheet of ventricular muscle. Although bidimensional cable equations were developed and implemented for the case of cardiac tissues, important limitations also apply to such equations. In general, one should bear in mind that, when unidimensional cable equations are applied, it is assumed that current changes only along the fiber and across cell membranes but that no current is lost inside the fiber, transverse to its main axis. Third, it needs to be emphasized that these equations apply to the case of current moving across ohmic parallel RC circuits. Cable equations were extended to describe the case of action potentials traveling at a constant velocity along uniform, unidimensional nerve fibers. Some investigators applied similar equations to the case of cardiac propagation. The conditions of uniformity and unidimensionality continue to apply.

Propagation of the Action Potential: "Sink" and "Source"

Consider a linear array of cardiac cells, as illustrated in Figure 4.11a. A depolarizing current pulse is applied to one end of the cell array, thus eliciting an action potential at that site. A voltage gradient is created, between the cell that has fired the action potential, and the other cells downstream. Electrical current will move along this gradient. The inward (depolarizing) current associated with the action potential upstroke in the active cell becomes a *source* of electrical charge to the cells downstream, which act as a current *sink*. These "receiving" cells are depolarized due to the arrival of positive charges. For cells that are far away from the source, the electrotonic potential is subthreshold, and its amplitude decays exponentially with distance (following

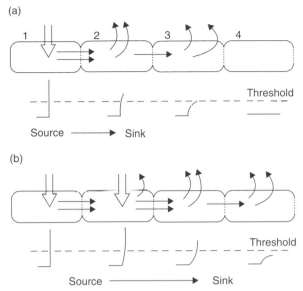

Figure 4.11 Distribution of intracellular charges during propagation of an action potential from depolarized (source) to resting cells (sink). (a) The source is located in cell 1. (b) The source has extended to cell 2.

cable properties). However, for cell 2, the current source causes sufficient depolarization to bring that cell to its threshold potential. In Figure 4.11b, the initiation of an action potential in cell 2 generates a new influx of inward current downstream in the array. Cell 2 now becomes a source of current for those cells that are further downstream, and the process repeats itself as the action potential travels along the fiber. Note that, as opposed to the case of a single myocyte where all inward current that enters the circuit discharges that cell's capacitor, in the case of the array, only a fraction of the current depolarizes each cell. A good proportion of the current is used to depolarize the cells downstream. In other words, there is a "loading effect" imposed by the cells downstream on the cell that is being activated. The loading effect draws charges away from the local capacitor (i.e., the capacitor at the site of excitation) and, consequently, prevents depolarization.

Current Load and the Concept of Liminal Length

When the membrane potential of a cell is brought above threshold, an inward ("all or none") depolarizing current will ensue. However, when the initial depolarization does not attain threshold, then an outward repolarizing current will result. Recall that the resting membrane potential is determined primarily by a background potassium conductance (I_{K1}, see Chapters 1 and 2). Therefore, when a given cell in an array is depolarized, its membrane potential moves away from the equilibrium potential for potassium (E_K). However, its

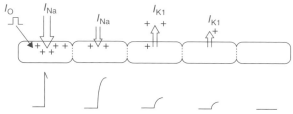

Figure 4.12 Local circuit currents established upon depolarization of cell 1 in a section of infinitely long cable.

potassium channels remain conductive, and thus outward flow of potassium ensues. As shown in Figure 4.12, this repolarizing current opposes the depolarizing influence of the current source (I_{Na} in most cases, see Chapters 1 and 2). Thus, in the case of the propagated action potential, there are both inward and outward currents moving at the same time on different points in the fiber. While at the site of excitation there is an influx of charge, at distal sites charges are leaving the fiber as the repolarizing currents oppose the depolarizing influence of the current source. In this regard, the current sink is not a purely passive element in the propagation circuit; it plays an important active role because it dynamically opposes the depolarization of the fiber.

In 1937, Rushton developed the concept of liminal length to describe analytically the interplay between depolarizing and repolarizing forces in the propagated action potential. In the case of a unidimensional cable-like structure, this concept defines the length of fiber that needs to be raised above threshold so that the depolarizing influence of the currents generated within that length exceeds the repolarizing influence of the fiber downstream. Rushton concluded that a propagated action potential ensues when the density of the depolarizing current overcomes the density of the outward current that is elicited away from the site of excitation. This is illustrated graphically in Figure 4.13. In the top graph, the ordinate represents the amplitude and polarity of the current flowing through the membrane. In the bottom graph, the ordinate shows the value of membrane potential at a particular site in the cable. In both panels, the distance (x) from the site of current injection is plotted on the abscissa. A surge of depolarizing current is delivered at $x = 0$. The amplitude of the depolarization decays with distance as predicted by the cable equations. Between points A and B, the depolarization is large enough to bring the membrane potential above the threshold for Na current activation. However, for cells to the right of point B, depolarization is subthreshold. In the top graph, the distribution of current is such that, while for the cells between points A and B an inward current is elicited (shadowed area), the cells downstream only respond with repolarizing current (hatched area). According to the liminal length concept, success or failure of propagation would be determined by whether the density of depolarizing current (i.e., the total shadowed area in Figure 4.13) can overcome the repolarizing current downstream.

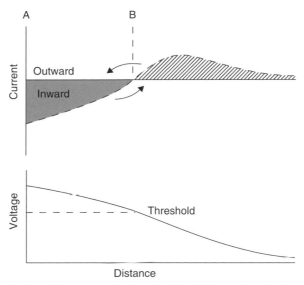

Figure 4.13 Liminal length for propagation (see text for detailed explanation).

Factors Regulating Action Potential Propagation in Cardiac Tissues

The concept of liminal length is useful as a didactic tool to explain the inter-action between sink and source forces during propagation of the action potential. One can summarize the process of propagation of the cardiac action potential as being dependent on (1) the balance between the magnitude of the current source and the magnitude of current needed to depolarize cells downstream and (2) the ability of the current to move from cell to cell through gap junctional channels. Conduction velocity and, in general, the success or failure of propagation can be affected by changes in either one of these factors. The amplitude of the current source is determined, for the most part, by the amplitude of the active inward currents. In the working atrial and ventricular muscle cells, as well as in the ventricular specialized conduction system, Na currents provide the largest fraction of the excitatory current. In the SA and AV nodes, on the other hand, inward current during the action potential upstroke is largely provided by the Ca channels. As reviewed in other chapters, pharmacologic manipulations that decrease the amplitude of these currents can drastically impair propagation or modify pacemaker synchronization.

Propagation can also fail because the tissue acting as a sink is no longer excitable. Administration of Na channel blockers (or Ca channel blockers in the case of nodal tissue) significantly impairs cell excitability. Thus, even if an action potential invades the cell acting as a current sink, that cell cannot become a source of current unless inward channels are available to produce all-or-none depolarization. In other words, administration of Na (or Ca) channel blocking agents has the double effect of decreasing the amplitude of the current source and impairing the responsiveness of the cells acting as the current sink. There are other conditions that affect cell excitability without impairing inward currents. A good example is the increase in background outward conductance that follows activation of ATP-sensitive K channels in cardiac cells during hypoxia (see Chapter 2). Indeed, the outward conductance opposes the depolarizing influence of the excitatory current. Thus, a cell whose ATP-sensitive K current was activated requires a larger excitatory input to generate in it an action potential. In addition, the resultant decrease in membrane resistance causes a decrease in the space constant (see Equation 4.3) and an increase in the liminal length, thus further impairing excitability.

Failure of propagation can also occur because of a loss of intercellular communication. Indeed, the heart is a functional syncytium, and excitatory current has to move from cell to cell across gap junction channels. Conditions such as an increase in proton concentration in the intracellular space (which is likely to occur during myocardial ischemia) can cause the closure of gap junction channels and, consequently, prevent electrical charges from moving from the source to depolarize cells downstream.

In summary, propagation is a highly dynamic process where the various electrical elements present in the cell participate, alternatively, as sources of current or as sinks; charges move in the direction of the more negatively polarized tissue to bring about cell depolarization and, if of enough intensity, an action potential. To successfully maintain propagation, current also must move from the source to the sink across permeable low-resistance pathways; as the charges return to the source through the extracellular space, the propagation of local circuit current is attained.

Concept of "Safety Factor" for Propagation

From the foregoing it is clear that, in a linear cable composed of electrically interconnected excitable cells, impulse propagation is determined primarily by the ratio between the current available to excite cells downstream (the source) and the current required by those cells to be excited (the sink). Among the factors that influence the source, we can include the maximum rate of rise of the action potential upstroke, the action potential amplitude, and, under certain conditions, the action potential duration. Passive membrane properties and cell-to-cell communication may also modulate the amount of excitatory current delivered by the source. On the other hand, the factors that influence the sink include the membrane resistance, the voltage threshold, and the difference between voltage threshold and membrane potential. Thus, the safety factor for propagation in a 1-D cable is proportional to the excess of source current over the sink needs. Slowing of conduction and block may result from a progressive decrease in the safety factor. Geometrical factors may lead to a mismatch between sink and source that will result in

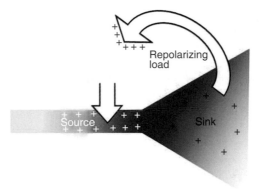

Figure 4.14 Sink-to-source mismatch resulting from changes in geometry of a conducting pathway. The large sink imposes a repolarizing load on the source which impairs propagation and may lead to block.

propagation disturbances. For instance, as illustrated in Figure 4.14, an action potential may effectively propagate through a cable but block at an expansion as a result of a sudden increase of the repolarizing load. Similar rules apply for the initiation of a propagated response. In this case, a liminal length of cable has to be excited simultaneously to overcome the repolarizing (loading) effect of resting cells.

Experimental studies as well as computer simulations have shown that either a decrease in cell excitability or an impairment of electrical coupling will lead to propagation block. Yet, the minimum conduction velocity that can be sustained prior to block is much slower when electrical communication is impaired. Mathematical simulations by Shaw and Rudy showed that if sodium conductance is decreased, conduction velocity decreases from 54 to 17 cm/s before conduction fails. However, if sodium conductance is left intact but intercellular resistance is increased (i.e., if electrical coupling is decreased), conduction velocity can reach extremely low values (0.26 cm/s) before failure occurs. This phenomenon is related to the fact that loss of electrical coupling also decreases the load imposed on the cell to be excited by the cells downstream, thus facilitating local activation, even if the electrical barrier between cells slows propagation velocity along the array of cells. In general, the characteristics of propagation slowing or failure vary depending on whether sink or source properties are affected. The latter is relevant to the propagation of action potential in relation to fiber orientation and the mechanisms of arrhythmias (see "Anisotropic Propagation").

While loss of electrical coupling eventually leads to propagation failure, the changes in conduction velocity are not always linear. In fact, in areas of discontinuity, partial uncoupling can improve propagation, as demonstrated by studies of Rohr and his collaborators showing a paradoxical improvement of impulse conduction by partial uncoupling. These authors showed that the large current load imposed by the tissue acting as a current sink can slow down propagation. Partial uncoupling can reduce the load, preserving charge within the area being excited and facilitating propagation from one cell to the next. Further impairment of coupling would eventually lead to propagation block.

Recent studies show that the key molecular complexes involved in cell excitability localize in close proximity with those relevant for intercellular communication. Indeed, both the sodium channels and the gap junctions preferentially localize to the site of end-to-end apposition between cells, within an anatomical structure called the intercalated disk. Clustering of sodium channels at the site of cell apposition could increase the inward current density at the site, thus increasing the availability of electrical charges for depolarization of the neighboring cell. The functional consequences of this spatial distribution of molecular complexes to propagation remain to be determined, but it is possible that it improves the margin of safety for propagation in the direction longitudinal to the axis of the cells.

Propagation in Two Dimensions and the Concept of Curvature

The foregoing discussion has centered on the characteristics of propagation in continuous and discontinuous unidimensional cables of electrically coupled cardiac cells. However, except for the Purkinje fibers and other subendocardial thin bundles and trabeculae, action potential propagation in the heart can hardly be considered unidimensional. When propagation of the impulse occurs in two, let alone three dimensions, additional factors come into play. For example, in two dimensions (2-D) the shape (i.e., curvature) of the wave front is thought to be a major determinant of the success or failure of propagation. The more convexly curved a wave front, the lower is its velocity of propagation. Beyond a certain critical curvature, propagation of the wave front cannot proceed. This concept of critical curvature is very much related to the existence in 2-D cardiac muscle of a liminal area for propagation, equivalent to the liminal length in a 1-D cable. In Figure 4.15, this is easily appreciated when one considers that the relative area of tissue to be excited (the sink) ahead of a convexly curved wave front (the source) is larger than the area forming the sink in front of an equivalent plane wave. Similarly, the ability of a curved wave front to propagate depends on the excitability of the tissue. If excitability is impaired, propagation block will occur even for more planar (less angled) wave fronts. In general, because a large curvature of the wave front causes a reduction in velocity, propagation is possible only for wave fronts whose curvature is less than critical.

Anisotropic Propagation

One of the fundamental characteristics of cardiac muscle is its structural anisotropy, which is a direct result of the rodlike shape of adult cardiac

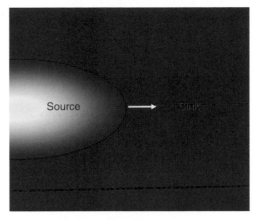

Figure 4.15 Propagation of a convexly curved wave front (source) is hampered by the large area that needs to be excited (sink) for propagation to continue.

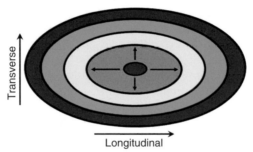

Figure 4.16 Idealized ellipsoidal wave fronts expected from point stimulation in the center of a rectangular 2-D sheet of anisotropic cardiac muscle. The long axis of the cardiac fiber is represented horizontally.

myocytes, the heterogeneous distribution of gap junctions on the surface of the membrane, and the orientation of cell bundles along the long axis of the cells. Thus, activation maps of 2-D cardiac muscle demonstrate that the activation fronts that emanate from suprathreshold stimulation by a point source at the center of the muscle are elliptic (Figure 4.16). As a consequence, any quantitative measurements involving spatial dimensions are, necessarily, directionally dependent (anisotropic). Parameters that are directionally dependent include, among others, space constant, conduction velocity, width of the wave front, and, of course, curvature. In the case of conduction velocity, an action potential generated in the center of a sheet of cardiac muscle travels faster in the direction that is parallel to the axis of the fibers than in the transverse direction. In fact, not only is conduction velocity directionally dependent, but also propagation may be more likely to fail in one direction than in the other. The direction in which propagation fails (i.e., longitudinal or transverse to the fiber axis) varies depending on the conditions used to challenge the propagation properties of the tissue. However, it seems clear that lines of propagation block that are associated with the anisotropic properties of the tissue can serve as a substrate for the generation of cardiac rhythm disturbances.

Propagation failure may occur preferentially in one direction or another, and the specific direction may vary depending on whether membrane properties, or intercellular coupling, are impaired. Early studies by Madison Spach and Mailen Kootsey in anisotropic ventricular muscle, under conditions in which there was uniform depression of active membrane generator properties (i.e., quinidine perfusion or ischemia), suggested that, as a result of a greater upstroke velocity (dV/dt_{max}) of action potentials propagating transversely in cardiac muscle, longitudinal conduction is more vulnerable to block. Studies by other investigators also showed that an increase in intercellular resistance leads to conduction block in a clearly anisotropic manner. In that case, however, propagation in the transverse direction failed first, while longitudinal propagation was maintained. In other words, when electrical coupling was compromised, the margin of safety for propagation was greater along the longitudinal axis of the fibers. Subsequent simulation studies suggested that, by reducing load, reduced intercellular coupling (as in the case of transverse propagation) augments the safety factor when the latter is reduced because of a depressed membrane (reduced source). However, at high levels of membrane depression, the augmentation of safety factor is insufficient to delay the onset of conduction failure. Under such condition, block is expected to occur earlier in the transverse than in the longitudinal direction of the fibers. In any case, it is clear that directional differences in the susceptibility to propagation block can set the stage for reentrant activity (anisotropic reentry).

Propagation in Three-Dimensional Cardiac Muscle

The myocardium is essentially 3-D, and thus a full understanding of propagation requires knowledge of what happens in the thickness of the atrial or ventricular wall, as the electric impulse moves transmurally. A number of studies have demonstrated that, for an impulse initiated by point stimulation of that surface, the activation fronts near the epicardial site of stimulation is elliptic, but becomes asymmetrical and has folds and undulations as it penetrates the wall. In addition, the ellipses in each plane rotate clockwise toward the endocardium. Such an extremely complex pattern of 3-D propagation is explained in part by the intricate anatomic structure of the ventricles, including rotational anisotropy. Thus, in addition to the elongated shape of and asymmetrical connections among myocardial fibers, which results in anisotropy of propagation, the muscle fiber axes rotate transmurally as much as 120° in some areas. Moreover, excitation patterns are also affected by the Purkinje fiber network in the subendocardium and by macroscopic discontinuities and connective tissue septa separating muscle bundles.

Propagation at Junctional Sites

Conduction velocity is not only heterogeneous within a tissue but also across cardiac tissues. Indeed, the heart is a highly complex 3-D structure, composed of various regions with drastically different propagation properties. Conduction block can occur at the site in which one region meets another simply because of the mismatch imposed by the geometrical and/or electric properties of the tissues. An interesting example is that of the Purkinje–muscle junction. A Purkinje fiber is a well-organized structure, where most of the current is densely packed within a group of cells that are oriented parallel to the fiber direction. The situation therefore arises where curvature effects come again into play because a small source of depolarizing current (the end of the Purkinje fiber) has to provide enough excitatory current to a large 3-D mass of tissue (the ventricular muscle) that is acting as a current sink (Figure 4.17a).

Studies conducted on this subject showed that the success of propagation is indeed challenged by this transition. If the transition is too abrupt (i.e., if the small strand opens abruptly into a large muscle mass), propagation is more likely to fail than if the transition is more graded (e.g., if several Purkinje–muscle junctions exist within a small area). Moreover, propagation in the antidromic direction (i.e., from muscle to Purkinje) is facilitated by the fact that a larger source needs to depolarize a smaller sink (Figure 4.17b). This

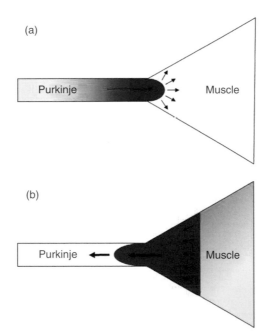

Figure 4.17 The funnel theory of propagation in an asymmetric sink:source system, e.g., the Purkinje–muscle junction. The safety factor for wave front propagation is smaller in the orthodromic (a: source larger than sink) direction than in the antidromic (b: sink larger than source) direction.

mismatch opens the possibility that unidirectional block may occur at the junction. For example, an increase in intercellular resistance at the junction would decrease the amount of excitatory current reaching the muscle during normal propagation. This decrease in the amplitude of the current source may be enough to prevent excitation of the tissue downstream. On the other hand, if propagation is moving in antidromic direction, the excitatory current may still be enough to elicit an action potential. This form of unidirectional block may serve as a source for the development of reentry. However, it was shown that further uncoupling may paradoxically suppress unidirectional block, as a result of the asymmetry of the effects of uncoupling on source and sink.

Heterocellular Interactions and Their Role on Propagation

The foregoing discussion on propagation is based on the assumption that each cell within the circuit is an excitable cardiac myocyte. Yet, in reality, the heart is a multicellular system where at least half of the cells are not myocytes. Among the non-myocyte cardiac cell populations, fibroblasts represent the largest fraction. This simple observation has attracted a lot of attention recently, as it has been demonstrated that myofibroblasts not only form functional gap junctions with their homologous neighbors, but also with closely apposed cardiomyocytes (i.e., heterocellular coupling), as shown in the left panel of Figure 4.18. Hence fibroblasts can serve as an electrical bridge between separated strands of myocytes. Therefore, since fibroblasts are not excitable cells, one would intuitively expect fibroblasts to behave as electrical sinks that

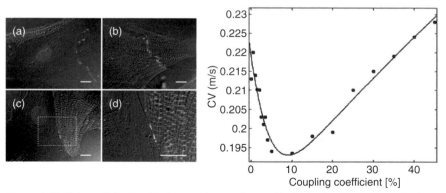

Figure 4.18 Heterocellular fibroblast–myocyte coupling and its biphasic effects on conduction velocity (CV). Left: Immunofluorescence samples showing Cx43-positive staining (green) between two myofibroblasts (a), between two myocytes (b), and between a myocyte and a myofibroblast (c, d—higher magnification of box in c). Myocyte-22 specific sarcomeric α-actinin in red and nuclei in blue. Scale bars, 10 μm. Right: Numerical results for CV vs. myofibroblast to myocyte coupling coefficient for pacing at 3 Hz. All simulations were performed for a myofibroblast/myocyte area ratio of 0.25. (Modified from Zlochiver *et al.*, *Biophys J* 2008, doi:10.1529/biophysj.108.136473).

never become current sources. From that standpoint, the expectation would be that fibroblasts should provide a substrate for very slow conduction and block. However, recent numerical and experimental studies on the effects of heterocellular coupling on conduction velocity (CV) have yielded very surprising results: the relationship between CV and degree of myocyte-to-fibroblast electrotonic coupling is in fact biphasic. As illustrated by the numerical results reproduced in the right panel of Figure 4.18, as heterocellular coupling increased gradually from zero, an initial decrease in CV is followed by an increase. In addition, low heterocellular coupling resulted in fragmented and wavy wave fronts (not shown here), but at high coupling wave fronts became smoother. These apparently paradoxical results, which also occurred experimentally in monolayers of cocultured myocytes and fibroblasts exposed to overexpression or silencing of Cx43, were explained as follows. At very low levels of coupling the wave front entering the myofibroblasts from the myocytes is insufficient to transmit enough depolarizing current downstream to other myocytes. Thus, at these levels the myofibroblasts behave as current sinks that hamper successful propagation. In the 2-D monolayer, the wave front finds alternative pathways and circumnavigates the myofibroblast. Therefore, conduction is maintained via these alternative pathways at the expense of overall CV, and is characterized by heterogeneous wave propagation. As coupling increases toward the threshold level, myofibroblasts drain more and more charge from their neighboring myocytes, resulting in further CV decrease, which explains the left half of the curve in Figure 4.18b. Above threshold, however, the excitation wave provides enough charge through the myofibroblasts to excite downstream myocytes. At this point the myofibroblasts switch from being charge sinks to become short-range charge transmitters that facilitate downstream excitation with increasing levels of coupling. Hence, wave fronts become smoother, and velocity increases, explaining the right half of the curve in Figure 4.18b. Therefore, the consequences of fibroblast–myocyte coupling in vitro are complex and would be expected to be more so in the in vivo heart. Such complexity is likely to have important clinical implications and is currently a matter of intense investigation.

Summary

This chapter focused on the study of the role of electrical coupling on pacemaker synchronization and impulse propagation in the heart. We introduced the reader to basic concepts of electrotonic propagation and local circuit currents and their role in ensuring sinus pacemaker synchronization for the generation of the cardiac impulse as well as for successful impulse conduction. Based on those principles, the concepts of phase resetting and mutual entrainment as well as the manner in which thousands of pacemaker cells in the sinus node synchronize to initiate together are cardiac impulse. In addition, the text brings attention to the fact that, although the unidimensional cable equations provide a good analytical tool to characterize the various electric elements involved in the propagation process, the heart is a highly complex 3-D structure, and its behavior commonly departs from that predicted by simple cable models. In this regard some of the possible mechanisms by which active propagation may fail are discussed. The concept of wave front curvature, with its potential to lead to conduction slowing, the property of anisotropic propagation and the case of propagation across the Purkinje–muscle junction, as well as the presence of heterocellular interactions between myocytes and non-myocyte cells, all serve to illustrate the fact that cardiac impulse transmission does depart from simple unidimensional models.

5 Rate Dependency of Discontinuous Propagation

The focus of this chapter is the study of rate dependency of discontinuous action potential propagation in cardiac tissues. In Chapter 4, the reader was introduced to basic concepts of electrotonic propagation and local circuit currents and their role in active pacemaker synchronization and impulse propagation. This chapter discusses the dynamics and ionic mechanisms of complex patterns of propagation, such as Wenckebach periodicity, which provides a framework for the understanding of cellular and tissue behavior during high-frequency excitation and arrhythmias. Given the structural intricacies of the various cardiac tissues and the complex nonlinear dynamics of cardiac cell excitation, it seems reasonable to expect that any event leading to very rapid activation of atria or ventricles may result in exceedingly complex rhythms, including fibrillation.

Continuous versus Discontinuous Propagation

As discussed in Chapter 4, when viewed microscopically, cell-to-cell propagation in the heart is stepwise with the electrotonic currents propagating to initiate in each cell a local "all-or-none" action potential as the impulse moves downstream in the bundle. This form of propagation is the result of the connection of each cardiac myocyte to neighboring cells through gap junction channels, whose resistance, r_j is higher than r_i. Yet, at the macroscopic level, the action potential appears to travel at a uniform and continuous velocity. In other words, in the case of a discretized but uniform cable of cells interconnected by low-resistance gap junctions (Figure 5.1a), the distance traversed by the action potential may be considered to be a linear function of time (Figure 5.1b), with a slope (dx/dt) that defines the velocity.

It is important to note, however, that, unlike the idealized system depicted in Figure 5.1, cardiac tissues are not uniform, and propagation through them

Basic Cardiac Electrophysiology for the Clinician, 2nd edition. By J. Jalife, M. Delmar, J. Anumonwo, O. Berenfeld and J. Kalifa. Published 2009 by Blackwell Publishing, ISBN: 978-1-4501-8333-8.

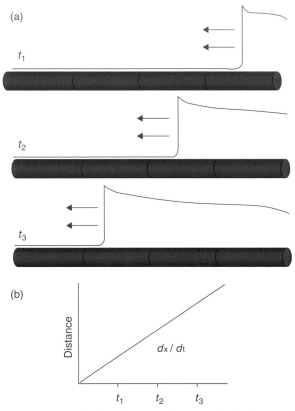

Figure 5.1 Continuous propagation of action potentials in an idealized homogeneous cable of cardiac cells. (a) Action potential wave front moves from right to left at constant speed. (b) Distance traversed by the action potential is a linear function of time elapsed. The slope dx/dt defines velocity.

is discontinuous, not only because of the presence of gap junctions but also because of differences in cell geometry, as well as nonuniform 3-D distribution of gap junctions connecting neighboring myocytes. In the normal heart, an important source of discontinuity is provided by the large anatomic and electrophysiological variations that exist within and between the various types of cardiac tissue. Severe discontinuities in action potential propagation can indeed occur at branching regions of cell bundles and at the junctions between tissue types as a result of these variations. A case in point is the atrioventricular (AV) conducting system. To reach the ventricle, an impulse originated in the atrium must propagate across the AV node and the His-Purkinje network. This impulse therefore must travel across several areas connecting tissues that may have very different properties from each other in terms of excitability, refractoriness, and cell-to-cell communication, as well as a great variability in the geometric arrangement of their respective component cells. However, severe discontinuities usually do not become manifest electrophysiologically unless active generator properties (i.e., excitability) are impaired or when premature impulses occur in partially recovered tissues. The wave front may thus find several obstacles in its path. As such, an electric impulse generated in the atria or ventricles may reach a junction (atrium-node, node-node, node-His, etc.) in which propagation is not possible because the tissue did not yet recover from a previous depolarization. The ensuing impulse may stop at such a junction and become extinguished or may renew its journey, but only after a delay imposed by the time necessary for recovery of excitability of all the tissues involved (see Figure 5.2).

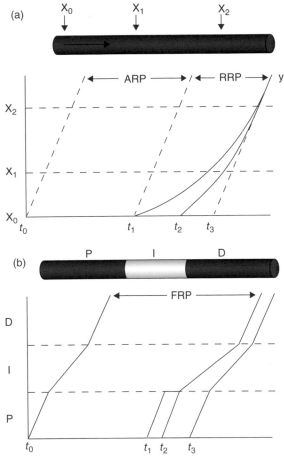

Figure 5.2 Impulse propagation across continuous (a) and discontinuous (b) cables. (a) X_o, site of impulse initiation; x_1 and x_2, sites of recording; t_n, times of impulse initiation; y, time of arrival at x_2; ARP, absolute refractory period; RRP, relative refractory period. (b) The impulses are initiated at a site (P) that is proximal to an intermediate area of depression (I), and the functional refractory period (FRP) is measured at the distal (D) element of the cable. (Modified with permission from Jalife, *Pacing Clin Electrophysiol* 1983; 6:1106–22.)

In the late 1950s, Arturo Rosenblueth, at the National Institute of Cardiology in Mexico City, defined the functional refractory period (FRP) as the time that must elapse after the propagation of an impulse in an excitable tissue before another impulse can propagate. The diagrams in Figure 5.2, adapted from one of Rosenblueth's papers, illustrate the laws of propagation across a continuous (panel a) and a discontinuous (panel b) unidimensional cables. In Figure 5.2a, the cable on top is considered to be continuous and homogeneous with respect to all properties of excitable tissues, including excitability, gap junction conductivity, and refractoriness. X_0 is the site of impulse initiation; x_1 and x_2 are the location of recording electrodes at two different positions along the cable. In the graph, the distance traveled by the impulse is plotted on the ordinate, and time is plotted on the abscissa. In this system, an impulse initiated at X_0 and time t_0 propagates across fully recovered tissue at a uniform velocity (i.e., the slope dx/dt is constant). A second impulse, initiated at the same site at a later time t_1, will travel at a gradually increasing velocity, until it meets fully recovered tissue (y).

If the monotonic curve t_1-y defines the conditions for propagation during the relatively refractory period (RRP) (Figure 5.2a), then in a continuous cable an impulse initiated at any time t_2 between t_1 and t_3 will encounter tissue less refractory and will travel faster and faster, but it could never reach any point $X < X_2$ at the same time delay or earlier than the impulse initiated at t_1. Thus, if two premature impulses are initiated at different moments during the RRP and reach $X < X_2$ at the same time, their concordance could not be explained by a simple acceleration of conduction in a continuous cable. The scenario illustrated in Figure 5.2b shows the conditions for propagation in a discontinuous cable composed of a central area of depressed excitability (I) separating two fully excitable zones (P, proximal; D, distal). As shown by the bottom graph, in this cable, velocity of propagation is not uniform (i.e., dx/dt is not constant) regardless of the timing of the stimulus. Moreover, the impulse initiated at t_1 is likely to have stopped for some time at some place in the depressed excitability region in the course of its propagation (i.e., its velocity was zero), so that it reached the D segment with the same time delay as the impulse initiated at t_2. This could not occur in a continuous system, in which the relationship between input and output (see Figure 5.3a), obtained during programmed P_1P_2 stimulation, with P_2 stimuli applied at progressively more premature intervals, must terminate on the left in a curve of diminishing slope. If, as in the case of Figure 5.3b, at any point the slope becomes zero or changes sign, i.e., if the impulse initiated at t_2 reaches $x > x_2$ at the same time or earlier than that initiated at t_1, the conditions for propagation must be different and the cable cannot be continuous. As illustrated in Figure 5.2b, the region that determines the FRP of the entire system is that where the recovery of excitability takes longer (I). In Figure 5.3a,b, the FRP corresponds to the minimum attainable D_1-D_2 interval.

These concepts indicate that the mechanisms of rate-dependent and intermittent block processes such as during Wenckebach periodicity in AV

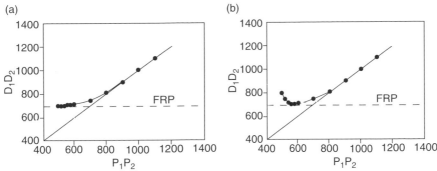

Figure 5.3 Input–output plots. (a) Continuous system, e.g., a cable of cardiac cells connected by gap junctions. Experiment is carried out by applying programmed stimulation to the proximal end of the cable at progressively shorter input (P_1P_2) intervals. Output (D_1D_2) intervals are plotted on the ordinate against the corresponding P_1P_2 intervals, both expressed in milliseconds. At long P_1P_2 intervals, D_1D_2 falls on the identity line. At short P_1P_2 intervals, P_2D_2 conduction time increases, and thus D_1D_2 falls above the identity line following an asymptote toward the functional refractory period (FRP). (b) In an inhomogeneous system (i.e., the AV node or a Purkinje fiber sucrose gap preparation), the D_1D_2 to P_1P_2 relation presents a hook at early intervals because the impulse stops for some time at a junctional site. Under these conditions, very short P_1P_2 intervals may yield very long D_1D_2 intervals.

transmission are readily explained by discontinuous propagation across non-homogeneous systems in which an impulse stops at some junctional site (Figure 5.2b) and resumes propagation after a delay imposed by the FRP of the less excitable element. In the early 1980s, we tested this concept using an experimental model of nonuniform propagation in which a Purkinje fiber was placed in a three-chamber tissue bath (Figure 5.4a). A narrow zone of depressed excitability was created by superfusing the central segment of the fiber with an ion-free sucrose solution. Continuous microelectrode recordings were obtained from the two segments in the outer chambers, which were super-fused with normal Tyrode's solution. Impulses initiated in the proximal (P) chamber propagated to the distal chamber with delays that depended on the frequency of activation and on the degree of conduction impairment imposed by the unexcitability of the central segment. Note in Figure 5.4a the disconti-nuity in the action potential upstroke of the D segment, which exhibits a double component. The first component corresponds to passive electrotonic spread from the unexcitable element, which leads to eventual excitation of the distal end. The latter was modulated by bridging the two outer segments with a copper wire connected to a potentiometer (i.e., a variable resistor) in such a way that a complete "local circuit" was established from the wire through the solution in the proximal bath, the membranes of cells in that bath, the intracellular space, the cell membrane, the solution in the distal bath and then back to the distal end of the wire. As shown in Figure 5.4b, by changing the resistance of the bridge it was possible to modulate the degree of block and control the P to D delay of electric impulses initiated in the proximal segment. Moreover, as shown by the different symbols in the plot relating

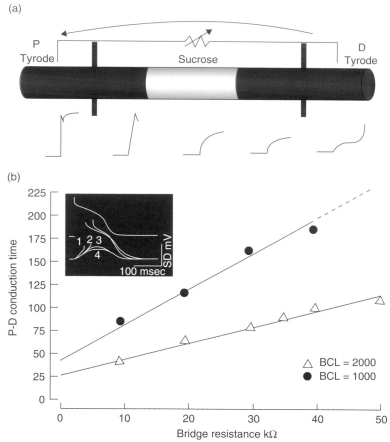

Figure 5.4 Dependence of conduction on the external impedance between proximal (P) and distal (D) segments of a calf Purkinje fiber in the sucrose gap. (a) Diagram of the preparations. The fiber is placed in a tissue bath divided into three compartments by two rubber membranes (dark vertical bars). The two outer segments are superfused with Tyrode's solution, and the central segment is superfused with ion-free sucrose solution. A variable resistor is used to bridge the sucrose chamber. (b) Ordinate: P-D conduction time expressed in milliseconds. Abscissa: Bridge resistance value expressed in kΩ. Triangles: P-D conduction time at a basic cycle length (BCL) of 2000 milliseconds. Circles: Data at BCL = 1000 milliseconds. The black lines were drawn by eye. The dotted line extending the top curve (BCL = 1000 milliseconds) indicates the development of Wenckebach periods with variable conduction times and followed by complete block. Top traces are transmembrane potentials from P; bottom traces are from D (inset). BCL = 1000 milliseconds. Four superimposed traces are shown at bridge resistance values of 20 kΩ (trace 1), 40 kΩ (trace 2), 50 kΩ (trace 3), and 60 kΩ (trace 4). Calibrations: 300 milliseconds and 50 mV. (Modified with permission from Jalife, *Circ Res* 1981; 49:233–47.)

conduction time to bridge resistance, the degree of conduction impairment depended on the basic cycle length (BCL) of stimulation.

Rate-dependent conduction block is a property of the AV conducting system, which is exemplified by the so-called "Wenckebach point." Rate-dependent block also occurs in experimentally depressed cardiac tissues as well as in diseased human ventricle. In many cases, periodicities in conduction were shown to correlate with changes in the amplitude of prepotentials recorded in fibers within or just beyond a region of low excitability. In Purkinje fibers, these changes may be the result of time-dependent changes in amplitude of electrotonic (subthreshold) depolarizations and active (suprathreshold) responses during diastole. The change in the magnitude of subthreshold events in nonhomogeneous or depressed atrial or ventricular myocardium reflects a concomitant delay in the recovery of excitability that, in turn, determines the frequency dependence of conduction. This hypothesis was tested in the model of discontinuous propagation as depicted in Figure 5.5. The superimposed tracings in Figure 5.5a illustrate the pattern of P:D propagation achieved at a critical BCL of stimulation of the proximal segment. The 6:5 typical Wenckebach pattern was stable as long as the conditions remained unchanged. In panel (b), when the BCL of P stimulation was

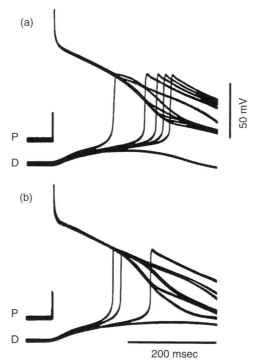

Figure 5.5 Two examples of second-degree block in the sucrose gap model (dog). P = proximal; D = distal transmembrane potential recordings; BCL = 1500 milliseconds and no bridge resistance between P and D. (a) Six superimposed oscilloscope sweeps show 6:5 block with "typical" Wenckebach structure, i.e., maximum increment of delay occurs after first P-D interval, with progressive decrease in subsequent beats. In panel (b), the four superimposed sweeps illustrate "atypical" Wenckebach and 4:3 block. In all cases, the distal activation delay is electrotonically mediated and is determined by the amplitude and rate of rise of the action potential "foot." (Reproduced with permission from Jalife, *Pacing Clin Electrophysiol* 1983; 6:1106–22.)

abbreviated, the pattern changed to atypical 4:3 Wenckebach periodicity. Thus, when the safety factor for conduction was reduced to a relatively low level (as in panel a), conduction aberrations emerged. As the frequency of stimulation increased further (as in panel b), there was further impairment of propagation due to changes in diastolic current requirements (sink) of depressed tissue as well as in the magnitude of current supplied (source) by the invading activation front.

Postrepolarization Refractoriness

Propagation of the action potential across cardiac tissue depends on the excitable properties of the cells and requires appropriately low values of intracellular and extracellular resistances. The sucrose gap preparation described earlier was used as a convenient method to illustrate the effects of changes in some of the parameters on propagation and its frequency dependence. As shown in the previous section, when the central segment of the fiber was superfused with low-resistance sucrose solution, connecting the two outer segments by a bridge provided a low-resistance extracellular pathway for the local circuit currents and restored P to D propagation. However, when the resistance of the bridge was set at a constant but relatively high value, P to D propagation became critically dependent on the interval of stimulation. This is illustrated in Figure 5.6, modified from an experiment in which a calf Purkinje fiber was placed in the sucrose gap chamber. At a BCL of 2000 milliseconds, action potentials (Pl) initiated in the proximal segment were transmitted to D at a constant P_1D_1 interval of 55 milliseconds (panels a–d). Test stimuli (P_2) applied after every 10th basic beat at progressively earlier intervals activated the distal segment with progressively longer P_2D_2 delay (panels a and b) until, at a P_1P_2 interval of 525 milliseconds (panel c), complete action potential block occurred. Yet, although action potentials no longer reached the distal segment, the local circuit (i.e., electrotonic) currents responsible for propagation did not die out abruptly at the site of block (i.e., the sucrose gap) but were manifest in the distal segment as a subthreshold depolarization, an appreciable distance away from that site. Note also that, as the distal response was delayed to longer and longer P_2D_2 intervals (panels a and b), the foot of the action potential in that segment became more apparent. When block occurred (panel c), this foot failed to bring the membrane potential to threshold and appeared as a depolarization that coincided with the P_2 action potential. Similar foot potentials were shown to occur in the AV node and other discontinuous systems when block occurred as a result of rapid pacing or premature stimulation. These subthreshold depolarizations are the electrotonic images of action potentials generated by tissues proximal to the site of block.

The time course of the recovery of excitability after an action potential propagated through a given heterogeneous pathway may be approximated by measuring the effective refractory period (ERP) of the pathway. ERP may

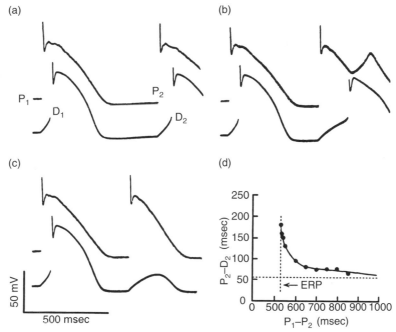

Figure 5.6 Postrepolarization refractoriness in a calf Purkinje fiber–sucrose gap preparation. Panels (a), (b), and (c) show analogue recordings. The proximal segment (P, top traces) was driven at a BCL of 2000 milliseconds. Single test stimuli applied after every 10th basic beat at progressively earlier P_1P_2 intervals yielded increasing delays in distal segment (D, bottom traces) activation. Complete P-D block (c) occurred at P_1P_2 of 525 milliseconds; P-D (effective) "refractoriness" outlasted action potential duration. Panel (d) illustrates complete scan of same experiment. ERP, effective refractory period. Horizontal broken line is control P_1D_1 interval at P_1P_2 2000 milliseconds and constant bridge resistance between P and D of 20 kΩ. Spikes were retouched. (Reproduced with permission from Jalife, *Pacing Clin Electrophysiol* 1983; 6:1106–22.)

be defined as the longest premature interval at which stimulation at a proximal site fails to generate a distal response (Figure 5.6d). When the pathway between P and D is highly discontinuous, the ERP can greatly outlast action potential repolarization. This phenomenon, known as postrepolarization refractoriness, is an invariable manifestation of discontinuous propagation. It occurs normally in the AV node but is also characteristic of all nonhomogeneous systems in which a local electrophysiological or structural alteration interferes with the normal transmission of the electric impulse.

Cellular Mechanisms of Discontinuous Propagation

An important question that arises from the foregoing discussion is whether the imbalance between sink and source properties underlying discontinuous propagation and postrepolarization refractoriness represents primarily an alteration in the active generator properties (e.g., inhomogeneous excitability) or in the electric coupling between cells or both. In this regard, the development of new optical techniques for measuring membrane potential with high spatial and temporal resolution enabled investigators to study propagation at the microscopic level as well as the role discontinuities in cell-to-cell connections in establishing imbalances between sink and source and leading to conduction block. We have investigated the role of tissue discontinuities in the two-dimensional activation spread in neonatal rat heart cell monolayers. The average cell dimensions in such monolayers were smaller than in adult canine myocardium, but the degree of cellular connectivity was similar. We measured the spread of the activation front (i.e., the action potential upstroke) using a high-resolution video camera to detect the fluorescence emitted by a voltage-sensitive dye embedded in the membranes of the cultured myocytes. Such a recording system enabled us to directly correlate the constructed activation maps with the cellular architecture, and the presence of discontinuities created by a linear lesion in the monolayer made using a sharp blade. As shown in Figure 5.7, the presence of the lesion created the substrate for slow conduction. Panel (a) shows the activation maps obtained when an electrical impulse was created on the right border of the monolayer above the lesion.

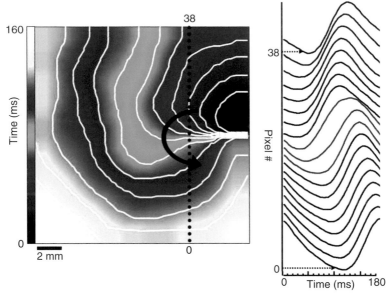

Figure 5.7 Discontinuous propagation created by the presence of a sharp obstacle in a 2-D sheet (a monolayer) of neonatal rat cardiomyocytes in an optical mapping experiment (Redshirt CDD camera, Di-8-ANEPPS). Left: Isochrone map of the spread of activation initiated at the point marked by the white asterisk (white lines are 10-millisecond isochrones). The white horizontal band at the center of the right border is the left edge of the obstacle. Impulses initiated at a cycle length of 215 milliseconds were forced to pivot around the obstacle at varying velocities for a total round time of 160 milliseconds. Right: 38 single-pixel recordings obtained along the dotted black line on the map. Note discontinuity in the action potential upstroke at the pivot point only (red tracings). (D. Auerbach and J. Jalife, unpublished.)

The electrical impulse was forced to circumnavigate, make a sharp turn, and pivot around the left edge of the lesion. As shown by the crowding of iso-chronal lines, conduction was exceedingly slow at the pivot point. In panel (b), optical action potential upstrokes recorded along the vertical column of pixels bounded by the broken lines exhibited an activation time. Hence, although the results presented in Figure 5.7 were somewhat different from those presented in the previous section (see Figures 5.5 and 5.6), they both point to sink-to-source mismatch as the underlying cause of the slowing of conduction and complex upstroke shapes. In one case, heterogeneities in active generator properties, brought about by the interposition of an unexcit-able element between two active sites, result in discontinuous propagation (Figure 5.5) and frequency-dependent block (Figure 5.6). In the other case, a sharp obstacle sets the stage for slow discontinuous propagation (Figure 5.7). In the latter case, depression of excitability increases the likelihood of block.

Unidirectional Block

Unidirectional block is essential for the development of reentrant arrhyth-mias, but its fundamental mechanisms are not well understood. At the end of the 19th century, Engelmann concluded that, under appropriate conditions, unidirectional block can occur in single skeletal muscle fibers, and he made the generalization that an impulse propagates more easily from rapidly con-ducting tissues to slowly conducting tissues than in the reverse direction. On the other hand, in 1914, George Mines suggested that one-way block may result from asymmetric decremental conduction in a depressed region. Later, in 1928, Schmitt and Erlanger exposed isolated turtle muscle strips to local-ized changes in the ionic environment but were unable to find any rules predicting the directionality of conduction. They therefore suggested that unidirectional block results from longitudinal dissociation in the area of depression and from the development of multiple pathways with differing conduction characteristics. Microelectrode recordings in apparently normal Purkinje fiber and muscle bundles usually show some degree of asymmetrical propagation, which is not surprising because one would expect absolute sym-metry of conduction only in a completely uniform and homogeneous cable (see Figures 5.1 and 5.2a). In the heart, such cable properties are probably the exception rather than the rule because 3-D interbundle connections, frequency, and distribution of gap junctions and branching are not uniform either along the His-Purkinje network or in the ventricular syncytium, and there are vari-ations in passive and active properties as well. Thus, it should be expected that any isolated segment of heart tissue would conduct more rapidly in one direction than in the other. Asymmetry may be exaggerated by agencies that depress excitability, including cold, pressure, high KCl, external electric block-ing currents, or ischemia. However, historically, unidirectional block suffi-ciently stable to allow detailed investigation was difficult to produce experimentally, and only a handful of examples were reported. In 1971, Paul

Cranefield, Herman Klein, and Brian Hoffman showed that it was possible to obtain unidirectional block, slow conduction, and reentrant activity in bundles of Purkinje fibers depressed by partial encasing of a false tendon in agar containing 47-mM KCl. The same year, Betty Sasyniuk and Carlos Mendez showed that, at the level of the Purkinje–muscle junction, the margin of safety for orthodromic impulse propagation is lower than in the antidromic direction, thus allowing the conditions for unidirectional block and reentry. As shown 10 years later by Jalife and Moe, unidirectional block could also be obtained when a Purkinje fiber bundle was positioned asymmetrically across a sucrose gap apparatus. If the proximal segment of the bundle is longer than its counterpart, action potentials will propagate in the proximal-distal direction, but they may be blocked in the opposite direction. Finally, numerical solutions for unidimensional cable equations representing a cardiac strand were carried out in 1980 by Ronald Joyner and his associates. These authors found major effects of asymmetry in cell diameter and electric coupling in the development of one-way block.

From the foregoing it is clear that the establishment of the unidirectional block that leads to reentrant and ectopic pacemaker arrhythmias seems to depend on a number of factors whose relative importance was not completely delineated. One common factor seems certain, however, and that is that there has to be some degree of spatial asymmetry in one or more electrophysiological parameters. In this regard, Stephan Rohr and colleagues demonstrated that spatially uniform reduction of electric coupling can lead to successful bidirectional conduction in asymmetrical discontinuous cardiac structures exhibiting unidirectional block. This study calls attention to the need for considering the interplay of structural and electrophysiological factors when attempting to establish the cause(s) of unidirectional block under a given set of circumstances.

Cellular Mechanisms of Wenckebach Periodicity

Rate-dependent heart block was first demonstrated by W. His in 1899 and subsequently studied in detail by K.F. Wenckebach in 1899. The so-called Wenckebach phenomenon in second-degree heart block occurs when the atrial rate is abnormally high or when AV conduction is compromised. In its "typical" manifestation, Wenckebach periodicity is characterized by a succession of electrocardiographic complexes in which AV conduction time (the PR interval) increases progressively in decreasing increments until transmission failure occurs. Following the dropped ventricular discharge, propagation is reinitiated, and the cycle is repeated (Figure 5.8). Several hypotheses were put forth to account for such an interesting cyclic phenomenon, and perhaps the most plausible is that originally proposed as early as 1925 by Mobitz, who brought attention to the fact that the progressive lengthening of the PR interval occurs at the expense of the subsequent RP interval (recovery time; see Figure 5.8a), which shortens concomitantly after every ventricular discharge.

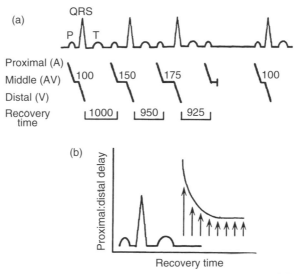

Figure 5.8 Schematic diagram of ECG recording illustrating the dynamics of Wenckebach periodicity. (a) Electrocardiogram and Lewis diagram of a 4:3 Wenckebach cycle. Numbers are in milliseconds. A, atrium; AV, atrioventricular node; V, ventricle. (b) Recovery curve. The upward arrows indicate timing of atrial discharges.

Consequently, the pattern must be associated with a progressive shortening of the time for recovery of ventricular excitability. As the AV conduction time increases progressively on a beat-to-beat basis, the impulse finds the ventricles less and less recovered, until failure occurs (Figure 5.8b). In the late 1950s, Rosenblueth (1958a,b) confirmed Mobitz's contention. His experiments in the canine heart further suggested that the progressive delay and eventual failure, leading to recovery and to the start of a new cycle, were in fact the result of discontinuous propagation across the AV conduction system.

Subsequent microelectrode studies in the 1960s using isolated rabbit AV node (by John Merideth *et al.* in Gordon Moe's laboratory) provided strong support to Mobitz's and Rosenblueth's hypotheses. In addition, Merideth and his collaborators demonstrated that the refractory period of the so-called "N" cells in the center of the AV node greatly outlasts the action potential duration (postrepolarization refractoriness), thus supporting Rosenblueth's conjecture that the FRP of the AV conducting system is determined by the time of recovery of the less excitable elements in that system (see Figure 5.4b). Sixteen years later, in 1974, Matthew Levy and his colleagues at the Mount Sinai Hospital in Cleveland used Mobitz's idea to derive their "positive feedback" model of AV node Wenckebach periodicity. In this model, the gradual shortening of the RP interval which results from the progressive PR prolongation can be considered a gradual increase in the prematurity of impulses crossing the AV node. Thus, as the RP abbreviates more and more, the AV node is less recovered, and the PR interval must increase with each beat, until failure occurs.

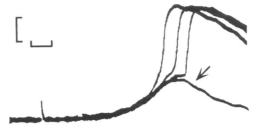

Figure 5.9 Example of 4 : 3 Wenckebach recorded from a cell in the NH region of an isolated atrioventricular node. Five superimposed traces are shown. Calibrations are vertical, 20 mV; horizontal, 20 milliseconds. (Reproduced with permission from Paes de Carvalho and de Almeida, *Circ Res* 1960; 8:801–9.)

In 1960, Paes de Carvalho and de Almeida published the first microelectrode recordings of Wenckebach periodicity in the AV node (Figure 5.9). Their study revealed no significant changes in the upstroke velocity of the action potential of the AV nodal cell that could explain the gradual increase in the activation time. Douglas Zipes, with Carlos Mendez and Gordon Moe, later proposed that, at the cellular level, the Wenckebach phenomenon could be explained in terms of electrotonically mediated delays in the excitation of the AV nodal cell. In fact, it is clear from the example of 4 : 3 AV nodal Wenckebach shown by the four superimposed traces in Figure 5.9 that the time course of the "foot" that precedes each of the superimposed active responses is essentially the same as that of the subthreshold depolarization (arrow) induced by the atrial impulse during the blocked beat. Because propagation through the N region of the AV node is highly discontinuous, during successful propagation the electric impulse stops momentarily at that region. As such, the progressive PR prolongation (Figure 5.8) is seen to result from a progressive decrease in the amplitude and rate of rise of the action potential foot as the relative prematurity of impulses crossing the AV node increases with the decreasing RP interval. Thus, as the RP abbreviates more and more, the N region is less recovered, which makes it more difficult for the action potential foot to attain threshold for an active NH response (Figure 5.9). Consequently, the PR interval must increase with each beat, until failure occurs.

From the foregoing it is clear that Wenckebach periodicity and postrepolarization refractoriness result from a relatively slow recovery of the excitability of cells within a conducting pathway. Slow recovery of excitability is an inherent property of the AV node as well as other cardiac tissues. Because Wenckebach periodicity is demonstrable as a frequency-dependent phenomenon, it seems reasonable to suggest that, in the setting of discontinuous conduction brought about by complex 3-D microanatomy, as well as heterogeneous distribution of intercellular connections, the underlying mechanism of such a cyclic behavior is related to time-dependent changes in the recovery of excitability of individual cardiac cells. In 1989, we tested this hypothesis in single, enzymatically dispersed guinea pig ventricular myocytes maintained in

(a)

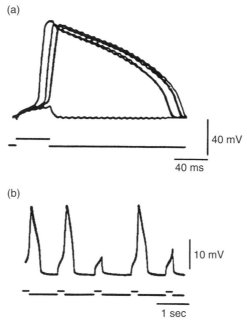

40 mV

40 ms

(b)

10 mV

1 sec

Figure 5.10 Wenckebach periodicity in single ventricular myocytes. (a) Five superimposed microelectrode recordings during repetitive stimulation at a basic cycle length of 1000 milliseconds. Note typical structure of Wenckebach periodicity with increasing delays at decreasing increments. (b) Time recording showing a 5:3 pattern of activation in a different cell. In both panels, the bottom trace is a current monitor. (Reproduced from Delmar *et al.*, *Circ Res* 1989; 65:761–74.)

HEPES-Tyrode solution. Whole-cell transmembrane recordings and depolarizing current pulse application were carried out using a single patch pipette. Cells were well polarized, and resting potentials were always more negative than –79 mV and gave rise to action potentials of the expected morphology. However, as shown in Figure 5.10, under conditions of repetitive stimulation with depolarizing pulses of suprathreshold but relatively low amplitude, it was easy to demonstrate a cyclic behavior in the excitation process of the cell. Such behavior closely mimicked the Wenckebach phenomenon demonstrated almost 30 years earlier by Paes de Carvalho and de Almeida in the rabbit AV node (see Figure 5.9). Figure 5.10a was obtained from a ventricular myocyte whose resting potential was –81 mV. Five superimposed traces are shown. Depolarizing current pulses, 40 milliseconds in duration and 0.15 nA in strength, were applied at a BCL of 1000 milliseconds. A 5:4 (stimulus: response) activation pattern was clearly manifest. In fact, the latency between the onset of the current pulse and the action potential upstroke increased in decreasing increments until failure occurred, thus reproducing very closely the typical structure of Wenckebach periodicity (see Figure 5.8). Figure 5.10b shows another example taken from a different cell. Constant current pulses (amplitude 0.25 nA; duration 200 milliseconds) were applied through the recording microelectrode at a constant cycle length of 1100 milliseconds. Under these conditions, alternations between 3:2 and 2:1 activation ensued. Note that, in both panels, the impulse failed always when the stimulus occurred several milliseconds after the repolarization phase of the action potential, thus emphasizing the importance of postrepolarization refractoriness in the development of Wenckebach periodicity.

Mathematical modeling can be used to study excitation block processes because it allows manipulations that would be impossible to carry out experimentally in single myocytes. In the 1970s, George Beeler and Harald Reuter from the University of Berne in Switzerland formulated a model of the cardiac ventricular cell. The model included formulation for four transmembrane ionic currents: the rapid Na current, responsible for the action potential upstroke; the Ca current, responsible for the plateau; a time-dependent potassium current (I_K) responsible for repolarization; and a time-independent potassium current (I_{K1}) that maintained the resting potential. Although the model is somewhat inaccurate and oversimplified in its representation of the electric activity of the cell, it is nevertheless a useful tool to study the frequency-dependent behavior of the myocyte. Figure 5.11 shows the simulated action potentials recorded when current pulses were applied repetitively

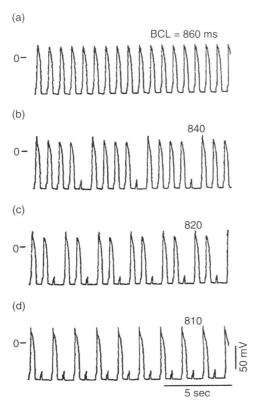

Figure 5.11 Computer simulations of Wenckebach periodicity using a modified version of the Beeler and Reuter model of a ventricular cell. Action potentials were elicited by repetitive application of depolarizing current pulses (amplitude, −1.4 μA/cm²; duration, 100 milliseconds) at varying cycle lengths. BCL, basic cycle length. (Reproduced with permission from Delmar et al., Circ Res 1989; 65:761–74.)

at various cycle lengths. Figure 5.11a shows a tracing with 1:1 response when the BCL was relatively long. Just as in the ventricular myocyte experiment, progressive abbreviation of the stimulus cycle length yielded patterns of frequency-dependent activation failure, including 5:4 (b), 3:2 (c), and 2:1 (d).

Recovery Curve

The tracings shown in Figure 5.11 suggest that the recovery of excitability after each action potential is indeed a function of the diastolic interval and that under certain conditions, refractoriness can outlast the repolarization phase. Figure 5.12 shows the results of additional computer simulations in which an S1S2 protocol was used to study the conditions for recovery of excitability as a function of the diastolic interval. In panels (a–c), a test pulse, S_2, of relatively long duration and low amplitude was applied at various coupling intervals after the last S_1 stimulus in a train of 10 (BCL = 1000 milliseconds). Clearly, the activation delay S_2V_2 increased as the coupling interval

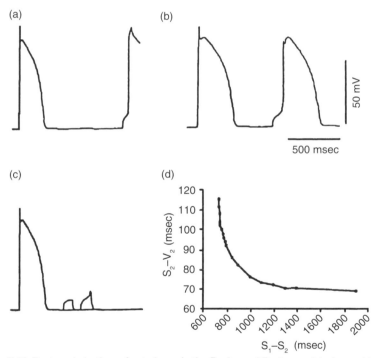

Figure 5.12 Postrepolarization refractoriness in the Beeler and Reuter model of a ventricular cell. A test pulse (S_2; amplitude, -1.4 $\mu A/cm^2$; duration, 100 milliseconds) was used to scan the diastolic interval after an action potential induced by S_1. (a) At a relatively long S_1S_2 interval, the S_2V_2 interval (measured from the onset of the stimulus to 50% of the action potential upstroke) was brief. (b) At shorter S_1S_2 intervals, the S_2V_2 was prolonged. (c) Two superimposed tracings show subthreshold responses at two different S_1S_2 intervals. (d) S_2V_2 as a function of S_1S_2. (Reproduced with permission from Delmar et al., Circ Res 1989; 65:761–74.)

decreased (cf. panel b to panel a) until activation failure occurred. Panel (c) shows two superimposed tracings demonstrating subthreshold responses at two different premature S1S2 intervals. In panel (d), a complete plot of S_2V_2 as a function of S_1S_2 shows a monotonic recovery curve, which is similar to those described for the AV node, and for multicellular preparations of isolated Purkinje fibers and ventricular muscle.

Recovery Curve Predicts Nonlinear Dynamics of Rate-Dependent Propagation

In principle, it is expected that any linear system should behave in a simple and totally predictable manner when one of its parameters is changed. For example, if the volume of a closed space is compressed progressively, the resulting pressure within that space will increase proportionately within a given range. Yet, in biology, it is very difficult, if not impossible, to find a completely linear system; nonlinearity is probably the rule, and the heart is no exception. Nonlinear dynamical systems, including those that are described by a small number of variables (e.g., action potential duration, latency, and excitability), can behave in complex ways.

From a mechanistic point of view, the common denominator in the occurrence of rate-dependent intermittent propagation (excitation) phenomena, including Wenckebach periodicity, may be a slow recovery time for membrane excitability after each activation. Slow recovery of excitability may be plotted in the so-called recovery curve as a means to make quantitative predictions about the patterns of propagation that should emerge when a discontinuous system is forced to conduct at relatively high stimulation rates. For example, in 1987, Alvin Shrier with his coworkers at McGill University in Montreal used the AV nodal recovery curve, obtained using an S_1S_2 protocol in patients undergoing electrophysiological testing, to predict patterns of first- and second-degree AV block induced by rapid pacing. Because the AV nodal recovery curve gives the conduction time through the AV node (i.e., the A_2H_2 interval), as a function of the recovery time from the last successful anterograde activation of the His bundle (i.e., the H_1A_2 interval), they used a simple numerical iteration of a monotonic function derived from the AV nodal recovery curve to demonstrate that, with increasing stimulation frequency, there was a decrease in the activation ratio, defined as the m/n ratio, where m = number of ventricular responses and n = number of atrial stimuli. Their results provided new insight in our understanding of the dynamics of rate-dependent heart block. Most importantly, they demonstrated that cyclic phenomena such as Wenckebach periodicity, reverse Wenckebach, and alternating Wenckebach are demonstrable in simple discontinuous systems without the need of invoking complex geometric arrangements in cell bundles or multiple levels of block. In fact, the results in single myocytes (see Figure 5.10) clearly show that Wenckebach-like phenomena are demonstrable in single cells, provided stimuli of appropriately low amplitude, and high frequency are used.

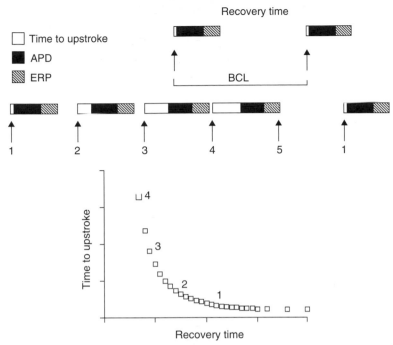

Figure 5.13 Dynamics of Wenckebach periodicity as derived from the recovery of excitability curve. APD, action potential duration; ERP, effective refractory period; BCL, basic cycle length. (Reproduced with permission from Jalife and Delmar, In: Glass L, Hunter P, McCulloch A, eds. *Theory of Heart.* New York: Springer-Verlag; 1991: 359–76.)

In the case of Figure 5.11, as the BCL was progressively decreased, the activation ratio, measured as m/n (m = number of cell responses; n = number of stimuli) changed from 1.0 (tracing a) through 0.8 (tracing b), 0.67 (tracing c), and finally 0.5 (tracing d).

As in the case of AV nodal Wenckebach, in single ventricular myocytes, cyclic excitation patterns during repetitive stimulation are predictable using the recovery curve. In Figure 5.13, we illustrate the dynamics of a 5:4 Wenckebach period in terms of the recovery curve of a normally polarized myocyte driven by repetitive stimuli of constant magnitude and cycle length. In this representation, the horizontal boxes represent the excitation and repolarization processes; the white boxes represent the interval between the onset of the stimulus and the action potential upstroke (time to upstroke); the black boxes represent the APD; and the dashed boxes represent the duration of postrepolarization refractoriness (ERP). Recovery time is the interval between the end of the preceding action potential and the occurrence of the next stimulus. The recovery curve is a plot of the time to upstroke as a function of the recovery time. In the middle diagram, the first pulse (labeled 1), which occurs at a relatively long premature interval, gives rise to an action potential whose time to upstroke in the recovery curve is relatively short. The second stimulus now occurs at a briefer interval within the recovery curve, and the action potential is further delayed. Because the cycle length is constant, the next recovery time is even briefer, which leads to an even longer delay. After the fifth stimulus, the recovery time is briefer than the refractory phase, and failure occurs. Subsequently (not shown) because of a long recovery time, a new cycle ensues, and the 5:4 Wenckebach pattern repeats once again.

Ionic Mechanism of Wenckebach in Ventricular and Atrioventricular Nodal Myocytes

The ionic mechanisms of the Wenckebach-like patterns observed in single ventricular myocytes were studied through a combination of current- and voltage-clamp techniques. Briefly, the results showed that both postrepolarization refractoriness and Wenckebach periodicity, in response to depolarizing pulses of relatively low amplitude, are the result of a slow recovery of cell excitability during diastole, which is determined by the slow deactivation of the delayed rectifier potassium outward current I_K. This is illustrated graphically by numerical simulations with the Beeler and Reuter model in the diagram presented in Figure 5.14. The top tracings represent the membrane potential; an action potential is followed by two subthreshold responses to a depolarizing current pulse of constant amplitude applied at two different intervals. The bottom tracing illustrates the time course of I_K conductance during the cardiac cycle, and the bottom arrows represent the time-dependent magnitude of the I_K opposing the depolarizing current pulse (I_p) at the two depolarizing instants. The conductance to potassium (G_K) increases gradually

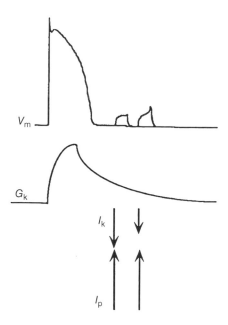

Figure 5.14 Proposed role of I_K in determining the time course of recovery of excitability in a single myocyte. Top: Transmembrane potential (V_m) simulated by the Beeler and Reuter model. Bottom: Changes in potassium conductance (G_K) during systolic and diastolic intervals. Arrows: Relative magnitudes of I_K and pulse current (I_p) at two different times during I_K deactivation. (Reproduced with permission from Jalife and Delmar, In: Glass L, Hunter P, McCulloch A, eds. *Theory of Heart.* New York: Springer-Verlag; 1991: 359–76.)

in the course of the action potential and becomes maximal during the plateau. On repolarization, G_K begins to decrease. Because of the slow time course of deactivation, most of the channel conductance decay occurs after repolarization has been completed. Yet, the diastolic potential remains constant because of the lack of driving force for I_K (i.e., the resting potential is at, or very close to, the K equilibrium potential). On the other hand, as illustrated in Figure 5.14, when a subthreshold depolarizing pulse is applied early in diastole, the membrane voltage displacement provides sufficient force for I_K, which tends to repolarize the membrane. The influence of G_K decreases at the longer diastolic intervals, which allows for an increase in the amplitude of the subthreshold response. Application of a pulse at a later interval should encounter I_K even more deactivated; thus depolarization should be greater and an action potential should ensue (not shown).

Additional results indicated that nonlinearities in the current–voltage relationship (rectification) of the inward-rectifying current, I_{K1}, played a major role in modulating the amplitude and shape of the foot potentials that precede the progressively more delayed active responses in the Wenckebach cycle as well as the subthreshold event that ensues when activation fails (Figure 5.5). Studies in isolated guinea pig ventricular myocytes have shown that postrepolarization refractoriness can occur at diastolic potentials even if the Na^+ current, I_{Na}, has had sufficient time to recover completely from inactivation, because of the slow gating kinetics of I_K. The identification of the proteins responsible for the rapid and slow components of I_K (I_{Kr} and I_{Ks}, respectively; see Chapter 2 for details on these transmembrane currents) in the early 1990s opened the door for further understanding of such postrepolarization refractoriness.

We recently gained insight into the possible mechanisms underlying I_{Ks}-induced failure of activation by using a heterologous expression system in the absence of other native cardiac-specific proteins that could confound the interpretation of the results. Accordingly one group of human embryonic kidney (HEK293) cells was stably transfected with Kir2.1, responsible for I_{K1} to set the resting membrane potential at about -70 mV. A second group of HEK293 cells was co-transfected with Kir2.1 and KvLQT1-minK, which is responsible for the I_{Ks}. The cells in each group were subjected to a whole-cell current-clamp S1-S2 stimulus protocol, as illustrated by the representative experiments in Figure 5.15. In panel (a), the applied stimulation protocol shows a square depolarizing pulse S1 (duration: 300 ms; frequency: 1–2 Hz) followed by an S2 of equal magnitude, but briefer duration (50 ms) with a varying S1-S2 intervals, with the minimum S1-S2 duration adjusted so that S2 does not encroach on the S1 response. As shown in panel (b), the amplitude and shape of the action potential-like response in cells expressing Kir2.1 alone was not affected by the timing of the S2 stimulus. This is because the I_{K1} channels maintained an I–V and conductance profile that was not affected by the timing of S2. In contrast, as shown in panel (c), a clear time dependency was demonstrated in cells expressing both Kir2.1 and minK-KvLQT1 genes:

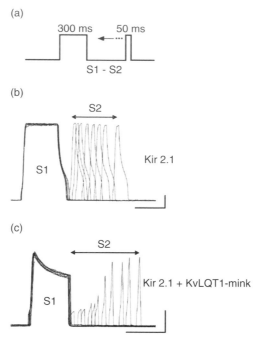

Figure 5.15 I_{Ks} slow deactivation underlies the molecular mechanism of postrepolarization refractoriness. Current-clamp data in HEK293 cells. (a) S1-S2 protocol. (b) Responses of a representative cell transfected with Kir2.1. (c) Response of a representative cell co-transfected with Kir2.1 and KvLQT1-minK. Scale bars: horizontal = 250 milliseconds; vertical = 25 mV. (Reproduced with permission from Muñoz *et al.*, *Circ Res* 2007;101: 475–83.)

progressively reducing the S1-S2 interval resulted in gradual changes in both the shape and amplitude of the S2 response, indicative of slow I_{Ks} deactivation inducing an increased membrane conductance concomitant with the S1-S2 interval abbreviation. Taken together, these results support the idea that both I_{K1} and I_{Ks} are important in the recovery of the current requirements for excitation during the diastolic interval.

Observations in single AV nodal myocytes, obtained by enzymatic dispersion of rabbit hearts, showed somewhat more complex cellular events and ionic mechanisms. As illustrated in panel (a) of Figure 5.16, the results in some AV nodal cells demonstrated that, when depolarizing stimuli of constant but critical magnitude are used to scan the diastolic interval, a monotonic recovery of excitability is clearly observed. However, as seen in panel (b_1), a few myocytes demonstrated a highly nonlinear time course of recovery after an action potential. Such nonlinear recovery included a period of supernormal excitability where the latency between the stimulus and the action potential upstroke was smaller at very early intervals than at long intervals. This was followed to the right by postrepolarization refractoriness and slow recovery of excitability during diastole. These two different types of time-dependent changes were responsible for the development of two different types of

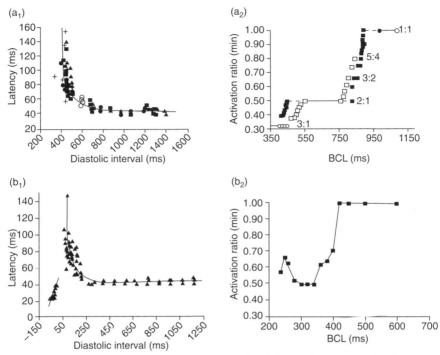

Figure 5.16 Rate dependence of activation patterns in relation to the recovery of excitability curve in two different rabbit atrioventricular (AV) nodal myocytes without (a_1 and a_2) and with (b_1 and b_2) supernormality. (a_1) Steady-state recovery of excitability plotted as time to upstroke (latency) vs. preceding diastolic interval during repetitive stimulation. Different symbols represent data for stimulation at varying basic cycle lengths (BCLs). The continuous line represents an empiric monotonic function that considers previous diastolic interval as the sole determinant of latency. (a_2) Open symbols show the ranges of stimulus:response ratios observed in the AV nodal myocyte whose recovery was monotonic (a_1). Data are plotted at various BCLs. The crosses are the stimulus:response ratios predicted by an iterative numerical procedure for the corresponding BCLs. (b_1) Non-monotonic steady-state recovery curve of a single AV nodal myocyte showing supernormal excitability (i.e., shorter than expected latencies at very early diastolic intervals). Lines were fitted by eye. (b_2) Activation ratio plotted as a function of BCL. In the presence of supernormality, the dependence of activation ratio on BCL does not decrease monotonically but jumps upward at very short BCLs. (Reproduced with permission from Hoshino *et al.*, *Circulation* 1990; 82:2201–16.)

stimulus:response patterns. First, when the myocyte was stimulated by repetitive depolarizing pulses and the recovery curve was monotonic (panel a_1), the response patterns were comparable to those observed during first- and second-degree AV block (panel a_2) (i.e., as the BCL of the stimulus was shortened, there was a monotonic stepwise change in the excitation pattern, from 1:1 through 5:4, 3:2, 2:1, and finally 3:1 [crosses]). The latter observation was confirmed using an analytical model that was devised on the basis of mathematical expressions that simulated the AV nodal recovery curve. Numerical iteration of those equations (open symbols) yielded stimulus:

response patterns that were similar to those observed during repetitive stimulation of the single myocyte (panel a_2). Second, in the presence of a nonlinear recovery (panel b_1), a monotonic change in the stimulus:response patterns was no longer present. As shown in panel (b_2), nonlinearities in such patterns were observed at stimulus cycle lengths between 200 and 300 milliseconds, where the activation pattern abruptly increased from 2:1 to 3:2 and then 6:11. Such cycle lengths corresponded to very short diastolic intervals in the recovery curve (panel b_1), where supernormality was present. Additional observations using voltage-clamp techniques suggested that at least three different ionic current systems are involved in AV nodal Wenckebach and complex rate-dependent excitation processes: the slow delayed rectifier potassium outward current, I_{Ks}, the time-independent rectifier potassium outward current I_{K1}, and the calcium inward current I_{Ca} (see Chapter 2 for details about these currents). The overall results may have important clinical implications because they provide a direct ionic basis for AV nodal Wenckebach periodicity and other heart rate-dependent AV conduction disturbances.

At first glance, these results in single AV nodal myocytes seem to contradict classical microelectrode studies in the isolated multicellular rabbit AV nodal preparation, in which the recovery of excitability curve did not demonstrate supernormality during repolarization. Yet, it should be kept in mind that the recovery curve constructed in the early study was from the N region of the AV node, and the analysis was limited to scanning the diastolic interval with intracellular stimuli; no attempt was made to determine whether these cells were excitable during the repolarization phase. Because AV node myocyte experiments clearly showed that, although latency to excitation increased monotonically at progressively earlier intervals until block occurred, a window of supernormal excitability was demonstrable during the repolarization phase (Figure 5.16b). The early studies failed to demonstrate supernormal AV nodal conduction in response to premature stimuli applied at a distant source. However, it is important to consider that conduction depends not only on the threshold for excitation but also on the ability of excited cells to depolarize their neighbors, the latter being determined by a number of parameters that include the rate of rise of the action potential, the degree of electric coupling, and the geometric arrangement of cell-to-cell connections. Thus, the possibility exists that, although present in the single cell, supernormal responses fail to propagate through the AV node.

Nonlinear Recovery and Complex Excitation Dynamics

These results support the idea that, despite their differences, many nonlinear systems with finite recovery time behave in much the same way. Provided that the relevant parameters, which in the case of the myocyte may be excitability, recover monotonically, the sequence of $n:m$ (stimulus:response) patterns that occur as the stimulation frequency is systematically altered can be predicted by the so-called "Farey tree" (see Figure 5.17a).

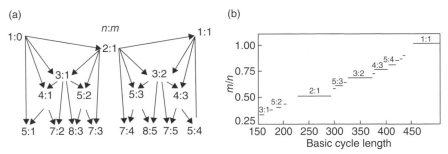

Figure 5.17 (a) Farey tree constructed for the first five generations. Starting from seed values 1:0, 1:1, and 2:1 on top line, a new line of activation ($n:m$) ratios is generated by adding the numerators and denominators of adjacent entries. The ratios in the third line are generated in a similar manner from those in the second line, and so on. (b) Devil's staircase obtained by plotting the m/n ratio as a function of basic cycle length (BCL). Theoretically, if the BCL is changed in infinitely small steps, there will be an infinite number of $n:m$ steps.

As shown in Figure 5.17a, for any two $n:m$ and $N:M$ neighboring stimulus:response patterns, there is always an intermediate $n + N:m + M$ stimulus:response pattern. Therefore, in the case of any given excitable system whose recovery is monotonic, when the stimulus cycle length is changed systematically in extremely small steps and then the resulting activation ratio (m/n) is plotted as a function of that cycle length, the resultant is an infinitely detailed staircase of $m:n$ steps (Figure 5.17b), known as the "devil's staircase."

However, as illustrated earlier for the single AV nodal myocyte, under certain conditions, cardiac tissues do not have a monotonic recovery of excitability (Figure 5.16b$_1$). Similarly, in multicellular Purkinje fibers, a relatively supernormal phase of excitability at early diastolic intervals is always present when the fiber is immersed in low KCl (<4 mM). Under these conditions, repetitive stimulation of such fibers may result in complex patterns of excitation. Careful and systematic experimental and numerical studies of such complex patterns showed that, under specific sets of circumstances, isolated cardiac cells and tissues can undergo transitions from regular and periodic to highly aperiodic (i.e., chaotic) behavior. Chaos theory, if used appropriately, may provide tools and insights into the laws that govern such behavior.

According to its mathematical description, chaos is an irregular, but nonrandom, behavior that may occur in nonlinear dynamical systems. A dynamical system is any system whose evolution is determined by the interplay of its intrinsic time-dependent variables (e.g., action potential duration and excitability); when such a time dependence is nonlinear, the system may undergo either ordered or chaotic behavior, depending on the value of the input parameter (e.g., BCL). In the chaotic regime, the system demonstrates irregularity as well as an exquisite sensitivity to initial conditions in such a way that it is impossible to make long-term predictions about its behavior. In other words, chaos theory deals with those systems in which periodic and chaotic patterns can emerge. The difference is merely in the value of a single parameter. Very small changes in this parameter can make a huge difference as to the ultimate behavior of the system. Note, however, that chaos is not simply disorder. It is more appropriately described as "order without periodicity." For instance, consider a chaotic sequence of numbers. The sequence appears random; however, each number in the sequence is determined exactly and exclusively by the numbers that precede it. This makes the sequence completely deterministic despite its lack of periodicity. By contrast, in a random sequence of numbers, the succession will be governed by a statistical probability distribution, will not be exactly determined, and may be different if sequenced again with the same initial conditions. Based on systematic studies in isolated cardiac Purkinje fibers, we proposed that the mechanism for the chaotic behavior demonstrated by isolated Purkinje fibers during repetitive stimulation was linked to the presence of supernormal excitability. The main arguments included (1) the recovery of excitability after an action potential is nonlinear and (2) during stimulation at a constant cycle length, there are negative feedback processes that are established among the action potential duration, the diastolic interval, and the latency of excitation, which result in specific patterns of activation.

Clearly, judicious use of nonlinear systems theory and of its mathematical tools allows one to gain insight into the principles that rule the regular and irregular behavior in cardiac tissues. This was convincingly demonstrated not only in isolated Purkinje fibers and Purkinje–muscle preparations but also in chick embryonic ventricular cell aggregates as well as in the human AV conduction system. Although no chaotic patterns propagation were found in the latter study, the investigators used the appropriate tools to investigate input–output responses of the AV node and made testable predictions on the basis of such tools. In 1992, a chaos-control strategy was used to stabilize arrhythmias induced by digitalis toxicity in isolated cardiac tissues. By applying electric stimuli at irregular times determined by chaos theory, the activity recorded locally was converted to periodic beating. Whether such control paradigms are applicable to the treatment of clinical arrhythmias remains speculative.

Role of Gross Anatomic Structure in Discontinuous Propagation

Although there are many studies demonstrating the effects of structural abnormalities on propagation in the atria and ventricles, the role of naturally occurring heterogeneities in the 3-D structure of cardiac tissues on propagation was the aim of study of a small group of investigators. Most such studies focused on the importance of atrial structure in clinical arrhythmias such as atrial flutter and fibrillation. However, although previous studies demonstrated the importance of the atrial structure in the initiation of reentry, the question of whether reentrant arrhythmias may be the result of preferential propagation through the complicated network of pectinate muscles in the atrial subendocardium with discordant activation of the subepicardium only recently began to be addressed.

The work of Spach and collaborators greatly advanced our understanding of the role of structural complexities in wave propagation in the atrial subendocardium. These investigators showed that "macroscopic" discontinuities (i.e., at size scale of ≥1 mm) in the muscle structure play an important role in the establishment of unidirectional block and the initiation of reentry. Their experiments demonstrated the role of anisotropy in unidirectional block at branch sites of the crista terminalis (CT) and pectinate muscles and at the junction between the CT and the limbus. In those experiments, the safety factor for propagation highly depended on clearly visible changes in the gross geometry of the muscular bundles involved. The size of such structural changes (>1 mm) is similar to that which is relevant to curvature effects leading to wavelet formation in isolated cardiac muscle and may be the mechanism underlying multiple wavelet formation during reentrant arrhythmias. In 1993, Richard Schuessler and his associates demonstrated discordant activation of the epicardium and endocardium, particularly in those areas of the atrium in which the wall thickness was >0.5 mm. Discordance increased with increases in the excitation frequency, which suggested that, during high-frequency excitation, discordant epicardial vs. endocardial activation may lead to transmural reentry, particularly in those regions in which the 3-D anatomy of the atrium is most heterogeneous.

We recently used video imaging and a voltage-sensitive dye to study the role of atrial structure on activation patterns and reentry. The results showed that the CT and pectinate muscles were sites of preferential propagation whose frequency dependence enabled disparity between endocardial and epicardial activation as well as reentry, with appearance of local block at junctional and branching points and epicardial breakthroughs. In addition, computer simulations using a model of a piece of atrial-free wall connected to a single pectinate muscle bridging the wall suggested that preferential propagation through the subendocardial atrial muscle bundles may destabilize reentry. Those initial results indicated that preferred propagation along the pectinate muscles contributes to complexity in cardiac arrhythmias. In a different set of experiments in isolated preparation of the sheep right atrium, we studied how the complexity of the propagation pattern across the pectinate network depends on the rate of activation.

The Phenomenon of Fibrillatory Conduction

As stated at the outset of this chapter, the structural complexities of the various cardiac tissues and the complex nonlinear dynamics of cardiac cell excitation establish the substrate for exceedingly complex rhythms when the rate of cardiac excitation exceeds critical levels. Studies in cultured cardiomyocyte monolayers, isolated atrial preparations, and whole hearts from several species ranging in size from mouse to pig have demonstrated that exceedingly rapid excitation even from a single source can result in ECG patterns that are indistinguishable from atrial or ventricular fibrillation, which suggests that at least some forms of fibrillation are highly organized and depend on the uninterrupted, periodic activity of a small number of high-frequency sources (see Chapters 8 and 9). The rapidly succeeding wave fronts emanating from such sources propagate throughout the atria or ventricles and interact with tissue heterogeneities, functional and anatomical, leading to fragmentation and wavelet formation, the end result being fibrillatory conduction. Apparently chaotic waves often recorded optically in intact hearts and attributed to fibrillatory conduction may be generated by sources located at a remote location in the same tissue. In this regard, it has been demonstrated that the intricate branching structure of the cardiac musculature provides a substrate for complex patterns of propagation during cardiac fibrillation. For example, as discussed in Chapter 8, it has been shown that during atrial fibrillation (AF) the excitation frequency in the left atrium (LA) may be higher than in the right atrium (RA). This is because, at least in some cases, AF results from activation by relatively stationary high-frequency sources of impulses, which undergo complex spatially distributed intermittent block patterns across interatrial pathways, e.g., from Bachmann's bundle (BB) through the CT and the branching network of pectinate muscles in the RA appendage.

To investigate in detail the response of the RA to incoming high-frequency excitation from the LA, we used an isolated coronary-perfused RA preparation and quantified the frequency-dependent nature of the propagation of wave fronts entering the RA from BB and the basis of fibrillatory conduction. Data from the endocardium of an isolated RA preparation are illustrated in Figure 5.18. The endocardium (right) is characterized by an intricate network of pectinate muscles (outlined for clarity) that branch out of the CT and tricuspid valve (TV) rim toward the RAA and across the cavity. A pacing electrode was used to stimulate BB and mimic LA-to-RA propagation. Brief pulses, 5-millisecond duration and twice diastolic threshold, were delivered at constant rates, varying from 2 Hz up to the fastest rate that allowed 1:1 capture of the tissue in the immediate vicinity of the electrode. The black arrows in Figure 5.18 indicate the general direction of propagation during pacing of BB at increasing frequencies of 2, 5, 6.3, and 6.7 Hz. As demonstrated by the color isochrone maps, as the activation frequency increased, 1:1 propagation across the CT and the grid of PM occurred with increasing delays that varied depending on the frequency and the location. For example, at 2.0 Hz the total activation time across the field of view was <30 milliseconds. However, at 6.7 Hz the most distal PM regions were activated with a delay as long as 120 milliseconds. As shown by the white asterisk, in this preparation, there was a breakthrough site emerging from the subendocardium, suggesting that propagation was complex not only on the endocardium but also on the entire thickness of the preparation.

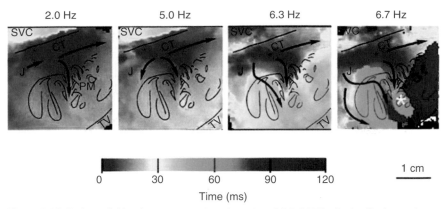

Figure 5.18 Endocardial isochrone maps at pacing rates of 2.0–6.7 Hz. During Bachmann's bundle pacing, the J region is excited first, followed by the crista terminalis (CT) and the pectinate muscle network. One-to-one propagation is maintained at all rates but conduction time increases in a frequency-dependent manner, with abrupt delays being manifest at 6.3 and 6.7 Hz. Arrows show direction of propagation; asterisk shows breakthrough site. TV, tricuspid valve. (Reproduced with permission from Berenfeld *et al.*, *Circ Res* 2002; 90:1173–80.)

To better understand the mechanisms of the complex pattern of propagation illustrated in Figure 5.18, we carried out a detailed analysis of the activation delays at equidistant pixel locations along the CT and PM at pacing rates between 2.0 and 6.7 Hz. Figure 5.19a shows a picture of the preparation to indicate the pixel locations. In Figure 5.19b,c, the top graphs show the conduction delay at each location. The superimposed optical action potentials in Figure 5.19b,c were taken, respectively, from pixels c1–c5 on the CT and p1–p6 on the PM in the center of the recording field. At frequencies between 2.0 and 5.9 Hz, conduction was relatively uniform across all pixels. However, at higher frequencies, activation time increased abruptly at specific locations of augmented structural complexity. For example, pixels c3–c5 were located at the region at which the CT underwent extensive branching into the PM region (Figure 5.19a). Thus, at c4, the conduction delay increased abruptly from 5 milliseconds at 6.3 Hz to 18 milliseconds at 6.7 Hz. Similarly, at c5, conduction delay jumped from 11 milliseconds at 6.3 Hz to 24 milliseconds at 6.7 Hz.

At the higher frequencies, the delays along the PM were much longer and exceedingly nonuniform. As shown in Figure 5.19c, at 2 Hz the delays between p1 and p6 were relatively short (total of ~10 milliseconds) and increased linearly across all pixels. Similarly, at 5.0 and 5.9 Hz, the delay between p1 and p6 increased gradually to 18 and 21 milliseconds, respectively. However, at the pacing frequency of 6.3 Hz, the action potential upstrokes in p4 and p5 became humped and there were disproportionately long step delays in p6 (red arrows). This pattern reflected the development of decremental conduction at p4 and p5, with p6 activation through a different pathway. This is more evident at 6.7 Hz (see also Figure 5.18) in that conduction block occurs in the p5-to-p6 direction, with p6 being activated much later from a different source.

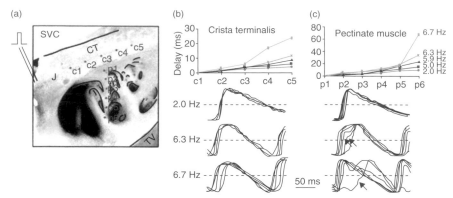

Figure 5.19 Frequency-dependent atrial activation. (a) Picture of right atrial endocardium of sheep heart showing locations of pixels c1–c5 on crista terminalis (CT) and p1–p6 on pectinate muscle. (b) Activation delay at c1–c5 relative to c1 (top); c1–c5 optical action potentials during rhythmic stimulation of Bachmann's bundle at 2.0, 6.3, and 6.7 Hz (bottom). Notice frequency-dependent increase in local activation time. (c) Activation delay at p1–p6 relative to p1 (top); p1–p6 action potentials for 2, 6.3, and 6.7 Hz during 1:1 propagation (bottom). The humps at p4–p6 (red arrows) reflect source-to-sink mismatch at the higher frequencies in this areas due to branching. Broken green line p5–p6 at 6.7 Hz denotes local block and change in direction of propagation, as shown by the subthreshold depolarization at p6 followed by an extremely delayed optical action potential (red arrow). Color code in panels (b) and (c) indicates frequency in Hz. TV, tricuspid valve. (Reproduced with permission from Berenfeld and Zaitsev, *Anat Rec A Discov Mol Cell Evol Biol* 2004; 280:1053–61.)

Close scrutiny of the anatomical structure of the preparation (Figure 5.19a) reveals that pixels p3 and p4 reside in an area with many small branches. Also, between p5 and p6, there is a connection to a thick PM emerging from above the TV rim. Thus, this complex structure may be a substrate for sink-to-source mismatch and low safety for propagation. Importantly, only major branch sites (with discontinuities in the scale > 1 mm) exhibited marked frequency-dependent increase in activation time.

During AF, the posterior left atrium of a large animal like the sheep AF can activate at frequencies as high as >7–10 Hz. Yet the RA is never activated at such high frequencies, which suggests that there must be a critical frequency at which the 1:1 input–output relation between the LA and RA breaks down. As shown by the local frequency maps presented in Figure 5.20a, rhythmic stimulation of BB at 5.0 Hz resulted in 1:1 activation of the entire right atrium and thus the output frequency was also 5.0 Hz. However, at 7.7 Hz, activation was no longer 1:1. Instead, a heterogeneous distribution of local activation frequencies that ranged from 3.5 to 7.7 Hz was established both in the endo-cardium and the epicardium. Composite results from five experiments are presented in Figure 5.20b. The local activation frequencies measured on the endocardium are plotted as a function of the pacing frequency. Clearly, below 6.7 Hz the response dominant frequency (DF) showed no dispersion in any of the experiments, which meant that activation in all regions was 1:1. Above

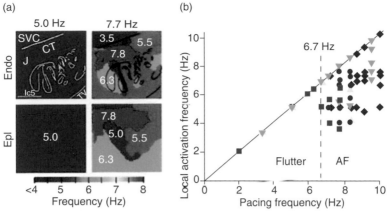

Figure 5.20 The breakdown frequency for fibrillatory conduction. (a) Endocardial and epicardial dominant frequency maps of same isolated right atrium preparation as in Figures 5.18 and 5.19 paced at 5.0 and 7.7 Hz. Note appearance of heterogeneous dominant frequency (DF) domains at 7.7 Hz. (b) Response DFs vs. the pacing rate (n = 5). Each symbol represents one experiment. Pacing Bachmann's bundle at rates below 6.7 Hz results in 1:1 activation. At higher rates, the number of domains increases but the DFs decrease. AF, atrial fibrillation. (Reproduced with permission from Berenfeld *et al.*, *Circ Res* 2002; 90:1173–80.)

the breakdown frequency of 6.7 Hz, there was a large DF dispersion manifest as multiple domains whose individual frequencies were either equal to or lower than the pacing frequency. Overall, these data demonstrate that stimulation of BB at frequencies below about 6.5 Hz results in 1:1 activation of the entire preparation, as it normally occurs during atrial flutter. Above that critical breakdown frequency, the response patterns are so complex as to result in fibrillatory conduction. These results support the idea that atrial flutter and atrial fibrillation may have a common reentrant mechanism and that the only difference between them is the frequency of the source responsible for the arrhythmia.

Summary

The focus of this chapter was the study of rate dependency of discontinuous action potential propagation in the heart. The chapter also discussed the dynamics and ionic mechanisms of complex patterns of propagation, such as Wenckebach periodicity and fibrillatory conduction, which provides a framework for the understanding of cellular and tissue behavior during high-frequency excitation and arrhythmias. Given the structural complexities of the various cardiac tissues and the complex nonlinear dynamics of cardiac cell excitation, it seems reasonable to expect that any event leading to very rapid activation of atria or ventricles may result in exceedingly complex rhythms, including fibrillation.

6 Basic Mechanisms of Cardiac Arrhythmias

Cardiac arrhythmias may arise from abnormalities in impulse formation (i.e., automatism), impulse conduction, or a combination of both (Table 6.1). Various forms of rhythm disturbances that are included within these categories were extensively studied in the experimental and clinical laboratories. Based on experimental data, it is possible to derive a set of rules that then can be used to identify the electrophysiological origin of the arrhythmia. Unfortunately, different cellular mechanisms may share some features, thus making the distinction difficult. Information regarding the clinical background of the arrhythmia (i.e., age, the presence of heart disease, medications, and electrolyte imbalance) may aid in the diagnosis of the underlying mechanisms. In addition, the characteristics of the onset and termination of the arrhythmia as well as their response to various maneuvers, pharmacologic agents, or electrical stimulation are commonly used to distinguish among the various cellular arrhythmogenic mechanisms. For instance, programmed electrical stimulation is used to establish the diagnosis of reentrant arrhythmias. In fact, in the past, the ability to initiate or terminate an arrhythmia by means of premature electrical stimulation was thought to establish the diagnosis of reentry. Recently, however, experimental observations revealed that arrhythmias other than reentry may eventually display similar properties. Subsequently, new and more specific criteria, such as entrainment or various resetting patterns were introduced to establish the diagnosis of reentry. Yet, in some cases, the ultimate diagnosis of reentry can only be determined by high spatial and temporal resolution mapping of the arrhythmia itself.

Similarly, the criteria for the diagnosis of non-reentrant arrhythmias, i.e., automatic or triggered, are not clearly defined. In addition to the classical electrocardiographic (ECG) manifestations and to the response of the arrhythmia to changes in heart rate, clinicians may require the use of pharmacologic

Basic Cardiac Electrophysiology for the Clinician, 2nd edition. By J. Jalife, M. Delmar, J. Anumonwo, O. Berenfeld and J. Kalifa. Published 2009 by Blackwell Publishing, ISBN: 978-1-4501-8333-8.

Table 6.1 Mechanisms of cardiac arrhythmias

Abnormal impulse formation	Alterations in the conduction of the impulse
Enhanced normal automaticity	Reentry
Abnormal automaticity	Reflection
Triggered activity (delayed and early afterdepolarizations)	

agents that hopefully are specific enough to affect only a given type of automaticity. Unfortunately, more often than not, this is not achieved.

Despite these and other shortcomings, we firmly believe that the understanding of cellular mechanisms is essential for a rational management of all types of cardiac arrhythmias. This chapter reviews the cellular mechanisms of arrhythmias with emphasis placed on those aspects that may be relevant to the analysis of their ECG manifestations. Arrhythmias observed in specific clinical settings (e.g., ischemia) will be discussed in more detail. In Chapter 7, we discuss concepts derived from the theory of nonlinear wave of propagation in generic excitable media and their contribution to our understanding of reentrant activity in the heart. Subsequently in Chapters 8 and 9 we deal specifically with mechanisms of atrial and ventricular fibrillation, to conclude in Chapter 10 with a general survey of some of the most prevalent inherited arrhythmogenic diseases.

Abnormal Impulse Formation

Enhanced Normal Automaticity

Sinoatrial (SA) nodal cells, as well as some cells in the atria, the atrioventricular (AV) node, and the His-Purkinje system possess the property of pacemaker activity or automaticity. Electric discharges in the form of action potentials may originate spontaneously in these cells even in the absence of any external input. As discussed in Chapter 1, automatic (i.e., pacemaker) cells show a gradual spontaneous decrease of the transmembrane potential during diastole. Diastolic or phase 4 depolarization (see Figure 6.1) brings the membrane voltage to threshold, giving rise to a new action potential, and so on. Enhancement of this type of activity may lead to sinus tachycardia as well as to a variety of ectopic tachycardias.

Ionic Basis

The ionic basis of spontaneous pacemaker activity is discussed extensively in Chapters 2 and 3. Briefly, phase 4 depolarization reflects a net inward current and results from the algebraic sum of several inward and outward currents as shown schematically in Figure 6.1. To recapitulate, the currents that seem to be involved in phase 4 depolarization include the following.

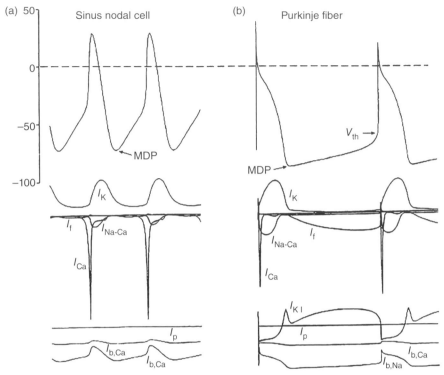

Figure 6.1 Ionic currents responsible for automatic activity. (a) Sinus nodal cell. (b) Purkinje fiber. Downward deflections from the zero line in the current traces indicate inward current; upward deflections from the zero line indicate outward currents. V_{th}, voltage threshold; MDP, maximum diastolic potential.

Outward Delayed Rectifying Potassium Current (I_K)

During an action potential, I_K becomes activated at a voltage positive to −40 mV and subsequently decays with repolarization. In the presence of an inward background current carried mostly by sodium, this decay in I_K leads to diastolic depolarization in pacemaking cells.

Hyperpolarization Activated, "Funny" Current (I_f)

This current is activated at relatively high levels of membrane potential (−40 to −60 mV), and it increases upon hyperpolarization. It seems to be more important for diastolic depolarization in Purkinje fibers than in SA nodal cells.

Transient Inward Calcium Current (I_{Ca-T})

This current operates at relatively high levels of membrane potential (−70 mV). It most likely contributes to the initial part of diastolic depolarization in SA nodal cells. I_{Ca-T} is insensitive to dihydropyridines but sensitive to nickel.

Long-lasting Calcium Inward Current (I_{Ca-L})
This current activates upon depolarization to −40 mV. It plays an important role during the late part of phase 4 depolarization and is the major ion carrier during the action potential upstroke in "true" pacemaker cells of the SA node and N cells in the AV node. I_{Ca-L} is blocked by dihydropyridines and by verapamil.

Time-independent Currents
Several time-independent currents, including the inward background current (I_b) carried by Na, the Na-K pump current (I_{pump}), the Na-Ca exchanger, the inward-rectifier current (I_{K1}), and the background Cl current (I_{Cl}), were also implicated in pacemaker activity. However, although it is generally accepted that the role of these currents varies with the membrane potential, their relative contribution to pacemaking activity remains somewhat controversial.

At the maximum diastolic potential (MDP) of SA nodal cells (approximately −60 mV), the initiation of diastolic depolarization seems to be the result of a progressive decay in I_K with contribution by the activation of I_f and the Na-Ca exchanger. I_{Ca-T} is activated midway through phase 4 and is followed by the activation of I_{Ca-L}. Because the MDP in Purkinje cells is more negative (−75 to −85 mV) than in nodal cells, it was suggested that I_f is the primary inward current causing diastolic depolarization in these cells. In the latter, I_{Ca-T} is supposed to be only partially activated during phase 4; both I_{Ca-T} and I_{Ca-L} are fully activated during the action potential upstroke.

Because of the differences in the contribution of Ca currents to phase 4 depolarization, it is not surprising that Ca channel blockers depress the automaticity of SN cells but have no significant effects on Purkinje cells. The opposite is true for lidocaine.

Enhancement of Automaticity
The normal rate of firing of SA nodal cells in the human heart is 60–100 beats per minute (bpm). So-called "subsidiary" pacemaker cells fire at slower rates (e.g., 40–60 bpm and 20–40 bpm in the AV junction and Purkinje system, respectively). The rate of discharge of pacemaker cells may increase as a result of several mechanisms, as shown in Figure 6.2: (1) an increment in voltage threshold (i.e., the voltage threshold becomes more negative, panel b); (2) a decrease in MDP (the membrane potential becomes less negative; panel c); and (3) an increase in the slope of phase 4 depolarization (panel d).

The rate of discharge of cells undergoing normal (i.e., phase 4 depolarization-related) pacemaker activity is controlled by the autonomic nervous system and is sensitive to various endogenous substances and pharmacologic agents as well as to electric stimulation. We will review each of these factors separately.

Autonomic Control
Stimulation of the vagus nerve leads to the release of acetylcholine (ACh), causing a muscarinic receptor-mediated opening of specific potassium

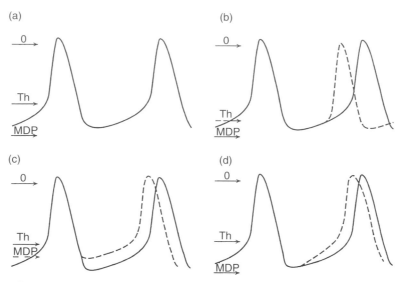

Figure 6.2 Mechanisms of enhanced normal automaticity. (a) Control. (b) Increased threshold (Th) voltage. (c) Decreased MDP. (d) Increased slope of phase 4 depolarization. The horizontal arrow in each panel indicates zero level of membrane potential. MDP, maximum diastolic potential.

Vagal effect

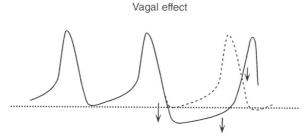

Figure 6.3 Effects of acetylcholine (ACh) on the membrane potential of an automatic cell from the sinus or the atrioventricular nodes. ACh leads to hyperpolarization, decrease in the slope of phase 4, and decrease in the action potential upstroke velocity. All these changes lead to a decrease in the rate of firing.

channels $[I_{K(ACh)}]$ on the cell membrane. The resultant increase in K permeability leads to hyperpolarization of SA or AV nodal pacemaker cells (Figure 6.3). Consequently, under the influence of ACh, there is an increase in the voltage difference between diastolic potential and voltage threshold. Thus, even in the absence of changes in the slope of phase 4 depolarization, there is a longer period of time for the membrane to reach threshold. ACh is also known to decrease I_{Ca-L} and I_f, leading to a decrease in the inward current responsible for both phase 4 and phase 0 (i.e., upstroke) of pacemaker cells. The combination of increasing I_K and decreasing I_{Ca-L} and I_f results in slowing of the firing rate of pacemaker cells.

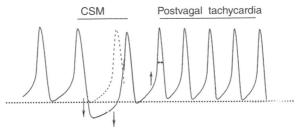

Figure 6.4 Effects of carotid sinus massage (CSM). This vagal maneuver prolongs sinus cycle length but leads to postvagal tachycardia upon its termination.

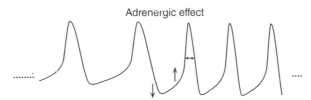

Figure 6.5 Effects of catecholamines on automatic cells.

The negative chronotropic effect of ACh is frequently used in patients both for diagnostic and therapeutic purposes. A supraventricular tachycardia resulting from enhanced normal automaticity is expected to respond to a vagal maneuver (i.e., carotid sinus massage) with a transient decrease in frequency. Once the carotid massage is interrupted, the rate of the arrhythmia is expected to progressively return to the initial value after transiently accelerating above that value (Figure 6.4). The latter phenomenon, known as "postvagal tachycardia," is in part due to the release of norepinephrine from sympathetic fibers in the vagus nerve and in part to other, yet-unknown mechanisms. If the arrhythmia is the result of a different mechanism (e.g., reentrant activity), vagal stimulation may have an all-or-none response, with either no effect or definitive acceleration of the tachycardia.

Adrenergic stimulation or blockade results also in characteristic changes in pacemaker activity. As discussed in detail in Chapter 3, β-adrenergic receptor stimulation leads to activation of adenylate cyclase and to subsequent increase in cyclic adenosine monophosphate (cAMP). cAMP activates protein kinase, which then phosphorylates ion channels. When phosphorylated, some channels are known to become more permeable. This is indeed the case for L-type Ca channels, and, in fact, catecholamines are known to increase the limiting conductance of I_{Ca-L} (but not I_{Ca-T}) without modifying the current kinetics. An increase in I_{Ca-L} leads to an increase in the rate of firing (Figure 6.5). In addition, β-adrenergic stimulation results in a positive shift of the activation curve of I_f, leading to an increase of the net inward current. Some investigators believe that the main function of I_f is to mediate the effects of β-adrenergic stimulation.

Under the influence of catecholamines, the rate of discharge of atrial cells and Purkinje fibers may be as high as 200 and 120 bpm, respectively. Accordingly, although rapid atrial tachycardias may result from enhanced normal automaticity, ventricular tachycardias (VTs) resulting from this mechanism are not expected to be very fast.

Metabolic Abnormalities

Enhanced normal automatic activity may occur in the presence of hypoxia as a result of Na-K pump inhibition. Low extracellular K concentration may also increase the slope of phase 4 depolarization and thus accelerate the rate of firing of normal pacemaker cells.

Overdrive Suppression

The hallmark of phase 4-dependent automaticity is overdrive suppression. As shown schematically in Figure 6.6, following a period of overdrive pacing, the slope of phase 4 depolarization of normal Purkinje fibers decreases, thus leading to a decrease in the rate of firing (suppression of automaticity). During the recovery time, there is a gradual return to the intrinsic firing rate (i.e., warming-up period). The degree of suppression and the recovery time are proportional to the rate of stimulation, as well as the time during which the stimulation was applied. Overdrive suppression plays an important role in the maintenance of sinus rhythm by continuously inhibiting the activity of subsidiary pacemaker cells.

Overdrive suppression is attributed to an intracellular overload of positive charges that result from the rapid succession of action potentials. During activity at a normal rate, each action potential results in a transient increase

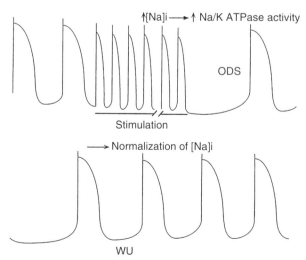

Figure 6.6 Overdrive suppression (ODS) and warming-up (WU) phenomenon in a Purkinje fiber.

in intracellular Na concentration. During the diastolic period, the intracellular ion concentration is restored by the activity of the Na-K pump. An increase in the rate of activation leads to an overload of intracellular Na. The activity of the Na-K pump is thus enhanced, which leads after a lag period of a few seconds to the restoration of the normal intracellular ionic concentrations by extruding Na from the cell and incorporating K from the extracellular fluid. Because the ratio between Na exiting the cell and K entering the cell is $3:2$, a net outward current is created by the activity of the Na-K pump (I_{pump}). This hyperpolarizing current neutralizes the currents responsible for phase 4 depolarization. The ultimate result is a decrease in the rate of the spontaneous firing, which is followed by a slow warm-up period toward control (see Figure 6.6).

It is important to note that cells whose MDP is low (i.e., normal sinus nodal cells or abnormally depolarized ventricular myocardial cells) are less sensitive to overdrive suppression. In these cells, most Na channels are inactivated so that the Na entrance during the action potential upstroke is significantly reduced.

Clinical Implications

Some cardiac arrhythmias are most probably the result of enhanced normal automatic activity. A typical example is represented by sinus tachycardia secondary to sympathetic stimulation associated with exercise, fever, and thyrotoxicosis. Note, however, that sinus tachycardia may also result from sinus nodal reentry. Atrial and ventricular accelerated rhythms show features that are consistent with enhanced normal automatic activity. In fact, some accelerated idioventricular rhythms are depressed by vagal stimulation and by adenosine. In addition, overdrive suppression was shown in some cases of accelerated idioventricular rhythms.

Escape rhythms originated in the ventricles are most likely the result of enhanced normal automaticity in the His-Purkinje system. Studies performed in patients with complete AV block showed that automatic foci arising from the ventricles undergo overdrive suppression and warm-up phenomena. In fact, a clear example of spontaneously occurring overdrive suppression is represented by cases of paroxysmal AV block. Exceedingly long pauses (i.e., suppression) are observed in cases of paroxysmal AV block in which the ventricular rate just prior to the occurrence of block is relatively high. This is in contrast to what is usually observed in cases in which complete AV block is preceded by a period of second-degree AV block with a relatively low ventricular rate.

The absence of overdrive suppression may indicate that the arrhythmia is the result of a mechanism other than enhanced normal automaticity. However, enhanced normal automatic activity may have a blunted response to overdrive as a result of entrance block. When cells undergoing normal pacemaker activity are protected from the surrounding activity, ectopic activity may arise in the form of parasystole. Because parasystolic foci are protected from the surrounding activity, they are not expected to show suppression or warm-up phenomenon; at least the effects of overdrive in these cases should be appreciably reduced.

Ectopic pacemaker activity initiated by depolarized cells also has relatively poor response to overdrive. In this case, the mechanism of the automatic rhythm is different from enhanced normal automaticity, as discussed in the next section.

Abnormal Automaticity

Normal contractile atrial and ventricular cells do not show spontaneous activity. However, abnormal automaticity may arise from these cells as a result of depolarization to levels between −60 and −10 mV. Depolarization-induced automatic activity was demonstrated in abnormal right atria in humans and in tissue surviving a myocardial infarct. Depolarization-induced automaticity may also be elicited in quiescent Purkinje fibers by lowering the extracellular K concentration, lowering the pH and the oxygen concentration in the bathing solutions, adding tetraethylammonium or Ba (the latter decreases the outward current and increases the slow inward current), or by simply applying constant depolarizing current as shown schematically in Figure 6.7. When the fiber is depolarized by a constant current pulse, the rate of firing of the cell dramatically increases (Figure 6.7a). The larger the depolarizing pulse, the higher is the automatic discharge rate (Figure 6.7b). The rate of discharge of

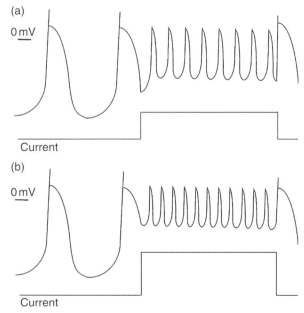

Figure 6.7 Depolarization-induced automaticity. (a) Relatively low level of depolarization. (b) Relatively high level of depolarization.

depolarization-induced automaticity is a function of both the MDP and the reversal potential of the pacemaker current. Thus, although progressive depolarization leads to a progressive increase of the activity, there is a level of depolarization (between −10 and +10 mV) above which all pacemaker activity ceases. The rate of discharge of depolarized cells is generally faster than that observed in enhanced normal automaticity and may be as high as 200 bpm.

Depolarization-induced automaticity may be interrupted by increasing the membrane potential. In addition, high extracellular K may also interrupt depolarization-induced automaticity even when the fibers remain depolarized.

Ionic Basis

One of the mechanisms that may explain the presence of automaticity in cells that normally do not show pacemaker activity is the development of net inward depolarizing current associated with a decrease in the K conductance. In most cases, depolarization-induced automaticity in ventricular myocardial fibers occurs at levels of depolarization at which the Na current is almost completely inactivated. Under these conditions, action potentials depend exclusively on inward currents carried through Ca channels. It is therefore not surprising that most cases of depolarization-induced automaticity can be suppressed by Ca channel blockers such as verapamil and manganese or by high K. The role of I_f in depolarized cells is not expected to be significant, although it may contribute to pacemaker activity when there is only a moderate level of MDP decrease. Accordingly, depolarization-induced automaticity is expected to be insensitive to Na channel blockers such as lidocaine.

Overdrive Suppression

An important distinction between enhanced normal and depolarization-induced automaticity is that the latter is less sensitive to overdrive pacing. As discussed earlier, one of the major contributors to overdrive suppression is the activation of the Na-K pump secondary to intracellular Na overload. Because most fast Na channels are inactivated as a result of the low membrane potential, the degree of Na-K pump activation is expected to be small. Yet, in these cells some degree of overdrive suppression may still occur as a result of an increase in intracellular Ca, leading to both an increase in K conductance and an increase in intracellular Na through transmembrane Na-Ca exchange. The increase in K conductance will create a hyperpolarizing current, which in turn will tend to neutralize the depolarizing effects of the pacemaker currents. On the other hand, the increase in intracellular Na concentration may ultimately activate I_{pump} and also lead to a hyperpolarizing current.

Clinical Implications

Depolarization-induced automaticity is thought to play a role in cases of elevated extracellular K and excess catecholamines or in the presence of low intracellular pH. Examples of arrhythmias that are probably caused by abnormal automaticity are ectopic atrial tachycardias as well as accelerated idioventricular rhythms and VTs that occur 24–72 hours after experimental myocardial infarction. Indeed, experimental studies indicate that abnormal automaticity may be responsible for some ventricular arrhythmias that are observed in the setting of acute myocardial infarction, specifically, during the first 15–30 minutes post-occlusion at which there is an increase in the local catecholamine concentration. In fact, as proposed in 1995 by Michiel Janse of the University of Amsterdam, areas surrounding the ischemic zone may be depolarized by increases in extracellular K. If, however, the concentration of K is too high, automatic activity is unlikely to occur. Another possible explanation for the presence of depolarization-induced automaticity is the development of so-called "injury currents," whereby the areas that are directly exposed to high K in the ischemic zone exert a depolarizing electrotonic influence on neighboring cells, which are exposed to normal concentrations of K. If such an influence is sufficiently large, it is conceivable that the latter cells may undergo depolarization-induced automaticity. In addition, because propagation of the impulse is severely delayed in the ischemic environment, maximum amplitude of the ischemic upstroke may occur during the diastolic phase of the surrounding cells, facilitating the development of depolarization-induced automaticity. These arrhythmias should theoretically be abolished by agents that increase the resting potential, such as activators of $I_{K(ACh)}$ in atrial cells or agents that increase Na-K pump activity. The arrhythmias may also respond to Ca channel blockers and, under some conditions, to Na channel blockers as well.

Triggered Activity

Triggered activity (TA) is the activity arising from membrane potential oscillations that occur during or immediately following an action potential. By definition, TA may not occur in the absence of a previous spontaneous or driven action potential. Triggered action potentials may be the source of a new triggered response, thus leading to self-sustaining TA. There are two distinct forms of TA: early afterdepolarizations (EADs), which occur during phase 2 or 3 of the action potential (Figure 6.8a,b) and delayed afterdepolarizations (DADs), which occur during the diastolic interval (Figure 6.8c). Because the two forms of TA are different in terms of their ionic mechanisms,

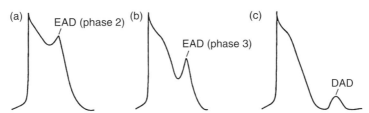

Figure 6.8 The initial event in triggered activity. (a) Early afterdepolarization (EAD) in phase 2. (b) EAD in phase 3. (c) Delayed afterdepolarization (DAD).

inducing agents, form of initiation and termination, and clinical implications, they will be discussed separately. We will start with the DADs for historical reasons because this type of oscillation was described earlier than the EADs.

Delayed Afterdepolarization-Induced Triggered Activity
Ionic Mechanisms
DADs were first demonstrated in Purkinje fibers exposed to toxic concentrations of digitalis. Inhibition of the Na-K pump by digitalis leads to an increase of intracellular Na, which promotes the release of Ca from the sarcoplasmic reticulum. In addition, the increased intracellular Na modifies the activity of the Na-Ca exchange in such a way that it makes it move Na out and Ca into the cell. The final result is a Ca overload in the cytosol. Increased intracellular Ca initiates a transient inward current (I_{TI}) through a Ca-dependent nonspecific ion channel (Figure 6.9). It is now clear that I_{TI} may be activated even in the absence of Na-K pump inhibition. In fact, the induction of DAD is associated with other conditions that cause intracellular Ca overload, including catecholamines, hypertrophy, ischemia, decrease in extracellular K, and

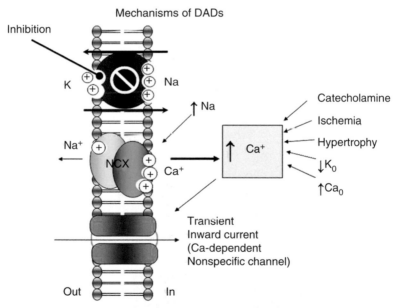

Figure 6.9 Pathophysiology of intracellular calcium overload. Inhibition of the Na-K ATPase (red) by digitalis results in intracellular sodium accumulation, which leads to increased entrance of calcium through the sodium-calcium exchange (NCX; blue) mechanism. This eventually overloads the cell with calcium and produces a transient inward current through a calcium-dependent nonspecific channel (orange) and to delayed afterdepolarizations (DADs). Other stimuli leading to intracellular calcium overload include catecholamines, ischemia, hypertrophy, reduced extracellular potassium, and increased extracellular calcium.

increase in extracellular Ca. Indeed, DADs can be consistently induced by β-adrenergic receptor stimulation, which in turn leads to sequential activation of the stimulatory guanine nucleotide binding protein (G_s), adenylate cyclase, cAMP, and protein kinase A (see Chapter 3). The ultimate result of this cascade is the phosphorylation of multiple ion channels, in particular the L-type Ca current, which leads to an increase in the intracellular Ca concentration and ultimately activation of I_{TI}.

Ischemia is a major cause of intracellular Ca overload. Ischemia-induced DADs are most likely mediated by the accumulation of lysophosphoglycerides, which are known to induce DADs even in the absence of ischemia. It is important to note, however, that any maneuver that tends to increase Na_i is expected to increase the activity of the electrogenic Na outward current I_{pump}, which acts to neutralize (and suppress) the depolarizing currents responsible for DAD.

Rate Dependence of Delayed Afterdepolarizations

One of the main characteristics of DADs is that they can be evoked by an increase in stimulation rate. In fact, the amplitude and number of triggered responses are direct functions of the rate and duration of stimulation. This is illustrated schematically in Figure 6.10. Each panel represents a Purkinje fiber exposed to toxic concentrations of a digitalis compound (e.g., ouabain). Stimulation at a relatively slow rate (Figure 6.10a) is followed by normal phase 4 depolarization but no triggered responses. Following a period of more rapid stimulation (Figure 6.10b), there are two small voltage oscillations during

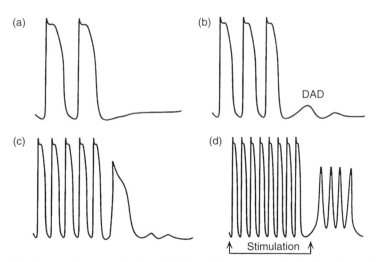

Figure 6.10 Delayed afterdepolarizations (DADs) and triggered activity resulting from inhibition of the Na-K pump. (a) No DADs following a train of stimuli at a relatively low frequency. (b) DADs but no triggered activity following a train of stimuli at intermediate frequency. (c) Triggered activity and DADs following a train of stimuli at high frequency. (d) Repetitive triggered activity following an even faster train of stimuli.

diastole. After a period of stimulation at an even higher rate (Figure 6.10c), the first DAD reaches threshold and generates a triggered response. Finally, a further increase in stimulation rate is followed by repetitive TA (Figure 6.10d).

There is an important distinction between DADs associated with Na-K pump inhibition and those arising from other mechanisms (e.g., catecholamine-induced DADs). In the latter, there is a window of stimulation rates that results in the initiation of DAD-induced TA. Rates that are faster than a certain limit may activate the electrogenic I_{pump}, which then neutralizes the DADs. In some cases, DAD and TA may occur following single premature stimuli. In those cases, there may be a direct correlation between the coupling interval of the premature (triggering) response and the coupling interval of the triggered response, i.e., the shorter the coupling interval of the triggering response, the shorter is the coupling interval of the triggered response.

Because DADs are sensitive to sympathetic stimulation, the inducibility of this type of arrhythmia in the clinical setting may vary with the autonomic status of the patient. Also, once a run of triggered responses is initiated, there is a gradual deceleration and, eventually, spontaneous termination of the arrhythmia. This is in contrast to what normally occurs with rhythms resulting from normal automaticity, in which the rhythm tends to accelerate as it recovers from overdrive suppression.

Triggered arrhythmias induced by DADs may be terminated by single stimuli. This was a rather disappointing finding at the time it was discovered because initiation and termination of an arrhythmia by premature beats were previously considered to be diagnostic of reentry. There are, however, some differences that may help make the distinction between the two mechanisms. The rate dependency of the coupling interval between the last paced beat and the first beat of the tachycardia may separate reentrant from triggered arrhythmias. In most cases of reentrant arrhythmias, the higher the rates or the briefer the coupling intervals of the initiating stimuli, the longer is the coupling interval of the first beat of the arrhythmia. Exceptionally, abbreviation of the coupling interval was described. On the other hand, in most cases of DAD-induced arrhythmia, the shorter the cycle of stimulation, the shorter is the coupling interval. Yet, there may be a paradoxical prolongation of the coupling interval at fast rates, which results from the induction of outward Na current. Thus, the response of DAD to pacing may not be the ideal feature to consider for the distinction between this type of arrhythmias and other mechanisms such as reentrant activity. Instead, the response to some pharmacologic agents may give valuable information.

Pharmacologic Interventions
Exogenously applied adenosine is used as a test for the diagnosis of DADs. There are two different adenosine receptor subtypes in the cardiovascular system, A_1 and A_2. The effects of adenosine on the heart are mediated via the A_1 receptors, whereas those in the vasculature are mediated via the A_2

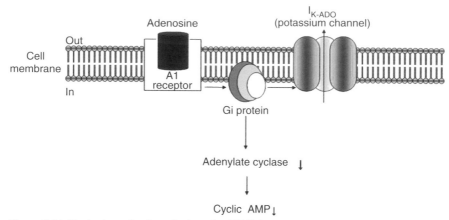

Figure 6.11 Mechanism of action of adenosine (ADO) (see text for details).

receptors. As illustrated in Figure 6.11, in the heart, binding of adenosine to the A_1 receptor leads to activation of the guanine nucleotide-binding protein, G_I, which, in turn, activates an inward-rectifying current I_{K-Ado} found only in the SA and AV nodes. Activation of G_i also results in inhibition of adenylate cyclase, which decreases intracellular cAMP and produces antiadrenergic effects. Overall, these results would be translated into slowing of heart rate and AV conduction. However, in patients these effects depend on the mode of administration and are modified by autonomic reflexes.

Because of the absence of I_{K-Ado} in the ventricles, adenosine has no direct effect on ventricular resting membrane potential, action potential amplitude, or duration or even levels of intracellular cAMP. However, adenosine may attenuate the adrenergic effects, both in the atria and ventricles.

Adenosine reduces I_{Ca} indirectly by inhibiting effects on adenylate cyclase and cAMP. Thus, adenosine may abolish DADS induced by isoproterenol and forskolin (adenylate cyclase activator) but does not alter DADs induced by Na-K pump inhibition. Adenosine was shown to have no effect on reentrant VT. In addition, adenosine may transiently decrease the rate of firing of normally polarized Purkinje fibers exposed to epinephrine. Therefore, the interruption of a ventricular arrhythmia by adenosine points toward catecholamine-induced DADs as the responsible mechanism.

Flunarizine decreases intracellular Ca through an unspecified mechanism and may abolish DADs induced by inhibition of the Na-K pump as well as β-adrenergic stimulation. In addition, flunarizine does not affect arrhythmias resulting from reentry or abnormal automaticity. Flunarizine may also block EADs induced by I_{Kr} blockade (i.e., administration of D-sotalol).

Clinical Implications
Arrhythmias induced by DADs can occur in patients with inherited mutations but structurally normal hearts (see Chapter 10). DADS may be facilitated by

isoproterenol, aminophylline, rapid pacing, and exercise. As discussed previously, they may be interrupted by adenosine as well as vagal maneuvers. Theoretically, they should also respond to drugs that reduce intracellular Ca overload (Ca channel blockers) and drugs that increase K conductance. Arrhythmias probably resulting from DADs include atrial tachycardias and VTs observed during digitalis toxicity, accelerated ventricular rhythms in the setting of acute myocardial infarction, some forms of repetitive monomorphic VT, reperfusion-induced arrhythmias and right ventricular outflow tract (RVOT) VT. Exercise-induced VT as in catecholaminergic polymorphic ventricular tachycardia (CPVT; see Chapter 10) and the so-called adenosine-sensitive VT are additional examples of DAD-related TA. There are two clinical groups of adenosine-sensitive VT: (1) so-called "Gallavardin tachycardia," which is a repetitive monomorphic tachycardia that occurs in normal hearts without apparent triggering circumstances; and (2) exercise-induced VT, which is a sustained monomorphic dysrhythmia induced by exercise or stress. In both cases, the QRS morphology is that of left bundle branch block plus left posterior hemiblock, indicating that the origin is the RVOT. Adenosine-sensitive VT may eventually arise from the left ventricle. Because of its consistent response to adenosine, this type of VT is thought to be the result of cAMP-dependent DADs.

Early Afterdepolarizations

EADs are oscillatory potentials (Figure 6.12) that may occur during the action potential plateau (phase 2 EADs) or during late repolarization (phase 3 EADs). Although both types of EADs may appear during similar experimental conditions (e.g., superfusion of a Purkinje fiber with quinidine or Cs and exposure to hypoxia plus epinephrine), they differ morphologically as well as pharmacologically and may be perturbed independently. Figure 6.12a illustrates

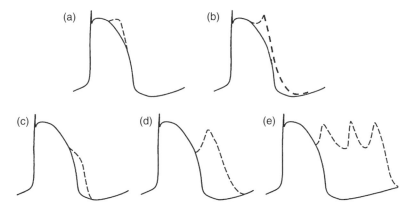

Figure 6.12 Early afterdepolarizations (EADs) and triggered activity. (a) Phase 2 EAD. (b) Phase 2 triggered activity. (c) Phase 3 EAD. (d) Phase 3 triggered activity. (e) Sustained triggered activity following a single action potential.

Table 6.2 Agents and manipulations that may lead to early afterdepolarizations

---

1. Slow rate (sinus bradycardia, complete AV block, etc.)
2. Stretch
3. Hypokalemia
4. Hypoxia
5. Acidosis
6. Low $[K]_o$
7. Low $[Ca]_o$
8. Low $[Mg]_o$
9. Class IA antiarrhythmic drugs (quinidine, disopyramide, procainamide)
10. Class IB antiarrhythmic drugs (lidocaine, tocainide, mexiletine)
11. Class IC antiarrhythmic drugs (flecainide, encainide, indecainide)
12. Class III antiarrhythmic drugs (amiodarone, sotalol, clofidium, bretylium)
13. Phenothiazine
14. Tricyclic and tetracyclic antidepressants
15. Erythromycin
16. Antihistaminics
17. Cesium
18. Amiloride
19. Barium

---

the appearance of a phase 2 EAD. Figure 6.12b shows an action potential triggered by a similar EAD in a hypothetical Purkinje fiber exposed to a class IA antiarrhythmic drug (e.g., quinidine). Panels (c) and (d) of the same figure show a phase 3 EAD (panel c) with its corresponding TA (panel d). Finally, panel (e) shows repetitive triggered responses.

EADs may be the result of decreased outward current, increased inward current, or both. As shown in Table 6.2, there is a wide variety of agents and conditions that were shown to induce EADs and TA.

Ionic Mechanisms
The transmembrane currents involved in the mechanisms of EADs may be divided into two groups: those that result in action potential prolongation and those that result in net inward current.

1. *Action potential prolongation.* Action potential prolongation may result from a decrease in outward current (i.e., I_K, I_{K1}, I_{pump}, and I_{TO}) or an increase of inward currents carried by Na (through the window current or a slowly inactivating Na current), Ca (through the Ca channels and a possible Ca window current), or the electrogenic Na-Ca exchange system. It is important to remember that, during the action potential plateau, membrane conductance is very low so that a relatively small change in net current can result in a significant change in membrane potential and consequently in an EAD.
2. *Net depolarizing current.* The inward current that is most likely responsible for the generation of EAD-induced TA is the L-type Ca window current.

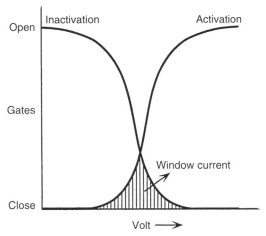

Figure 6.13 Schematic representation of voltage dependence of opening and closure of the activation and inactivation gates of the Ca channel. There is a window of voltage (stippled area) where current may flow as a result of the incomplete states of opening and closure.

Window currents are steady-state currents that arise within a narrow voltage range where the activation and inactivation gates of the Ca channel overlap (see Figure 6.13). Within such a window of voltage, channels may undergo transformational changes from inactivated to closed and to open states. Thus, Ca channels that inactivate during the action potential upstroke may reopen as the action potential repolarizes toward the voltage range of the L-type Ca window current. With a relatively small shift of the potential toward more negative levels, such as that produced by K channel blocking agents (i.e., quinidine and Cs), channels could be activated from a closed state.

Note that sustained triggered action potentials cannot be distinguished from action potentials observed during depolarization-induced automaticity. In the latter, however, activity may start in the absence of a previous normal action potential.

Pharmacologic Interventions Leading to Early Afterdepolarizations
Hypokalemia leads to a decrease in the conductance of the cell membrane to K ions. Thus, hypokalemia results in prolongation of the action potential duration (APD). In the presence of bradycardia, which also leads to action potential prolongation, hypokalemia is an important predisposing factor for the induction of EADs and TA. Also, microelectrode experiments in isolated Purkinje fibers showed that the incidence of quinidine-induced EADs increases when the stimulation frequency is decreased. There is also an inverse relationship between EAD incidence and extracellular K concentration.

However, at very low levels of extracellular K, there is an increase in the automatic activity of Purkinje fibers. Thus, when the extracellular K concentration is very low, Purkinje fibers tend to beat spontaneously at relatively fast rates, which leads to abbreviation of the action potential and suppression of EADs.

Quinidine and N-acetyl procainamide block I_K (at higher concentrations they also block I_{K1}) in a reverse use-dependent manner, i.e., both drugs prolong the APD and the effect is more prominent at slow rates. Consequently, both drugs are proarrhythmic in that at slow activation rates they induce EADs and TA. Quinidine also blocks inward currents (i.e., Na window current, I_f, I_{Na}, and I_{Ca-L}). Because the effects of quinidine on Na current are use-dependent, it is reasonable to speculate that, at low activation rates, the blocking effect on K currents will predominate and thus facilitate the induction of EADs. In Purkinje fibers, quinidine-induced EADs show the following characteristics (Figure 6.14): (1) both phase 2 and phase 3 EADs are readily observed; (2) in both cases, the lower the stimulation rate, the higher the incidence of EADs; however, phase 3 EADs occur at lower rates when compared to phase 2 EADs (Figure 6.14a); (3) the lower the extracellular K concentration, the higher is the incidence of EADs and the faster is the rate of stimulation at which EADs may occur (Figure 6.14b); and (4) increasing the extracellular Mg concentration abolishes the triggered action potential at all frequencies with no major changes in the incidence of EADs (Figure 6.14c). This effect is thought to be the result of a membrane-stabilizing action of Mg, which shifts the threshold of Ca current toward more negative values. Thus, even in the presence of EADs, Ca channels fail to reach threshold and thus TA does not ensue.

The role of L-type Ca window current in the genesis of EADs arising during the plateau of the action potential (phase 2 EADs) was supported by experiments using the Ca channel agonist Bay K8644. Bay K8644 increases I_{Ca} by increasing the open time of L-type Ca channels, which leads to increases in the duration of the action potential and induction of EADs. In addition, nifedipine and verapamil exert an inhibitory effect on TA with minor effects on APD or EAD appearance. Catecholamines, on the other hand, may enhance EADs by augmenting the Ca current. However, the increase in heart rate that results from adrenergic stimulation along with the increase in K current may act to reduce the APD and thus abolish EADs and TAs.

Table 6.3 summarizes some of the distinctive features of arrhythmias arising from all forms of automatic activity. The combination of the response to external stimulation and pharmacologic agents may help in the recognition of several types of arrhythmias.

Clinical Implications: the Long QT Syndrome and Associated Arrhythmias
DADs and EADs as well as reentry are thought to be involved in the mechanisms of life-threatening ventricular arrhythmias in patients with the long QT syndrome. Specifically, these patients may develop a peculiar type of

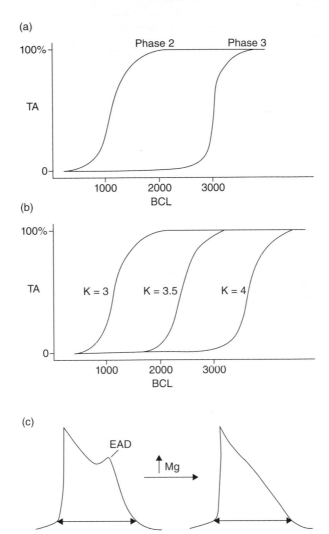

Figure 6.14 Some characteristics of triggered activity (TA). (a) Rate dependence of TA induced during quinidine superfusion. Although both phase 2 and phase 3 triggered responses increase at relatively long basic cycle lengths (BCLs), it is clear that phase 2 triggered responses occur at relatively higher rates. (b) Rate dependence of TA in the presence of various concentrations of extracellular K (in mM). The lower the extracellular K, the higher is the rate at which TA occurs. (c) Effect of Mg on early afterdepolarization (EAD) and TA. Mg abolishes TA without modifying the duration of the action potential.

polymorphic VT. Such VTs are characterized by an undulating shift in the QRS axis of the ECG and have therefore been called "torsades de pointes" (Figure 6.15), which translated from the French means twisting of the tips. The long QT syndrome and other inherited arrhythmogenic ion channel diseases are discussed in detail in Chapter 10.

Table 6.3 Characteristics of ectopic activity resulting from all four types of automatic activity

	Enhanced automaticity	Abnormal automaticity	DAD	EAD
Following pauses	Escape rhythms Suppression	NE	↑	↓
Following overdriving	Warming up	Weak suppression	↑	↓
β Stimulation	↑	↑	↑	↑/↓
β Blockade	↓	↓	↓	↑/↓
Ca blockers	↓/NE	↓	↓	NE
Adenosine	NE	NE	↓	NE

NE, no effect; ↑ increase; ↓ decrease; DAD, delayed afterdepolarization; EAD, early afterdepolarization.

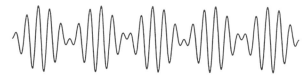

Figure 6.15 Schematic representation of "torsades de pointes" type of polymorphic ventricular tachycardia as seen in the electrocardiogram.

Alterations in the Conduction of the Impulse: Reentry

In its simplest definition, "reentry" is the circulation of the cardiac impulse around an obstacle, leading to repetitive excitation of the heart at a frequency that depends on the conduction velocity and the perimeter of the obstacle (Figure 6.16). According to the original description of George Mines in 1914, reentry occurs around a fixed anatomic obstacle and the physical disruption of the surrounding circuit will interrupt the activity. The initiation of the reentrant activity depends on the occurrence of unidirectional block so that activation occurs only in one direction within the circuit.

It is clear from Figure 6.16 that the rotation time around the circuit should be longer than the recovery period of all segments of the circuit. This excess time required for the impulse to successfully complete a rotation may result from a relatively large circuit, a relatively slow conduction velocity of the impulse, or the relatively short duration of the refractory period. Hence, the wavelength, which may be calculated roughly as the product of the refractory period times the conduction velocity, must be shorter than the perimeter of the circuit. An excitable region will separate the front of the impulse from its own refractory tail (i.e., excitable gap) and circus movement re-excitation will ensue. The classical scheme used to describe reentrant activation is displayed in Figure 6.17, where a Purkinje fiber is shown to be attached to the ventricular myocardium by two terminal branches. In such a scheme, the first prerequisite for reentry is met, i.e., the presence of a predetermined circuit. There is a region of impaired (slow) conduction in one of the terminal branches (shaded

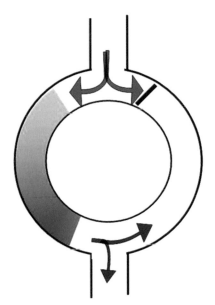

Figure 6.16 Classical representation of circus movement reentry around an obstacle. Reentry is initiated by downward unidirectional conduction through the left branch. The wavelength of the circulating impulse (red and orange area) is shorter than the length of the circuit. Physical interruption of the ring at any site will terminate the reentrant activity. Arrows indicate direction of propagation. Crossbar indicates unidirectional block.

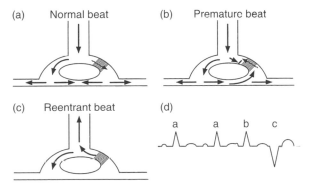

Figure 6.17 Schematic model of circus movement reentrant activity. The model represents a small Purkinje fiber and two terminal branches attached to the ventricular muscle. There is a region of impaired conduction ("damaged area") on the right terminal branch. (a) During a normal beat (i.e., sinus beat), conduction over the damage area is slow but the impulse still reaches the ventricular muscle distal to that area. (b) In the presence of a premature beat (i.e., accelerated sinus rate or supraventricular extrasystole), there is unidirectional block in the damaged area. Propagation fails in the anterograde direction on the right side, but retrograde propagation succeeds. (c) The reentrant impulse returns to the initial common pathway and results in an extrasystole. (d) ECG manifestation of the extrasystole. The letters "a," "b," and "c" refer to events in panels (a), (b), and (c), respectively.

area in the right branch), which also recovers slowly from previous excitation (this region may represent an area of ischemia where the conditions for both slow conduction and excessively long recovery time are usually encountered). This region may set the stage for the unidirectional block that is needed for the initiation as well as the slow conduction that is appropriate for the maintenance reentry. Panel (a) represents activation of the tissue when the Purkinje fiber branches derived from the main trunk are excited by a beat of sinus origin at a relatively slow frequency. Because of the presence of the area of impairment, there is some delay in the activation of the right branch. Yet the impulse moves slowly through that area and eventually reaches the attached myocardium. The result, as recorded by an ECG (panel d) would be a normal QRS complex. Panel (b) illustrates the dynamics of propagation across the same anatomic circuit during premature activation (e.g., as a result of sinus nodal tachycardia, an atrial extrasystole, or an electric stimulus that follows the previous impulse very closely in time). Under these conditions, the tissue in the slow conduction region is not yet fully recovered from previous excitation and anterograde block ensues. Over the left branch, however, the impulse moves unimpaired to activate the ventricular myocardium. That same impulse then continues retrogradely to excite the already recovered right branch. Panel (c) shows the impulse reaching the initial site of activation after exciting the entire right branch. The ECG manifestation of this process would be in the form of a ventricular extrasystole (complex "c" in panel d).

Reentry is responsible for a variety of arrhythmias, including supraventricular and ventricular extrasystoles, atrial flutter, AV nodal reciprocating tachycardias, supraventricular tachycardias associated with accessory AV pathways, bundle branch VTs, and monomorphic VTs associated with myocardial infarction. There is also strong evidence to suggest that more complex arrhythmias such as atrial fibrillation, polymorphic VT, and ventricular fibrillation are the result of reentrant mechanisms.

The classical model of anatomically determined reentry is directly applicable to certain specific cases of tachyarrhythmias. These include supraventricular tachycardias occurring within the AV node or using accessory pathways and bundle branch reentrant tachycardia. However, other types of reentrant arrhythmias require somewhat different mechanistic explanations. For example, the cellular basis of closely coupled ventricular extrasystoles initiated somewhere in the Purkinje fiber network can be explained by the so-called "reflection" mechanism (see Figure 6.18a). On the other hand, many tachyarrhythmias that originate in the myocardium (atrial or ventricular) require mechanisms whereby reentrant activation may occur as vortices of electric excitation rotating over an area of myocardium in the absence of a predetermined obstacle or circuit (Figure 6.18b). Accordingly, the impulse must circulate around a region of functional block. Until recently, the most widely accepted hypothesis to explain such functionally determined reentry was the so-called "leading-circle" hypothesis, with its two variants of "anisotropic" and "figure-of-eight" reentry. Over the last several years, a different postulate for vortex-like reentry, the "spiral wave reentry" hypothesis has become much more widely accepted. It is derived from the theory of wave propagation in excitable media and attempts to provide a unifying explanation for the mechanisms of monomorphic and polymorphic VTs as well as

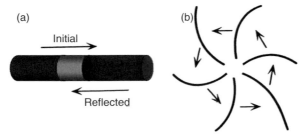

Figure 6.18 Reentry occurring in the absence of a predetermined circuit. (a) Reflection where reentry occurs over a single pathway. An action potential generated on the left side (initial) blocks at an area of depressed conductivity (yellow). Its electrotonic effects are capable of initiating an action potential on the right end of the fiber with sufficient delay to allow reflection back to the initial site. (b) Functional reentry in the 2-D myocardium. Curved lines are isochrones indicating consecutive positions of the wave front. Arrows indicate direction of propagation.

fibrillation. The concept of spiral wave activity is presented in detail in Chapter 7. For the sake of historical continuity, and to introduce the reader to such complex phenomena, the remainder of this chapter focuses on the characteristics of reflection, circus movement reentry, and leading-circle reentry and on some of the tests used in clinical electrophysiology that attempt to distinguish reentrant from other mechanisms of tachyarrhythmias.

Reflection

The presence of a region of severely impaired conduction (but not complete block) in a linear pathway (e.g., a Purkinje fiber or a thin muscle trabecula) may give rise to reentrant excitation even in the absence of an anatomic circuit (see Figure 6.18a). In the reflection model of reentry, back and forth activation occurs over the same pathway. Because of the simplicity of the experimental model, reflection was used to analyze in detail the effects of various conditions (stimulation rate, antiarrhythmic agents, ischemia, etc.) on the manifestation of reentrant activity, specifically, single reentrant excitation or extrasystoles.

A convenient approach to study reflection is the sucrose gap preparation (see Chapter 5). As shown in Figure 6.19, the sucrose gap preparation consists of a linear Purkinje fiber bundle that has been excised from the endocardium of a dog or sheep ventricle and placed in a three-compartment tissue bath. Each compartment is perfused independently. The central chamber is perfused with an ion-free solution containing isotonic (~300 mM) sucrose. The cells in the central segment thus become unexcitable, even though they remain connected to the cells of the two outer segments. In Figure 6.19, an external bridge (a silver chloride wire with variable resistance determined by a potentiometer) is used to connect the extracellular fluid or the outer chambers. Such a bridge is used to modulate the degree of conduction block across the central compartment.

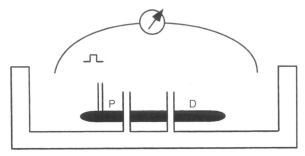

Figure 6.19 Sucrose gap model. A Purkinje fiber (black area) is placed on a three-compartment chamber. Ion-free sucrose solution is perfused continuously in the central chamber, while Tyrode's solution is perfused in the two outer chambers. Stimulation is delivered to the proximal side (P), and recordings are obtained both from P and distal (D) sites. An external wire with variable resistance connected to both outer chambers restores the electrical circuit that is broken by the sucrose in the central chamber.

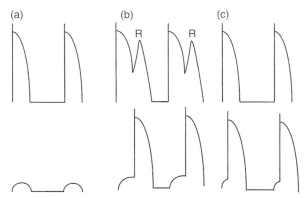

Figure 6.20 Conduction delay, block, and reflection in the sucrose gap model. Each frame shows two responses initiated in the proximal (P) segment of the fiber. (a) High degree of block. There is complete failure of activation of the distal (D) segment. (b) Intermediate level of block. The delay in activation of the D segment is long enough to allow recovery of the P segment and reflection (R), whereby each propagated response reactivates the P segment, giving rise to reflections in a bigeminal pattern. (c) Low degree of block. There is a slight delay between P and D responses.

In Figure 6.20, we present the results of a sucrose gap experiment in a linear Purkinje fiber. In all three panels, the top recordings are from the proximal segment; the bottom recordings are from the distal segment. When the proximal end of the fiber is stimulated, action potentials would normally propagate toward the central segment. However, cells in the central segment (the gap) are not excitable because they are surrounded by an extracellular space that contains only trace amounts of ions, including Na ions. Thus, as shown in Figure 6.20a, in the presence of virtually ion-free sucrose solution, an action potential is unable to propagate through these cells. Yet the local circuit current generated at the site where the action potential stops is sufficient to depolarize passively (i.e., electrotonically) the unexcitable cells to induce a subthreshold response. As discussed in Chapter 4, and also apparent from Figure 6.20, electrotonic current decays rapidly with distance. Yet, if the length of the gap is relatively small (~1 mm), and an electrical bridge is placed between P and D as depicted in Figure 6.19, enough current may reach the distal segment to bring the membrane of those cells to threshold and initiate an action potential after an appreciable delay. As shown in Figure 6.20b, proximal-to-distal activation is successful. However, please note that it is the sink-to-source ratio that determines whether propagation is successful, and also the time required for excitation of the distal segment. Thus, when the sink-to-source ratio enables successful propagation and the time for distal activation is appropriately slow, the distal action potential occurs at a time when the proximal segment already recovered. Thus, the distal segment becomes the source and reactivates the proximal segment (i.e., there is reflection, R). In Figure 6.20c, when the resistance bridging the gap is further decreased, the time for distal activation decreases, which prevents the occurrence of reflection.

Rate Dependency of the Extrasystoles

In the example of reflection presented in the previous section, the amount of source current depends on various factors, including the amplitude and maximum upstroke velocity (V_{max}) of the proximal action potential. On the other hand, the requirement of current for excitation (i.e., the sink) is determined by the excitability of the distal segment. Because both source and sink are sensitive to changes in the activation rate, the manifestation of reflected beats is also a sensitive function of the activation rate. In general, the higher the stimulation rate (proximal activation rate), the slower is the proximal-to-distal activation time. Because reflection occurs only with intermediate levels of block, a gradual increase in the stimulation rate usually leads to absence of arrhythmias at low rates (i.e., conduction is too good), to high incidence of arrhythmia at intermediate rates (i.e., conduction is appropriately slow), to absence of arrhythmia (i.e., there is complete block). This is represented in Figure 6.21. In panel (a), the rate of stimulation is slow enough to allow for rapid 1:1 propagation from proximal-to-distal segments. In panel (b), the rate of stimulation of the proximal site was increased. Although propagation continues to be 1:1, there is a delay in the activation of the distal segment, which is long enough to result in reflection. Indeed, each of the proximal responses is reflected back to the proximal segment, giving rise to a bigeminal rhythm. Finally, at even higher rates (panel c), proximal-to-distal propagation fails, and the pattern becomes 2:1. Blocked beats are obviously not followed by reflection. However, because the conduction time of the propagated responses is relatively fast (following a blocked beat, there is a longer time for recovery), reflection does not occur after conducted beats either.

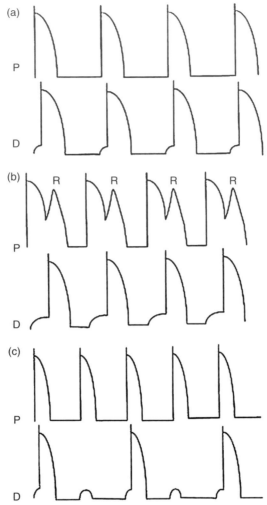

Figure 6.21 Frequency dependence of conduction and reflection in the sucrose model. (a) Low stimulation frequency. Propagation from proximal to distal (P:D) is 1:1, and the delay between P and D is relatively short. (b) Intermediate stimulation frequency. Propagation from P:D is still 1:1; however, the delay in activation is long enough as to allow for reflections in a bigeminal pattern. (c) High stimulation frequency. Propagation from P:D is now 2:1. In addition, because the propagated action potentials have a relatively low frequency, conduction time between P and D is short, thus preventing the occurrence of reflection.

Antiarrhythmic Agents and Rate Dependency of Extrasystoles

A variant of the sucrose gap preparation is the ischemic gap preparation, in which the central compartment is perfused with Tyrode's solution containing a combination of high K, low pH, and low oxygen, instead of sucrose. As shown in Figure 6.22, the main effect of the ischemic solution is to depolarize

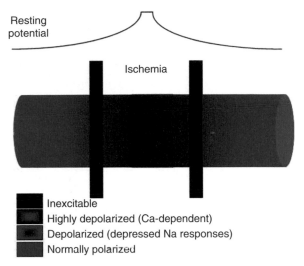

Figure 6.22 Distribution of resting potential and excitability in the ischemic gap model. Although the whole central compartment is perfused with "ischemic" solution, only a central segment (black) is fully depolarized and unresponsive. The electrotonic influences of neighboring cells lead to a distribution of resting potentials and excitability states.

the cells in the central segments until rendering them unexcitable. Because of the mutual electrotonic influence between central and outer segments, cells that are close to the borders of the central segment may show various levels of depolarization. The ischemic gap reproduces the rate dependency of extrasystoles observed in the sucrose gap. In addition, it allows for the study of agents, which may selectively affect cells at various levels of depolarization. Thus, a drug that depresses Ca currents is expected to abolish the active responses of cells in the central segment that are depolarized (i.e., all Na channels are inactivated and the action potential depends on Ca currents) and yet not completely unexcitable. The result will be a widening of the zone of unexcitability with a significant impairment in conduction. Similar effects may result from the addition of a drug that suppresses Na currents. In the context of the rate dependency of reflection, we may analyze the effects of various agents.

In Figure 6.23 we have plotted data from a hypothetical experiment in which the percentage of reflected impulses that result in extrasystoles (50% represents bigeminy) is plotted as a function of the stimulation rate. At slow and fast rates, the percentage of extrasystoles decreases. Maximum manifestation of the arrhythmia occurs at intermediate stimulation rates. The addition of quinidine, which is expected to block Na channels and thus increase the amount of cells that are unexcitable, leads to a shift in the rate dependency of the extrasystoles. Thus, the highest percentage of extrasystoles occurs at rates that are lower than those observed during control. Furthermore, the effect of quinidine may be considered antiarrhythmic when compared with

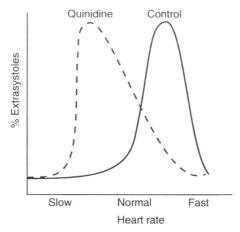

Figure 6.23 The effect of quinidine on rate dependence of reflection. The percentage of reflected responses (i.e., extrasystoles) is plotted as a function of the stimulation frequency. Peak manifestation of the extrasystole occurs at slower frequencies following the exposure to quinidine.

control at high stimulation rates and arrhythmogenic when considering the slower stimulation rates.

Thus, the reflection model has been very useful for the interpretation of more complex in vitro or in vivo models of arrhythmias as well as clinical studies. In summary, because the arrhythmia is influenced by the rate-dependent changes in conduction, drugs that affect heart rate may indirectly increase or decrease the incidence of extrasystoles. On the other hand, drugs that decrease conduction speed across the ischemic gap will shift the peak incidence of extrasystoles toward slower rates, whereas drugs that increase conduction speed will show an opposite effect. Consequently, both types of agents may result in arrhythmogenic or antiarrhythmic effects, depending on the initial conditions and the heart rate. Finally, determining the rate dependence of extrasystoles may have prognostic value because arrhythmias present at slow rates may be more susceptible to drugs that depress conduction.

Circus Movement Reentry

Undoubtedly, the concept of circus movement reentry, in which a cardiac impulse travels around a predetermined circuit or around an anatomic obstacle, can be successfully applied to a variety of clinical situations. Two clear examples of reentrant arrhythmias based on the circus movement mechanisms are supraventricular tachycardias observed in patients with Wolff–Parkinson–White (WPW) syndrome and bundle branch reentrant VT, which is more commonly seen in patients with idiopathic dilated cardiomyopathy. All concepts derived from the original idea of circus movement reentry may be found in these two types of arrhythmias, as follows:

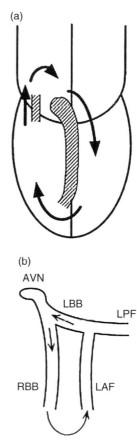

Figure 6.24 Examples of anatomical reentry. (a) Reentrant circuit in the presence of an atrioventricular accessory pathway. (b) Reentrant circuit using the branches of the intraventricular conduction system, in this case the right bundle branch and the left anterior fascicle of the left bundle. AVN: Atrioventricular node; LBB: Left bundle branch; LPF: Left posterior fascicle; RBB: Right bundle branch; LAF: Left anterior fascicle.

1. *Need for an intact predetermined anatomic circuit.* As shown schematically in Figure 6.24a, in the case of the WPW syndrome, the circuit is formed by various types of structures, including the atrium, the AV node, the His-Purkinje system, ventricular muscle, and an accessory AV pathway. In the case of bundle branch reentry (Figure 6.24b), the circuit is composed of the main bundle branches and the interventricular septum. The need for the integrity of the circuit is demonstrated by the fact that physical interruption of the circuit at any point leads to the interruption of the arrhythmia.

2. *Need of unidirectional block for the onset of the activity.* In most cases, unidirectional block occurs in the region of longest refractory period (see Chapter 5) and is the result of an increase in heart rate. Unidirectional block may occur as a result of various conditions, including (1) increase in sinus rate, (2) rapid or premature atrial pacing, (3) retrograde activation from a ventricular extrasystole, (4) autonomic influences, (5) antiarrhythmic drugs, and (6) ischemia.

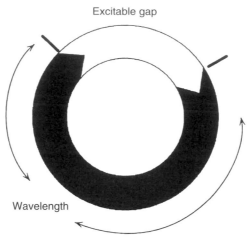

Figure 6.25 "Ring-type" model of circus movement reentry.

3. *Facilitation by slow conduction in part of the circuit.* In the case of WPW, the arrhythmia may begin after significant prolongation of the anterograde AV nodal conduction time. The activation of the ventricles occurs at the time when both accessory pathway and atria are recovered. This leads to retrograde activation of the accessory pathway and initiation of reentrant arrhythmia.

4. *The wavelength of the impulse is shorter than the length of the circuit.* As shown in Figure 6.25, there is a segment within the circuit that remains excitable during reentrant activity. The presence of an excitable gap has major significance for various reasons: (1) the reentrant activity will likely be stable in the presence of an excitable gap because the reentrant wave front will find only fully recovered tissue in its path; and (2) the activity may be entrained and/or interrupted by means of external stimulation (see section "Leading Circle Model"). An externally initiated impulse may invade the circuit during the excitable gap and thus advance the activation front. Depending on the timing or the rate of external stimulation, the wave front may be advanced enough to collide with the repolarizing tail and thus terminate the activity. (3) Agents that prolong the refractory period may not affect the reentrant process unless the prolongation of refractoriness totally obliterates the excitable gap.

Functionally Determined Reentry

Circus movement reentry is based on propagation around a 1-D circuit or ringlike structure. Although the model is entirely applicable to arrhythmias such as those observed in the presence of AV accessory pathways, it may not represent a realistic model for reentrant arrhythmias occurring in the atrial or ventricular myocardium. Reentrant activity may indeed occur in the absence of a predetermined circuit. Furthermore, the electrical impulse may rotate around a region that is anatomically normal and uniform but functionally discontinuous.

The first description of reentrant excitation in the heart in the absence of anatomic obstacles was presented in 1924 by Garrey in his description of experimental studies of circus movement in the turtle heart. Garrey's observations suggested that point stimulation of the atrium was sufficient to initiate a regular wave of rotation around the stimulus site. Subsequently, in 1946, Norbert Wiener and Arturo Rosenblueth, at the National Institute of Cardiology in Mexico, developed the first mathematical model of circus movement reentry, which supported waves of rotation around a sufficiently large barrier, but they could not demonstrate reentry in the absence of an obstacle. This prompted Wiener and Rosenblueth to suggest that perhaps Garrey may have unwittingly produced a transient artificial obstacle near the stimulation site.

Leading Circle Model

In 1973, Maurits Allessie and his associates at the University of Limburg in Maastricht, the Netherlands, provided the first direct experimental demonstration that the presence of an anatomic obstacle is not essential for the initiation or maintenance of reentry. These authors studied the mechanism of tachycardia in small pieces of isolated rabbit left atrium by the application of single premature stimuli. Using multiple electrode mapping techniques, they demonstrated that the tachycardias were based on rotating waves (Figure 6.26) and suggested that such waves were initiated as a result of unidirectional block of the triggering premature input. Transmembrane potential recordings demonstrated that cells at the center of the vortex were not excited but developed local responses. It was hypothesized that such depolarizations led to some degree of refractoriness and served as a functional obstacle around

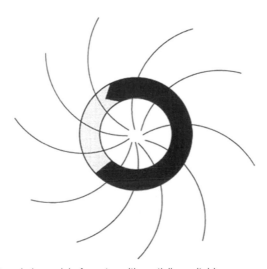

Figure 6.26 Leading circle model of reentry with partially excitable gap.

which the impulse rotated. These observations were the basis for the development of the "leading circle" concept of circus movement reentry.

According to the leading circle concept, in the absence of an anatomical obstacle, the dynamics of reentry are determined by the smallest possible loop in which the impulse can continue to circulate. Under these conditions, the wave front must propagate through relatively refractory tissue, in which case there will be no "fully excitable gap" and the wavelength will be very close to the length of the circuit. Thus, there are several differences between circus movement reentry occurring around fixed anatomic obstacle and leading circle reentry:

1. Because in leading circle reentry there is no anatomically determined circuit, there is no theoretical possibility of interrupting the arrhythmia by disrupting the circuit.
2. The absence of a fully excitable gap makes the arrhythmia unstable, i.e., relatively small variations in the electrophysiological characteristics of the tissues involved (e.g., a small increase in the refractory period) may result in a change in the cycle length of the arrhythmia or, eventually, termination of the activity. Also as a result of the absence of an excitable gap, this leading circle reentry would be expected to be insensitive to electrical stimulation. Thus, entrainment and annihilation of the arrhythmia by externally applied stimuli are theoretically very unlikely.
3. Finally, when compared with reentrant activity around an anatomic obstacle, leading circle-type reentry is expected to have a shorter cycle length.

As will be discussed in detail in Chapter 7, although the leading circle idea paved the way for major advances in our understanding of functional reentry, over the last several years, many of its original predictions were proved to be inaccurate. In addition, the model of the leading circle seems incompatible with some of the major properties of functionally determined reentry that are commonly observed experimentally in normal cardiac muscle, including the phenomenon of reentry "drift," which results in beat-to-beat changes in the location of the rotation center.

Anisotropic Reentry

More recent work implicated microscopic structural complexities of the cardiac muscle in the mechanism of reentrant activation in both atria and ventricles, particularly in relation to the orientation of the myocardial fibers, the manner in which the fibers and fiber bundles are connected to each other, and the effective electric resistivities that depend on the fiber orientation. Indeed, it is well known that action potential propagation in the heart is determined not only by the electrical properties associated with cell excitability and refractoriness but also by the high degree of anisotropy in cell-to-cell communication resulting from the specific parallel arrangement of the

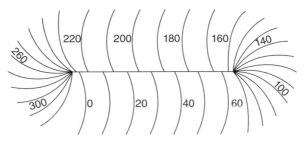

Figure 6.27 Anisotropic reentry.

fiber bundles and the paucity of the transverse electrical connections between them (see Chapter 4). Consequently, propagation velocity in the cardiac muscle is three to five times faster in the longitudinal axis of the cells than along the transverse axis. In addition, asymmetry in the safety factor for propagation may result in conduction block occurring first in one direction (i.e., unidirectional block). Thus, it was suggested that structural anisotropy may set the stage for heterogeneity of functional properties and thus lead to the initiation and maintenance of reentry (Figure 6.27). Mapping studies using multiple extracellular electrodes showed that, in the setting of myocardial infarction, reentry may occur in the surviving rim of epicardial tissue. Under such conditions, the wave circulates around a functionally determined elongated region of block, the so-called line of conduction block. Based on line-of-block orientation, it was thought that anisotropic propagation played a major role both in the initiation as well as in the maintenance of reentry in ventricular tissue surviving a myocardial infarction. In addition, propagation velocity is exceedingly slow at the edges of the lines of block (the pivoting points), which was also attributed to anisotropic propagation.

Thus, anisotropic reentry may be considered a model of functionally determined reentry, in which both initiation and maintenance of the activity is based on the histological properties of the tissue. However, the true role of anisotropic propagation in determining the reentrant circuit remains unclear. First, the line of block does not follow strictly the direction of the fibers. Furthermore, in most published examples of so-called anisotropic reentry, there are beat-to-beat changes in the direction of the line of block that cannot be attributed to transient changes in anisotropy. Most importantly, recent experimental studies demonstrated that, in reentrant circuits occurring around a thin linear anatomic obstacle produced by a laser beam, the slowest propagation was observed at the pivot points regardless of the actual orientation of the fibers (see Figure 6.27). Finally, the anisotropic properties of the tissue were also implicated in the establishment of an excitable gap. This was recently challenged by computer simulations in which the rotation period and the excitable gap were not significantly modified by the addition of anisotropy to the circuit. Therefore, we believe that, although anisotropic propagation may play a role in arrhythmogenesis, there are other aspects of wave propagation

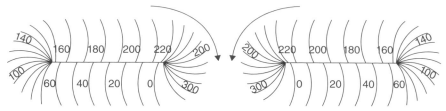

Figure 6.28 Figure-of-8 reentry in anisotropic cardiac muscle.

such as wave front curvature (see Chapter 7) and macroscopic tissue structure that must be taken into consideration to better understand 2-D and 3-D reentry in the myocardium.

Figure-of-8 Reentry

Figure-of-8 reentry was recognized as an important pattern of reentry in the late stages of myocardial infarction. In most cases, two counter-rotating waves coexist at a relatively short distance from each other (Figure 6.28). As described for the case of single reentrant circuits, each wave of the figure-of-8 reentry circulates around a thin line or arc of block. The region separating the lines of block is called the common pathway. A detailed description of the common pathway is of great practical importance because there is evidence that such a pathway could be a strategic region for surgical or catheter ablation in this type of reentry. In fact, unlike other forms of functionally determined reentry, figure-of-8 reentry may indeed be interrupted by physical disruption of the circuit. Several experimental studies attempted to describe the characteristics of propagation in the common pathway. However, the properties of the common pathways are still not clearly defined. The common pathway effectively behaves like an isthmus limited by two functionally determined barriers. In addition, there are two wave fronts that interact in the common pathway. As a result, propagation may be determined by a combination of factors other than those analyzed in most experimental studies such as anisotropy. The study of propagation across an isthmus and the influence of wave front curvature may have significant implications in the understanding of the properties of the common pathway, as will be discussed in Chapter 7.

Use of Programmed Electric Stimulation to Study Mechanisms of Arrhythmias

The idea of electric stimulation for the study of the mechanisms of supraventricular arrhythmia began in the late 1960s by the group of Durrer. The concept was later extended for the study of ventricular arrhythmias. Currently, programmed stimulation became an important tool in the diagnosis of supraventricular as well as ventricular arrhythmias, and the features that are usually considered for the diagnosis of reentry in clinical arrhythmias are (1) the demonstration of continuous local electric activity; (2) the inducibility by programmed electric stimulation; (3) the inducibility by programmed stimulation that is not influenced by isoproterenol; (4) the inducibility from specific sites; (5) in most cases, the relationship between coupling interval of the initiating stimulus and the coupling interval of the first tachycardia beat; (6) the possibility of entrainment by means of external stimulation; and (7) the visualization of reentrant activation by means of high-resolution intra-operative mapping techniques.

It is important to note, however, that, although programmed stimulation is used primarily for the study of phenomena occurring in the complex 2-D and 3-D structure that is the ventricular muscle, the explanations for all observed responses are based on a 1-D model of reentry. In fact, both resetting responses to single stimuli and entrainment are explained using the imaginary model of a well-defined circuit that has a central area of block, with a possible sector of slow conduction and with specific entrance and exit pathways. The real substrate for ventricular arrhythmias may greatly differ from this simplistic model. Yet, many of the responses fit very well with this useful 1-D model as will be discussed in this section.

Early studies indicated that the ability to initiate or terminate an arrhythmia by premature stimulation was clear indication of a reentrant mechanism. However, other types of electrophysiological abnormalities (i.e., DAD-induced TA) may respond similarly to premature stimulation. In addition, resetting of the arrhythmia by a premature stimulus may occur not only in reentrant arrhythmias but also in triggered and automatic rhythms. Thus, more specific description of the effect of single and multiple stimuli to reentrant process is necessary to firmly establish the diagnosis.

Resetting

As shown in Figure 6.29, the application of a single stimulus, S_2, during an episode of tachycardia may be followed by a compensatory pause. In other words, the interval between the beat of that tachycardia (R_1) just before S_2 and the next beat of the tachycardia, R_3, is equal to (R_1R_1) × 2. In this case, the tachycardia was not reset by S_2. When the introduction of S_2 results in R_1R_3 < (R_1R_1) × 2, the rhythm is said to be reset. The explanation for this response is as follows. Resetting may occur with reentrant arrhythmias, automatic rhythms, and triggered responses. When the conduction time from the stimulus to the advanced electrogram is longer than the tachycardia cycle length, it is termed "orthodromic resetting" because the stimulated impulse is supposed to traverse the tachycardia circuit in the same direction as the spontaneous tachycardia. It is thought that orthodromic resetting is the hallmark for reentrant tachycardia with excitable gap and suggests that the pacing site is proximal to the region of slow conduction.

As illustrated diagrammatically in Figure 6.30, the resetting response of the return cycle (first cycle of the tachycardia following S_2) as a function of the coupling interval of S_2 can be either flat (panel a), increasing to the left (panel b), or bimodal (panel c), depending upon the electrophysiological

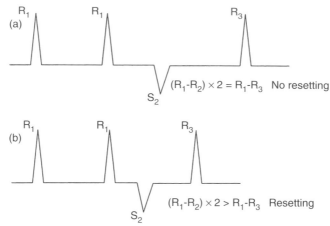

Figure 6.29 ECG manifestation of resetting a reentrant tachycardia. (a) A single stimulus (S_2) was delivered during the tachycardia, and it was followed by a pause, giving rise to an interval (R_1R_3) between the last beat of the tachycardia (R_1) and the first return beat (R_3), which is equal to twice the cycle of the tachycardia ($2 \times R_1R_1$). This type of return cycle indicates that the tachycardia was not reset by the stimulus. (b) The S_2 is now followed by a shorter pause so that R_1R_3 is briefer than $2 \times R_1R_1$. This response of the return beat indicates the presence of resetting.

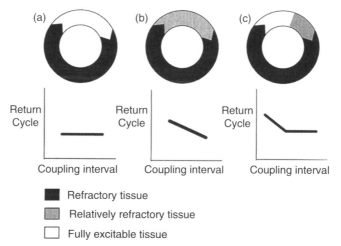

Figure 6.30 Types of return curve and proposed electrophysiological substrate. In each frame the top panel illustrates the characteristics of the circuit. White area indicates excitable gap, black area indicates absolute refractory period, and shaded area indicates relatively refractory period. The bottom panels show the plot of the return cycle as a function of the coupling interval of the external stimulus. (a) A flat curve indicates the presence of excitable gap and absolute refractory period and the absence of relatively refractory period. (b) A descending curve indicates the presence of an absolute refractory period and relatively refractory period and the absence of fully excitable gap. (c) A mixed curve indicates that the system has all three components (i.e., absolute and relatively refractory periods as well as fully excitable gap).

characteristics of the tachycardia circuit. As shown in panel (a), flat response indicates that stimuli of varying interval always fall within a fully excitable gap. When the return cycle increases as the S_1-S_2 shortens, it is an indication that the earlier the stimulus, the more refractory the tissue in circuit is and the more delay there is in propagation. Thus, a curve with negative slope is said to be characteristic of a variant of the leading circle type of reentry in which there is no fully excitable gap but instead there is partially excitable gap. Finally, as shown in panel (c), a mixed response in which very early S_2 stimuli are followed by increasing type of response, while later S_2 presents a flat type of response, is explained by the presence of reentrant circuits in which the excitable gap has two components: fully excitable and partially excitable.

In most cases, reentrant arrhythmias have specific responses to single stimuli. In general, the coupling interval of the first beat of the tachycardia shows an inverse relation to the interval of the initiating stimulus. Thus, as a rule, the earlier the applied stimulus, the longer is the coupling interval of the first beat of the tachycardia. Progressive slowing of conduction of the stimulated impulse over the reentrant circuit is considered to be the cause of such a response. This type of response is usually opposite to what is expected from rhythms originated from DAD-induced TA.

Entrainment

In the setting of reentrant rhythms, "entrainment" is defined as the continuous resetting of a tachycardia. There are four criteria commonly used for the confirmation of entrainment. It is important to note, however, that the absence of these criteria does not rule out the possibility of reentry. The first two criteria are based on the characteristics of the surface ECG. The third and fourth criteria are based on the characteristics of intracardiac electrograms. According to the first criterion, the morphology of the first beat of the tachycardia following the pacing train should be identical to that of the beats during tachycardia, but its cycle length should be the same as that of the paced beats. This criterion is based on the idea that, if one applies the stimuli at an appropriate region of the circuit, then each stimulated response will (1) generate a fusion beat, i.e., a beat that results from the activation initiated by the stimulus plus the activation from the reentrant impulse of the previous rotation, and (2) regenerate the rotating impulse for the next rotation. Thus, following the last stimulus, the QRS will show no fusion (activation will be originated only from the reentrant circuit), but the cycle length will still be that of the pacing train. The second criterion is that pacing at varying cycles yields varying degrees of fusion. This criterion is based on the concept that the faster the pacing rate, the larger is the contribution of the paced impulse to the activation of the heart and the larger is the degree of fusion. The third criterion is that, pacing at a relatively high rate (close to the rate that could terminate that tachycardia), localized conduction block may occur so that a given region will be activated from a different direction and with a shorter conduction time by the next impulse. The third criterion includes the termination of the arrhythmia. The fourth criterion is the intracardiac electrographic manifestation of the second criterion. Because of the changes in the degree of fusion, it may happen that two points are activated in reverse order at low (low degree of fusion) compared with high (high degree of fusion) frequencies.

At present, the ability to entrain a tachycardia remains the most useful information to demonstrate reentry and must be sought when attempting to ascribe a specific mechanism to an arrhythmia. However, the inability to reset or entrain does not exclude reentry as the mechanism.

Summary

The rate of increase in our knowledge of cardiac electrophysiology accelerated dramatically over the past 30 years. A wide variety of basic mechanisms is already well described in the experimental laboratory. Furthermore, the field was enriched by concepts derived from other disciplines, including molecular biology, cell biology, biochemistry, biophysics, and computer modeling. Yet, although several tools were developed for the identification of the cellular mechanisms of clinical arrhythmias (pharmacologic agents, pacing, etc.), the understanding of the mechanisms and the appropriate treatment of such arrhythmias continue to be very difficult tasks. In this chapter, we reviewed well-established concepts and provided some insights into the appropriate tools to diagnose an arrhythmia in the clinical arena, which should reflect in our ability to provide a more rational therapeutic approach. The future development of new 3-D mapping techniques as well as the long-term recording of spontaneously occurring rhythm disturbances will probably broaden our knowledge and offer new clues for diagnosing and managing cardiac arrhythmias.

7   Rotors, Spirals, and Scroll Waves in the Heart

In the context of cardiac electrophysiology, the term "rotor" applies to the organizing source (driver) of functional reentrant activity. It is the structure immediately surrounding the pivot of a rotating wave in two or three dimensions. On the other hand, a "spiral wave" is the two-dimensional wave of excitation emitted by a rotor and whose front is an involute spiral with increasing convex curvature toward the rotation center. The three-dimensional equivalent of a spiral wave is a "scroll wave." Here rotor and functional reentry are used interchangeably. It may be argued that functional reentry (i.e., a rotor) and anatomical reentry (i.e., reentry around an anatomical obstacle) may have the same underlying mechanism. In fact, when a rotor that drifts across excitable cardiac tissue encounters and interacts with an unexcitable obstacle (e.g., a scar or a natural arterial orifice), it anchors to it and begins to rotate around it. Thus, functional reentry may turn into anatomical reentry.

Rotors are a common feature of reentrant arrhythmias in atria and ventricles, including atrial tachycardia (AT), atrial fibrillation (AF), ventricular tachycardia (VT), and ventricular fibrillation (VF). Actually rotors are common to many biological, chemical, and physical excitable media and their dynamics have been the subject of intense research throughout the scientific world. In the heart, despite their vastly different structures and ionic currents of the atria and ventricles, not only are the dynamics of rotors and spiral waves similar but also, as has been shown in some species, both chambers share the presence of a left-to-right gradient of electrical activation frequencies, suggesting that the left heart plays the leading role in maintaining fibrillation. To provide some clues about the mechanisms of rotors, this chapter adopts a point of view that differs from the traditional electrophysiological outlook in cardiology. The approach is based on ideas derived from studies in other excitable media, particularly

Basic Cardiac Electrophysiology for the Clinician, 2nd edition. By J. Jalife, M. Delmar, J. Anumonwo, O. Berenfeld and J. Kalifa. Published 2009 by Blackwell Publishing, ISBN: 978-1-4501-8333-8.

homogeneous excitable media, and makes use of dynamical systems' theory as a means to explain accurately the behavior of rotors and spiral waves in the myocardium. The experimental results discussed are those derived from studies in which high-resolution mapping approaches were used to record from large areas of the surface of the atria or ventricles during spiral wave reentrant activity. To aid in the presentation, we make use of simplified diagrams based on those experimental results and on computer simulations obtained using 2-D and 3-D models of cardiac excitation. The objective is twofold: (1) to introduce briefly our current knowledge on the dynamics of rotors and spiral waves as a phenomenon of self-organization in a wide variety of excitable media and (2) to set the stage for a discussion on subsequent chapters on the contribution of rotor theory to the understanding of the mechanisms of two of the most dangerous cardiac arrhythmias, AF and VF.

Self-Organization in Excitable Media

Advances over the last 20 years in the understanding of vortex-like rhythms (i.e., functional reentry) came from studies that apparently have nothing to do with the heart. Indeed, vortex-like activity is not unique to abnormal cardiac rhythms. As illustrated in Figure 7.1, phenomena that have very much in common with spiral wave reentry in cardiac tissue (panel a) are also observed in other chemical and biological systems, such as autocatalytic chemical reactions (panel b), the brain and retina (panel c), and Ca^{2+} waves in *Xenopus laevis* oocytes (panel d).

The common feature of all the above systems is excitability because, just as in myocardial tissue, in any of these systems, a local excitation above a certain threshold results in the initiation of a propagating wave akin to the cardiac action potential (Figure 7.2). These systems are called excitable media and are governed by a mathematical description that is very similar to the well-known models of cardiac propagation. We should point out, however, that there are enormous differences in time and space scales in the various excitable media; e.g., conduction velocity of Ca^{2+} waves in the oocyte is ~30 µm/s, whereas in the heart muscle the normal velocity of action potential propagation is ~0.3–0.5 m/s.

Yet, in all types of excitable media that were studied thus far, it was demonstrated that a particular perturbation of the excitation wave may result in phenomena of self-organization with the appearance of vortex-like activity (Figure 7.3). During such activity, the excitation wave acquires the shape of an Archimedean spiral and is called a spiral wave or vortex, organized by its rotor. As in the case of functional reentry, spiral waves do not require a discontinuity, and their rotation period is close to the refractory period of the medium. The hypothesis that functional reentry is the result of a rotor giving rise to vortices of electric waves was formulated many years ago. Only recently, however, was this hypothesis supported by direct evidence. Such evidence was obtained using a newly developed high-resolution optical

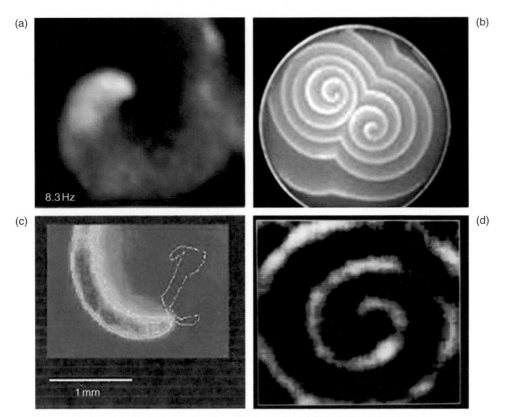

Figure 7.1 Spiral waves in four different excitable media. (a) Electrical spiral wave in a monolayer of neonatal cardiomyocytes recorded using the voltage-sensitive dye Di-8-ANEPPS and a high-resolution video camera. (Reproduced from Muñoz et al., Circ Res 2007; 101:475–83.) (b) Two counter-rotating spiral waves in the Belousov–Zhabotinsky reaction (Reproduced from http://www.apple.com/science/insidetheimage/bzreaction.) (c) Meandering spiral wave of retinal depression. (Reproduced from Gorelova et al., J Neurobiol 2004; 14:353–63.) (d) Spiral calcium wave pattern in Xenopus laevis oocyte. (Reproduced from Lechleiter and Clapham, Cell 1992; 69:283–94.)

mapping technique that enables direct visualization of the excitation wave in cardiac muscle (Figure 7.3).

Lessons about Cardiac Reentry from the B-Z Reaction

The Belousov–Zhabotinski (B–Z) reaction represents the cleanest and best understood example yet of oscillatory chemical reaction occurring under conditions that remain far from equilibrium. The reaction is basically a catalytic oxidation of an organic substrate (malonic acid) by bromate in water at low pH. The catalyst in the reaction is one iron held in the redox indicator, ferroin, which changes color from red to light blue and back to red as the reaction progresses (Figure 7.4), and allows the direct observation of the

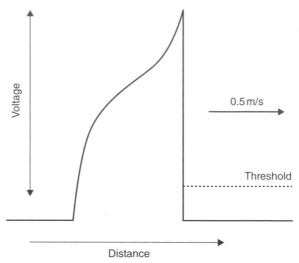

Figure 7.2 Snapshot of a cardiac action potential propagating from left to right at a speed of 0.5 m/s.

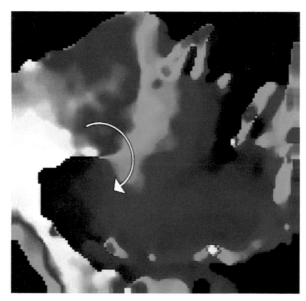

Figure 7.3 Snapshot of spiral wave rotating clockwise on the left atrial appendage of an isolated sheep heart during sustained atrial fibrillation induced by rapid pacing in the presence of acetylcholine. Each color in this phase map represents a different phase of the excitation–recovery process. Green is the wave front; red, yellow, and purple indicate different phases of recovery (repolarization); and blue is rest (i.e., the excitable gap). The activity was recorded using a voltage-sensitive dye (Di-4-ANEPPS) and a CCD video camera.

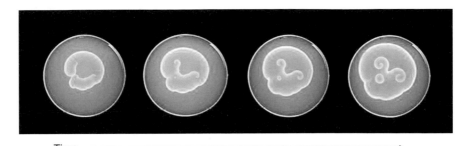

Time

Figure 7.4 Initiation of spiral waves in the Belousov–Zhabotinski reaction. Left, initiation of a circular wave by touching the solution with the tip of a hot wire. A few minutes later, the propagating wave may be interrupted by touching it again with the hot wire or if the wave front finds heterogeneity in the medium. As a result of the fracture of the wave front, a pair of self-sustaining counter-rotating spiral waves is initiated. (Reproduced from http://www.apple.com/science/insidetheimage/bzreaction.)

process when prepared in a petri dish or test tube. The most interesting feature of the reaction is that, like any other excitable media, it can exist as an oscillator that changes color periodically or may be changed to a quiescent but excitable state (red) by a small adjustment in the concentration of one of its components (sulfuric acid). Under the latter conditions, a single perturbation consisting of briefly dipping a silver wire in the solution triggers an outwardly propagating concentric circular blue wave arising from the "leading" or pacemaker center. As illustrated by the sequential snapshots in Figure 7.4, perturbing the blue wave front with the silver wire now breaks the wave front, which begins to curl at the wavebreak and initiates a long period of stable activity in the form of two counter-rotating reentrant waves circling at a constant period. Hence, the B–Z reaction and the cardiac tissue seem to be analogous in various crucial aspects of their behavior: (1) both are nonlinear systems; (2) under appropriate conditions, both can undergo self-sustaining oscillations; (3) both are excitable in the sense that an adequate stimulus can bring the system to its threshold for initiation of non-decremental wave propagation; (4) once activated, both systems undergo a refractory period during which no new activity may be initiated; and (5) similar laws of diffusion apply in both for the propagation of information from one region to another; in the case of the heart, electrochemical gradients provide the driving force for the depolarization wave to move from one cell to its neighbors; in the B–Z reaction the exchange involves concentration gradients established between regions in which certain molecules were recently synthesized and neighboring regions in which synthesis did not yet occur.

There is a difference, however, that may seem obvious enough to raise skepticism about the relevance of the chemical model to the study of wave propagation in cardiac tissue: unlike the B–Z reaction, the heart is a highly inhomogeneous and discontinuous anisotropic medium. Nevertheless, the behavioral similarities of the two systems are so pervasive that they prompted a number of investigators to use the B–Z reaction as a basis for developing numerical and analytical models to make predictions about dynamics of wave propagation in 2-D and 3-D cardiac muscle. The most remarkable of such predictions is that normal cardiac muscle can indeed sustain rotors and spiral wave activity (see Figure 7.3).

The Concept of "Wavebreak"

One way of visualizing such a wave is to think of it as a broken wave front that curls at its broken end and begins to rotate. This is illustrated in Figure 7.5, where a wave front that propagates in an excitable medium (e.g., the posterior wall of the left atrium) finds an obstacle in its path (e.g., a scar or a bundle of connective tissue). Whether the wave front will be broken by the obstacle will depend on the characteristics of that obstacle as well as on the excitability of the medium. As shown in Figure 7.5a, an obstacle with rounded

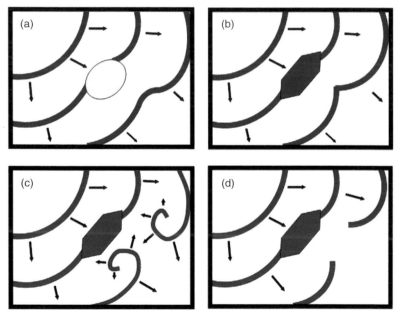

Figure 7.5 Schematic representation of the interactions between propagating waves and obstacles of different shapes and at different levels of excitability. (a) At a normal level of excitability, the red wave reaching the rounded obstacle (yellow) separates in two daughter waves that circumnavigate the borders of the obstacle and fuse again at the opposite side. No wavebreak occurs. (b) Still normal excitability. The wave now breaks as a result of the sharp borders of the hexagonal obstacle (blue). However, the broken wave fronts rapidly fuse without initiating spiral wave activity. (c) At lower levels of excitability, the broken wave front curls and initiates a pair of counter-rotating spiral waves (figure-of-8). (d) Finally, at even lower levels of excitability, the broken wave fronts are unable to rotate. Instead, they propagate decrementally until they disappear.

edges usually is not sufficient to break the wave. In Figure 7.5b–d, an obstacle with sharp edges does produce a "wavebreak" under three different conditions of excitability. In Figure 7.5b, the excitability is high. After reaching the obstacle, the wave breaks into two separate fronts whose broken ends rapidly fuse, reforming a single wave front. In Figure 7.5c, when the excitability is relatively low, the broken ends are unable to fuse, but, as in the example of the B–Z reaction, they begin to curl to initiate two counter-rotating spiral waves ("figure-of-8" reentry). In Figure 7.5d, when the excitability is much lower, the two wave fronts shrink as they propagate distally, undergoing decremental conduction until they disappear.

As shown in Figure 7.6, under normal conditions, during the propagation of linear (panel a), circular (panel b), or even elliptical waves, the wave front

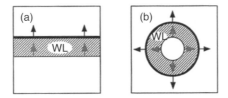

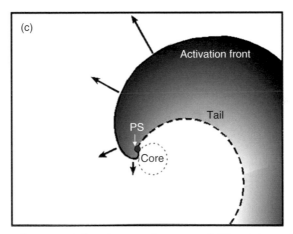

Figure 7.6 Schematic representation of propagating waves of different shapes in a homogeneous isotropic medium. In each panel, the thick black edge represents the wave front; the dashed area represents the repolarizing tail. Black arrows indicate the direction of propagation of the wave front, and dashed arrows indicate the direction of the wave tail. The distance between the wave front and tail of repolarization is the wavelength (WL). (a) Planar wave initiated by stimulation of the entire bottom border of the preparation. (b) Circular wave initiated by stimulation of a point in the center of the array. (c) Spiral wave. The wave front has variable curvature and conduction velocity. The trajectory of each point on the wave front varies according to its position. Outer points follow diverging trajectory, and inner points follow a converging trajectory. The red dot shows the phase singularity (PS) formed at the wavebreak. Note that all phases of the excitation–recovery cycle converge and the wave front and wave tail meet at the PS. The PS is the rotor which in this case follows a circular trajectory around the core.

is always followed by a refractory tissue represented by a recovery band of finite dimensions. The distance between the front and its tail of repolarization is the wavelength (WL) of excitation and is roughly equivalent to the product of the action potential duration (APD) and the velocity of propagation of the wave front. Obviously, the velocity of propagation of planar and circular waves is relatively constant at all points along the entire wave front. Under these conditions, the edge of the wave front and the edge of the wave tail never meet each other. In contrast, spiral waves show a unique phenomenon whereby the wave front and its repolarizing tail touch each other at the wavebreak (panel c), which forms a phase singularity (PS). The phase singularity is the pivot point (i.e., the rotor) of the wave front. Its continuing rotations around the core give rise to spiral wave activity.

Because of the continuously changing curvature of a spiral wave front, its dynamics of propagation are not intuitively obvious. Theoretical studies have used geometrical arguments to predict the manner in which spiral wave activity may occur in any given excitable medium. The idea is that individual points on the wave front (see Figure 7.6c) do not follow linear trajectories, but their evolution (movement) depends on their present location on the wave front. Thus, points located far from the core will tend to move in such a way that their trajectories will diverge. On the other hand, near the center the trajectories of individual points converge toward the core. The formation of a wavebreak is related to the concept of curvature and critical curvature for propagation, as will be discussed.

Under the appropriate conditions, a wavebreak may follow a rotating trajectory forming a rotor that gives rise to a spiral wave. Wavebreaks, rotors, and spiral waves may also occur at the intersection of a wave front with the tail of another propagating wave even in the absence of anatomic or functional discontinuities.

The Ever-Increasing Curvature of a Spiral Wave Front

As discussed in Chapter 4, the propagation velocity of a wave front in a 2-D or 3-D medium very much depends on its curvature; waves whose fronts are concave ("negative" curvature, Figure 7.7b) propagate faster than planar waves (Figure 7.7a), but the velocity of planar waves is faster than that of convex waves ("positive" curvature, Figure 7.7c).

For wave fronts of positive curvature, there is a value of curvature at which propagation is impaired. Such a "critical curvature" corresponds to conditions in which the wave front (the source) is insufficient to overcome the load imposed by unexcited tissue ahead (see Chapter 4). The value of the critical curvature varies with the excitability of the medium. Thus, at relatively low excitability, the critical curvature will decrease so that only wave fronts with less pronounced curvature may propagate. Spiral waves consist of curved wave fronts. Unlike planar waves or waves initiated by a point source in which the curvature is uniform throughout the wave front, in the case of spiral

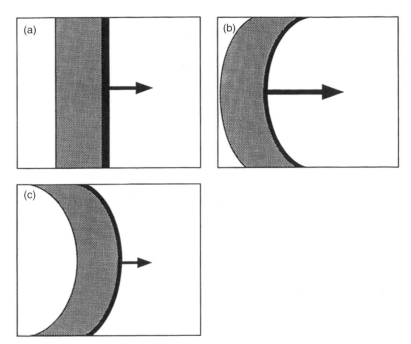

Figure 7.7 Cartoons showing the effects of curvature on wave propagation. Conduction velocity of a planar wave is (a) slower than that of a wave with negative curvature, but (b) faster than that of a wave with positive curvature (c).

waves the curvature progressively increases toward the center (Figure 7.6c). Thus, at the very tip of the spiral wave (PS in Figure 7.6c), the curvature reaches a critical value. At the core, cells develop small subthreshold electrotonically mediated depolarizations.

Wavebreaks and "Singularities"

Most models of functionally determined reentry describe the center of rotation as a region that remains refractory throughout the rotation period. In the leading circle model (see Chapter 6), the center of the rotation is seen as a region that remains refractory because of the depolarizing effects of the surrounding waves. However, experimental observations contradict such an explanation. For instance, in many examples of functionally determined reentry there are beat-to-beat changes in the position of the center of rotation; in other words the rotor "drifts." This indicates that during drift, the wave front must invade the core during the rotating activity. In addition, even if the core is partially depolarized by the surrounding waves, the excitability of the core need not be depressed. In fact, tissue slightly depolarized may show an increase rather than a decrease in excitability. More importantly, from the theoretical point of view, the generation of a core does not depend on the

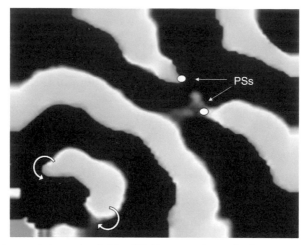

Figure 7.8 Rotors and phase singularities (PSs) in a monolayer of cultured neonatal rat ventricular cardiomyocytes obtained in an optical mapping experiment. The phase map shows two counter-rotating rotors generating spiral wave fronts that propagated upward until they encounter a local discontinuity (partially refractory cells), resulting in a wavebreak with the formation of two PSs. Red: wave front; yellow and green: different phases of recovery; blue: rest.

generation of a refractory region. The determining factor in the formation of a core is the wavebreak that results in the formation of a "phase singularity" (PS), also known as a "singularity point." As discussed earlier for Figure 7.6 and demonstrated by the experiment presented in Figure 7.8, the PS is a point during functional reentry where all phases of the excitation–recovery cycle, including wave front and wave tail, converge. The figure shows examples of stationary rotors (curved arrows) and PSs in a monolayer of neonatal rat cardiomyocytes recorded using a potentiometric dye (Di-8-ANEPPS) and a high-resolution CCD camera. Two stationary counter-rotating wave fronts on the lower left of the optical field generated spiral wave fronts that propagated upward but encountered a functional obstacle (i.e., small area of transient refractoriness) that resulted in wavebreaks and PSs, which became the pivot points of two new secondary counter-rotating waves. Similar phenomena are found during cardiac fibrillation in the presence of rotors and fibrillatory conduction (see Chapters 8 and 9).The circling of the PSs gives rise to spiral waves whose front has an involute spiral shape with increasing convex curvature toward the rotation center. Because propagation velocity decreases as the convexity of the rotating wave front increases (i.e., its curvature increases) toward the core, it follows that the velocity must be critical (i.e., zero) at some distance from the very center of the core. Indeed, according to the theory of spiral waves, the core is a region of excitable tissue that remains unexcited but is eminently excitable. Therefore, the center of rotation is not a true zone of block. The dynamics of propagation of a curved wave front and the existence of the PS explain the origin of the core.

Lines of Block in Anisotropic Reentry

As discussed in Chapter 6, functionally determined reentry occurring in the surviving rim of epicardial tissue after a myocardial infarction is characterized by activity that rotates around relatively long and thin areas of block. High-density mapping studies showed that these lines or "arcs" of conduction block may indeed be the result of a central region of "true" block as well as lateral regions in which there is very slow conduction velocity. The anisotropic properties of the tissue were implicated in the origin of these lines of block. Indeed, in the original description of anisotropic reentry, the lines of block were thought to depend on fiber orientation. Yet, in many examples, the angle of the line of block showed beat-to-beat variations, thus making fiber orientation a less likely explanation for these phenomena. Furthermore, propagation of the impulse around the line of block was clearly nonuniform. In general, propagation velocity was shown to be extremely slow at the pivot points. Again anisotropy was thought to be responsible for such a condition. However, the orientation of the lines of block may not always be parallel to the long axis of the fibers so that propagation at the pivot point may occur either in the longitudinal or in the transverse direction. These observations indicate that anisotropy should not be considered the major contributor for the establishment of the lines of block or for the conduction properties around such lines. According to the theory of wave propagation in excitable media, the center of a spiral wave may indeed have an elongated shape even in the absence of anisotropy (Figure 7.9). Theory predicts that depending on the excitability of the tissue, the core may be circular, elongated, or linear or may adopt a Z-shape. In addition, conduction of the wave around functional and anatomic obstacles with sharp edges (i.e., the pivot regions) must be slower as a result of the curvature effect, and velocity should be zero at the PS. This

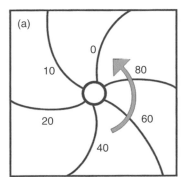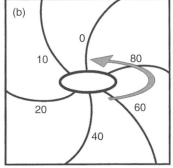

Figure 7.9 (a) Schematic representation of spiral wave activity with a circular core formed in an isotropic medium. (b) Anisotropy in cardiac muscle results in spiral wave activity with an elongated core. Curved gray arrows indicate the direction of the rotation; curved lines are isochrones; numbers are in milliseconds starting from an arbitrary zero line.

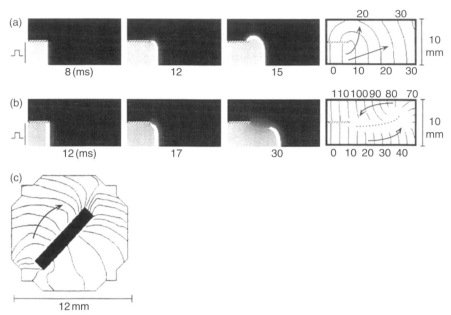

Figure 7.10 Simulated wave propagation around a linear obstacle in a 2-D Luo and Rudy model illustrates the phenomenon of "vortex shedding." (a) Under conditions of normal excitability, the wave curves at the edge of the obstacle and then continues to activate the rest of the array. (b) Under conditions of depressed excitability (decreased G_{Na}), the curvature imposed by the obstacle on the wave front is pronounced enough to fail to propagate around the obstacle. As a result, the wave front detaches from the obstacle and propagates as a wavelet (or wavebreak) in a linear direction. On reaching the high-resistivity right border of the array, the wave front is then able to propagate upward and the activation process is completed. Note that, although there were no heterogeneities in the array (except for the barrier), propagation around the obstacle in the presence of low excitability described a trajectory that is compatible with the presence of a line of block. (c) In the whole heart, other investigators found that propagation is slower at the pivot points of a sharp obstacle compared with the propagation along the obstacle. This is in spite of the fact that propagation around the edges of the obstacle occurs along the fiber orientation and is expected to be faster than propagation in the transverse direction.

theoretical prediction was confirmed in isolated tissue experiments in the presence of a linear barrier produced by a cut (Figure 7.10b) as well as in experiments using Langendorff-perfused rabbit hearts in which a linear lesion was produced by a laser beam (Figure 7.10c). In both cases, conduction around the edges of the obstacle was slower than at any other region of the preparation even though propagation around the edge of the obstacle occurred in the longitudinal direction. Thus, the theory of wave propagation in excitable media offers an explanation for the formation of the line of block and for the regions of slow propagation around it, which differs from the classical view in which anisotropic propagation plays major role.

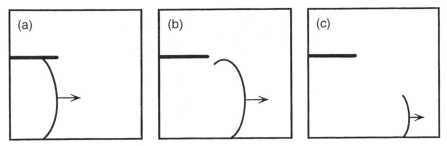

Figure 7.11 Simulation performed with a 2-D Luo and Rudy array to demonstrate decremental conduction of a wavelet occurring at the edge of an obstacle as a result of critical curvature for propagation. See text.

Spiral Waves and Wavelets

Functional reentry may be defined as a phase singularity rotating around an unexcited core and generating spiral waves. Self-sustaining spiral wave activity may be initiated simply by creating a wavebreak even though not all wavebreaks develop into spiral waves. As illustrated in Figure 7.11, whether in cardiac muscle or in other types of excitable media, wavebreaks may follow various types of trajectories. Relatively small changes in the excitability of the medium may dramatically alter the dynamics of propagation of wavebreaks. Figure 7.11 shows a situation in which the excitability of the medium is relatively low. As in Figure 7.5, a wavebreak is formed after the detachment of the wave front from a sharp-edged obstacle. In panel (a) of Figure 7.11, a wave front is initiated at the bottom half of the medium. The wave moves from left to right. In panel (b), the wave detaches from the obstacle in the center of the medium. The wavebreak then propagates to the right to form a "wavelet" that moves forward at decreasing speed (panel c). As it propagates, the wavelet contracts and then disappears.

Thus, the dynamics of wavebreaks are not only the basis for functionally determined reentrant activity but they may also explain more complex spatial and temporal activation patterns such as those observed as a result of the coexistence of multiple wavelets, as in AF and VF. The dynamics of propagation of wave breaks differ from those of a regular wave front in that wave breaks may interact with each other so that collision need not lead to mutual annihilation but rather to the formation of a new wave break, thus self-perpetuating the activity.

The concepts of wave front curvature and wave break also contributed significantly to our understanding of the mechanisms of initiation of reentry, the presence of the so-called excitable gap, drifting and anchoring of vortices, and the effects of externally applied waves.

Wavebreak Precedes the Initiation of Reentry

The essential step in the initiation of reentrant activity is the formation of a wavebreak. Wavebreaks may occur as a result of the interaction of the wave

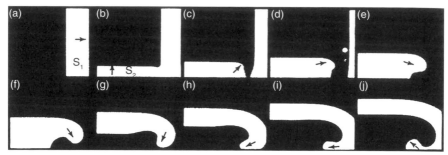

Figure 7.12 Initiation of spiral wave activity by cross-field stimulation in a homogeneous excitable medium. White area represents excitation, and black area represents resting potential. Arrows indicate the direction of the wave front. (a) Basic (S_1) planar wave propagating from left to right. (b) Premature (S_2) planar wave initiated perpendicularly from the bottom border of the array. (c) The S_2 wave front breaks into the refractory tail of S_1 and develops a pronounced curvature. (d–j) Curling of the wave front and initiation of a clockwise-rotating spiral. Frame-to-frame intervals are 16 milliseconds for panels (a–e) and 24 milliseconds for panels (f–j).

front with an anatomic or a functional obstacle. This is not much different from what was originally considered the mechanism for initiation of reentrant activity. The difference, however, is the recent notion that reentry may be initiated in totally homogeneous (anatomically and functionally) media. The only condition is the existence of a transient heterogeneity in the system, which in the heart may be induced by the application of two appropriately timed (S_1 and S_2) stimuli, each from a different site, a protocol known as "cross-field" stimulation. As shown in Figure 7.12, cross-field stimulation consists of initiating a basic (S_1) plane wave followed closely by the initiation of a premature (S_2) plane wave perpendicularly to S_1. In the example of Figure 7.12a,b, S_1 was initiated from the left side, and S_2 was initiated from the bottom of a 2-D sheet of cardiac cells in a computer simulation. Because the wave front of S_2 was initiated before the repolarizing tail of S_1 disappeared, S_1 acted as an effective barrier for S_2 propagation along the right edge of the medium. As a result, the S_2 wave front was broken at that edge forming a phase singularity around which the wave front curled to initiate a rotor (panels d–j). Results from experiments in vivo as well as in vitro demonstrated that, when premature cross-field stimulation is used, both the location of the rotor and the type of rotation can be controlled by the parameters of stimulation, which is what the theory predicts.

Excitability and Core Size

The center of functionally determined reentrant activity may vary in size and shape, depending on the excitability of the medium. The mechanism by which low excitability leads to a larger core may be derived from the results shown

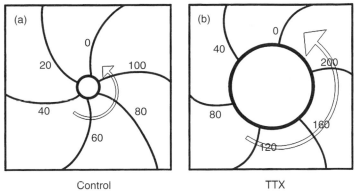

Figure 7.13 Effect of tetrodotoxin (TTX) on the size of the core of a stationary spiral wave. (a) Control. (b) During superfusion with TTX, an increase in the core size results in doubling of the rotation period. Curved arrows indicate direction of propagation; curved lines are isochrones; numbers are in milliseconds from an arbitrary zero time.

in Figures 7.5 and 7.6. At relatively low levels of excitability, the trajectory of the wavebreak tends to open. In fact, the lower the excitability, the less pronounced is the critical curvature. Accordingly, only the portions of the spiral wave front with lesser curvature are able to propagate. This leads to an opening of the trajectory of the wavebreak and of the whole wave front. In the case of spiral waves, changes in the trajectory of the wavebreak are directly reflected by changes in the size of the core. Figure 7.13 compares control conditions (panel a) with those prevailing when the excitability is reduced. The lower the excitability, the more open will be the trajectory of the wavebreak and the larger the size of the core (Figure 7.13). As a consequence, the path length of the spiral tip around the core will be increased, and thus the rotation period will be prolonged. Obviously, decreased excitability will lead to decrease in overall conduction velocity as a result of reduced availability of Na channels at any value of curvature. These predictions were corroborated in experiments in which the size of the core of a stationary spiral wave in isolated cardiac muscle was significantly increased by the addition of small concentrations of the Na channel blocker tetrodotoxin (TTX).

The Excitable Gap

Slowly rotating spirals with a large fully excitable gap are demonstrable even in totally homogeneous isotropic excitable media. In such cases, the necessary condition for the presence of an excitable gap is in fact the presence of a steep positive curvature near the tip of the spiral wave front.

Consequently, there are reductions in both the local current density and the ability of the wave front near the tip to excite tissue ahead of it. Hence, the conduction velocity is also reduced. This means that slow rotation is possible even in the presence of a fully excitable gap. A direct demonstration of the

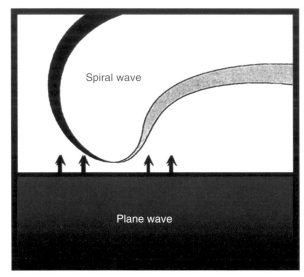

Figure 7.14 Interaction between a spiral wave and a planar wave generated by external stimulation.

existence of an excitable gap is the fact that externally induced propagating waves with lower curvature are able to invade the core region during spiral wave activity (Figure 7.14).

During stationary spiral wave activity, the core contributes to the formation of the excitable gap by electrotonically inducing premature repolarization in tissue located at distances as long as 1 cm from it. Indeed, computer simulations and experiments have confirmed that during stationary reentry, the action potential duration of cells near the center of rotation is shorter and conduction velocity is slower when compared with a situation in which the array is activated by planar waves at the same rate of the spiral. The electrotonic effect of the core on APD and conduction velocity (i.e., wavelength) is illustrated in panels (a) and (b) of Figure 7.15. The substantial shortening of APD and wavelength clearly explain why it is possible to induce stationary spiral waves in very small hearts such as those of mice and why the activity may reach rates that may be much higher than any achievable rates at which 1:1 (stimulus:response) activation is maintained during pacing. In addition, the presence of an excitable gap in those conditions indicates that, in general, the duration of the action potential is briefer during spiral wave activity than during planar waves.

Figure-of-8 Reentry and the Common Pathway

Figure-of-8 reentry (Figure 7.16), first described by El-Sherif *et al.* in a healed myocardial infarction model, is equivalent to two counter-rotating spirals separated by a relatively small distance.

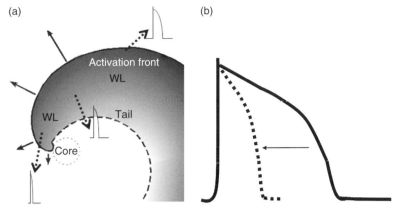

Figure 7.15 Diagrammatic representation of the effects of wave front curvature on conduction velocity and electrotonic effects of the core on action potential duration (APD) during spiral wave activity. (a) The increasing curvature of the wave front results in progressive reduction of conduction velocity toward the center (black arrows represent vectors whose magnitude is proportional to local velocity). Near the center, the velocity is critical and the core cannot be invaded and rotation ensues. Concomitantly, the APD and the wavelength (WL) are reduced progressively more toward the center as a result of repolarizing electrotonic influence exerted by the core and thus are exceedingly short at the spiral tip. Broken arrows point to APDs at three different locations. (b) Schematic representation of the repolarizing influence exerted by the core on APD in its immediate surroundings.

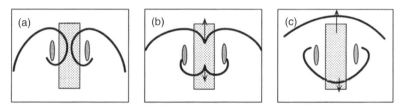

Figure 7.16 Propagation pattern in the common pathway of figure-of-8 reentry formed by two contiguous counter-rotating spirals in a computer simulation. In each frame, the activation wave front is depicted in black. The cores are represented by gray ellipses. Arrows indicate the direction of propagation at each point of the wave fronts. The dashed area represents the common pathway. (a) The common pathway is invaded by two curved wave fronts. (b) Collision of the wave fronts leads to the formation of two new wave fronts with negative curvature. As a result of the negative curvature, propagation both in the orthodromic (down-ward) and antidromic (upward) directions is faster than normal. (c) A few milliseconds later, the fused wave front develops positive curvature, which slows down propagation in both directions.

In the case of pairs of counter-rotating spirals occurring in homogeneous tissue, the common pathway is a region in which the activity largely depends on the interaction between the wave fronts arising from each spiral. Thus, the common pathway may show varying propagation patterns and velocities, depending upon the curvature of the resultant wave fronts. As shown schematically in Figure 7.16, computer simulations using homogeneous matrices of simulated cardiac cells demonstrate the interaction between two curved wave fronts at the level of the common pathway. First, as the two spiral tips develop their rotating course, there is a region in which both wave fronts collide and fuse (panel b). Subsequently, propagation of the two fused wave fronts continues toward the ends of the collision line (arrows). Conduction velocity in the orthodromic (downward) and antidromic (upward) directions is accelerated by the presence of a negative curvature. A few milliseconds later (panel c), however, the fused wave front in the orthodromic direction develops a positive curvature and propagates more slowly. The interaction between the waves and the resulting changes in conduction velocity may vary, depending on the distance between the cores.

Experimental measurements of conduction velocity in the region of the common pathway using optical mapping showed higher values during reentrant activity compared with the conduction velocity of planar waves. Yet, it is important to note that, in clinical cases of reentrant tachycardia, conduction velocity of the common pathway may be affected by pre-existing local heterogeneities of the tissue. However, even in completely homogeneous systems, conduction velocity is greatly influenced by the interaction of two curved wave fronts. Hence, conduction velocity during figure-of-8 reentry may be expected to be faster or slower than that during the propagation of a planar wave, depending on the site of measurement. Interestingly, a lesion that bridges the centers of the spirals through the "common pathway" should lead to interruption of the activity. Finally, according to the theory of rotating spiral waves, figure-of-8 reentry in 3-D myocardium may indeed represent the surface activation of a more complex structure, such as a U-shaped scroll wave or the coexistence of two counter-rotating scroll waves spanning a ventricular wall from endocardium to epicardium.

Drifting Spirals

Because the core remains excitable during spiral wave activity, it is not surprising that small changes in the conditions of the spiral wave tip (i.e., small changes in the excitability of the tissue) may lead to shifts in the trajectory of the wavebreak with activation of the core area. This is schematically shown in Figure 7.17. In panel (a), a spiral wave rotates around a core located at point 1 in a simulated cardiac cell array. A few rotations later, in panel (b), the core moved to the bottom left quadrant.

To move from one point to the other, the wave front must have invaded and moved through the original core. Under such conditions, the phase singularity at wave front tip necessarily loses its stationary cyclic trajectory (either circular or elliptical) and may either undergo a cycloidal motion (Figure 7.18a) within an enclosed area (meandering spiral) or follow a rather linear pathway (drifting spiral; Figure 7.18b). It would be difficult to reconcile drifting with other proposed mechanisms of functional reentry, including leading

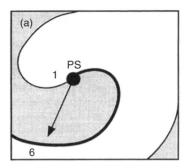
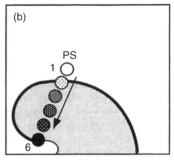

Figure 7.17 Drifting spiral wave. (a) The phase singularity (PS) driving the rotating activity is originally at point 1 and begins to drift downward and to the left (arrow). (b) After a few rotations, the PS has moved from its point of origin at 1 to point 6 on the bottom left quadrant and forced the spiral wave activity to drift with it.

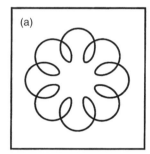
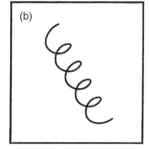

Figure 7.18 Drifting rotors may have various types of trajectories. (a) Flowerlike trajectory of a meandering rotor. (b) Cycloids in a more linear trajectory (drift).

circle and anisotropic reentry. On the other hand, drifting was demonstrated for rotors occurring in various types of excitable media as well as in computer simulations. The following are some of the characteristics of drifting rotors occurring in 2-D cardiac tissue:

1. Drifting may occur spontaneously in isolated cardiac preparations. Computer simulations showed that there are parameter ranges at which drift is expected to occur even in the absence of gradients or heterogeneities. In most experimental cases, however, asymmetries in the form of spatial gradients either in APD or conduction velocity are found that may be responsible for the drift.
2. Computer models and experimental studies showed that, in cases of APD gradients, the direction of the drift is toward the longer APD. On the other hand, in the presence of conduction velocity gradients, the direction of the drift is toward the region of slower conduction velocity.
3. Drift may occur at the interface between regions with different electrophysiological characteristics: when the rotor sits in between two regions

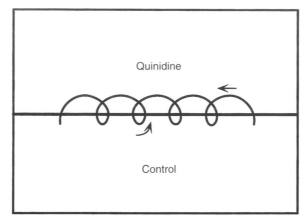

Figure 7.19 Diagrammatic representation of drift occurring at the interface between a region of prolonged action potential duration (APD) (top half) and a region of short APD (bottom half). In the actual experiment (not shown), APD prolongation on the top half of a small piece of cardiac tissue was induced by superfusion with quinidine. The trajectory of the phase singularity is more linear in the region of prolonged action potential, thus forcing the counterclockwise rotating spiral wave to move from right to left.

of different (i.e., normal and slow) conduction velocities, the drift is parallel to the interface in a direction that depends on the chirality (i.e., sense of rotation) of the spiral (Figure 7.19).

4. Drift velocity in isolated myocardium is approximately 10–30% of the velocity of propagation of a planar wave.
5. Because the heart represents a finite excitable medium, drifting spirals tend to have a short life. Collision of drifting spirals with unexcitable boundaries may result in annihilation of the activity.
6. Even in the presence of gradients, drifting spirals may suddenly turn into stationary spirals when they anchor to anatomic discontinuities. Furthermore, even in the presence of relatively strong gradients, spiral waves may be stationary if the core is anchored to a relatively large discontinuity.
7. During drift, spiral waves give rise to a Doppler effect (Figure 7.20), whereby the activation rate ahead of the core is faster than that behind the core. Doppler effect is responsible for the occurrence of complex activation patterns recorded electrocardiographically during drifting spiral wave activity.

Drifting Spirals and Electrocardiographic Patterns

Drifting spirals may result in complex electrocardiographic (ECG) patterns and may explain the transition between polymorphic and monomorphic tachycardias. The use of high-resolution optical mapping techniques enabled the demonstration that drifting spiral waves give rise to irregular

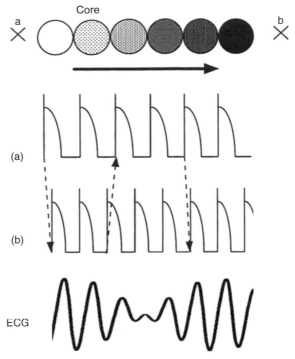

Figure 7.20 Doppler effect of spiral drift. Points "a" and "b" represent two fixed recording sites bounding the trajectory of a moving rotor. As shown by the respective action potentials, the activation rate produced by the rightward movement of the core is slower on the left recording site (a) than on the right recording site (b). There are six action potentials in panel (a) and eight action potentials in panel (b). The activation sequence changes on a beat-to-beat basis as shown by the arrows and results in a torsades-like pattern in the ECG.

spatiotemporal patterns of activation that result from a Doppler effect. The Doppler effect is a ubiquitous phenomenon in nature that is caused by the movement of any wave source with a consequent shift in the periodicity of the wave front, depending on the observation point. This is illustrated in Figure 7.20. In this example, as the spiral wave rotates, the core moves from left to right. Recordings of the electric activity at fixed points behind (site "a") and ahead (site "b") of the core show different activation periods, which depend on both the rotation period of the spiral and the velocity of the drift. Notice that the coexistence of two slightly different activation rates creates a situation in which there is a constant shift of the sequence of activation. It was demonstrated that these variations in the sequence of activation are accompanied by specific ECG patterns, including torsades de pointes.

Doppler Effect and Torsades de Pointes

Astronomers use the Doppler effect to estimate the relative velocity of stars or galaxies, and, for many years, physiologists have relied on the same phenomenon to calculate blood flow and other physiological variables. In cardiac electrophysiology, the Doppler effect provides a new means to explain the mechanism of irregular patterns of activation during reentrant activity. Indeed, as shown in Figure 7.20, during drift there are at least two dominant cycle lengths, a short one ahead and a long one behind the core. In isolated cardiac muscle, we found that the drift velocity is approximately 10% of the wave propagation in the same direction, which results in a difference in activation rates of ~20%. When the drift occurs in only one direction at a constant velocity, the ratio of activation ahead over activation behind the core is also constant (4:3, 5:4, etc.). Accordingly, the activation sequence may change periodically throughout the episode. For instance, during the first and second action potentials shown in Figure 7.20, activation occurred earlier in point "b" (placed on the left) than in point "a" (placed on the right). However, a few beats later, the sequence of activation completely reversed.

For more than 40 years, the ECG pattern observed in cases of torsades de pointes puzzled electrocardiologists and electrophysiologists. In fact, it is difficult to explain why the QRS axis gradually changes in a rather predictable manner in each episode of the arrhythmia. Early experiments were able to mimic the ECG pattern by pacing a canine heart with two electrodes placed one in each ventricle and using a slightly different stimulation frequency. Since then, the idea that two separate pacemakers may be responsible for the episodes of torsades de pointes was prevalent. Yet, the idea that two separate pacemakers may be activated at the same time and have similar but yet different rates made this hypothesis unlikely. On the basis of Doppler shifts observed during drifting spiral waves, we proposed a new way to explain the polymorphism in the ECG. The idea is that a single spiral wave migrating in one direction at a constant velocity will give rise to two slightly different frequencies. Thus, the global ECG appearance of the activity should be a gradual and periodic change in the direction of the QRS axis, similarly to that induced by dual pacing (see the schematic ECG of Figure 7.21). The interesting feature, however, is that, in the case of a drifting spiral, both frequencies

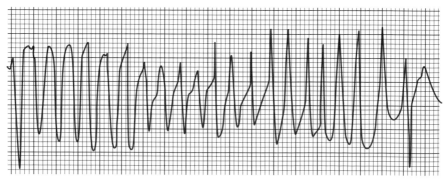

Figure 7.21 Example of torsades de pointes type of ventricular tachycardia (VT) obtained in a human heart.

are produced by a single wave source. More recent experiments using both isolated cardiac tissue and Langendorff-perfused hearts demonstrated that indeed a single drifting spiral wave gives rise to ECG patterns that very much resemble those observed during torsades de pointes (Figure 7.21).

Furthermore, in some cases, a single spiral wave can drift throughout the ventricles at very high and variable speeds. Under these conditions, the ECG pattern of activation may be totally irregular and difficult to distinguish from VF.

Anchoring and the Transition from Polymorphic to Monomorphic Activation

Drifting spirals are fleeting. The brief life span of drifting spirals is the result of either spontaneous termination or transformation into a stationary spiral as a result of anchoring. Even normal preparations of cardiac tissue contain heterogeneities such fibrosis, scars, or small branches of the coronary arteries that may act as anchoring points. In the case of 2-D preparations, even small (~1–2 mm) discontinuities may serve as an anchor of a drifting spiral wave. Theoretical studies suggested that, in a 2-D medium, a drifting spiral wave may anchor to a given obstacle if the size of that obstacle is at least as large as the size of the core (Figure 7.22). As will be discussed, the latter statement does not necessarily apply to reentry in 3-D media. Anchoring of a drifting spiral may express in the ECG as the transition from polymorphic to monomorphic tachycardia.

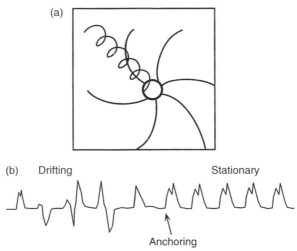

Figure 7.22 Anchoring of a spiral wave underlies the transformation of a polymorphic tachycardia into a monomorphic tachycardia. (a) Diagrammatic trajectory of the core during drift (from top to bottom and left to right) and anchoring (in the right bottom corner of the array) of a spiral wave. (b) Schematic ECG recording showing the transition between polymorphic and monomorphic ventricular tachycardia (VT).

Effects of Externally Applied Waves on Spiral Wave Dynamics

It is well known that electrical pacing may either terminate or change the rate and/or ECG appearance of reentrant ventricular tachycardia. However, the dynamics of interaction of reentrant waves with waves initiated by external pacing are poorly understood. Prevailing concepts on the effects of pacing on reentrant activity (i.e., resetting and entrainment) are based on models in which propagation occurs in 1-D rings of cardiac tissue. Because reentrant activation in the ventricles may occur also in two or three dimensions, such concepts might be insufficient to explain the mechanisms of pacing-induced effects. Recent studies used numerical and biological models of cardiac excitation to explore the phenomena that may take place as a result of pacing during functionally determined reentry. According to the theory of nonlinear waves, three major types of phenomena may take place in any given excitable medium as a result of the interaction of two propagating waves: collision, fusion, and wavebreak. As illustrated schematically in Figure 7.23, the result of the interaction between two waves depends on the shape of the individual waves as well as on the region of the wave that is affected by such an interaction (i.e., the wave front or the wave tail). The interaction between two planar wave fronts propagating toward each other is shown in panels (a) and (b). In this case, head-on collision (panel b) results in mutual annihilation of the waves. In panels (c) and (d), the interaction between a planar wave front and a wave front with positive curvature leads to fusion (marked with F) at each end of the collision line. The two newly formed wave fronts have a pronounced negative curvature (i.e., the wave front is concave), which results in faster conduction velocity in the upward and downward directions. Panels (e) and (f) illustrate the kind of interaction that occurs between two orthogonally propagating waves initiated one shortly after the other by the method or cross-field stimulation. In panel (e), a planar wave front (S_1), initiated by simultaneous stimulation of the leftmost column of cells, propagated toward the right border of the matrix. Shortly thereafter, a second planar wave (S_2) was initiated by simultaneous stimulation of all the cells in the top row. The S_2 wave intersected the repolarizing tail of S_1. As a result, a wavebreak took place at the intersection point. The broken wave front then developed into a rotating spiral wave (panel f). Hence, a broken wave front develops into a rotor, which is the sine qua non condition for the formation of spiral wave activity, although its persistence as such depends on the presence (or lack thereof) of other waves as well as on its interaction with the borders of the medium. Collision, fusion, and wavebreaks occur during the interaction between self-sustaining spiral waves and waves initiated by external stimulation.

Depending upon the initial position of the wavebreaks, the result of the stimulation may be termination, multiplication of the spiral (i.e., simultaneous occurrence of two or more spiral waves), or shift in the core position.

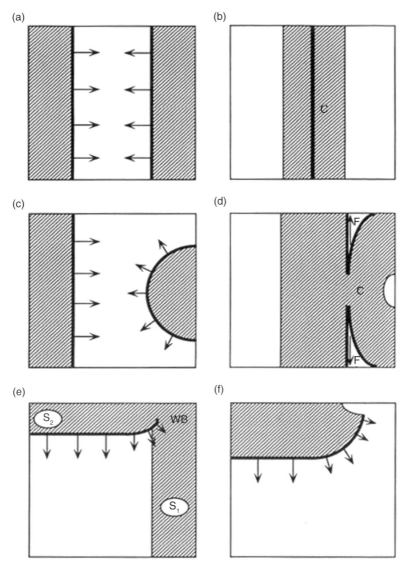

Figure 7.23 Schematic representation of the interaction between pairs of propagating waves of varying shapes and time relations. The wave front is represented by a thick black line. The repolarizing tail is represented by a dashed area. Arrows indicate the direction of propagation. The length of the arrows is proportional to the propagation velocity. (a,b) Interaction between two planar wave fronts that were initiated from opposite sides of the array. The collision (C) of the two wave fronts is followed by interruption of the propagation. (c,d) Interaction between a planar wave front initiated from the left and a curved wave front initiated from the right. Collision is followed by fusion (F) and formation of new wave fronts with negative curvature and high conduction velocity. (e) Interaction between a planar wave front initiated by stimulation of the top border and the repolarizing tail of a planar wave initiated sometime earlier from the left border. The right part of the wave front finds an increasing degree of refractoriness, which results in decreasing degree of penetration and finally breakage (i.e., wavebreak, WB) of the new wave front. (f) Spiral wave activity resulting from a WB.

Multiplication and shift of the spiral core are attended by changes in rate and morphology of the arrhythmia. Both numerical predictions and experimental results support the hypothesis that whether a pacing stimulus will terminate a reentrant arrhythmia or modify its ECG appearance depends on whether the interactions between the externally induced wave and the spiral wave result in the de novo formation of one or more wavebreaks. The outcome depends on the stimulus parameters (i.e., position and size of the electrodes and timing of the stimulus) as well as on the position of the newly formed wavebreak(s) in relation to that of the original wave. Thus, although more simplistic models of reentry were used for the analysis of the effects of pacing on reentrant excitation, the outcome of pacing may be the result of interaction that is more complex than that predicted by 1-D models.

Three-Dimensional Scrolls

The foregoing provides an overview of the general characteristics of reentrant activity in two dimensions. However, accurate understanding of the mechanisms of reentrant arrhythmias in the whole heart requires knowledge about the manner in which electric waves propagate in three spatial dimensions. Hence, the next logical step in the study of vortex-like reentry is the extension into the 3-D myocardium. Myocardial tissue is essentially 3-D, and it is important to understand what happens in the thickness of the atrial or ventricular wall when vortex-like reentry occurs. Of course, only experimental studies can provide a definite answer to this question, and, to our knowledge, present-day technology has not developed to the point at which 3-D propagation in the heart can be recorded with sufficient temporal and spatial resolution to provide reliable information about the detailed mechanisms of the arrhythmias. However, some qualitative features of 3-D reentry can be predicted from theoretical analysis, assuming that the analogy between functional reentry and spiral waves will hold in three dimensions.

Three-dimensional vortices were predicted in numerical experiments using anisotropic cubical models of 3-D excitable media described by reaction–diffusion equations such as the FitzHugh–Nagumo equations and were first observed by Arthur Winfree in 1973 in thick layers of the B–Z reaction (a chemical excitable medium). Figure 7.24a–d shows sequential frames of the simplest 3-D vortex obtained using the FitzHugh–Nagumo model. Because of its shape, such a vortex is called a scroll wave. The rotation axis of the scroll wave is shown by a vertical dashed line. In this example, the scroll wave rotates in a clockwise direction, and in each cross section perpendicular to the rotation axis, one may see an identical spiral wave. The activation pattern generated by the rotating scroll wave on the surfaces of the cube depends significantly on the orientation of the rotation axis with respect to the surface. When the axis is parallel to the surface, one would observe an elongated breakthrough area from which planar waves emanate. The rotating spiral wave can be observed only from the top and the bottom of the cube.

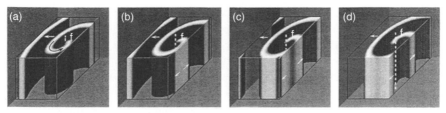

Figure 7.24 Three-dimensional vortex-like reentry in the form of a simple scroll wave obtained in computer simulations using the FitzHugh–Nagumo (FHN) model. The model consisted of an array of $48 \times 48 \times 48$ FHN elements connected to each other through a diffusion term. The cuboidal array was anisotropic in that the element size in the x-axis was twice as large as that in the y- and z-axes. Panels (a–d) are sequential snapshots of counterclockwise rotating excitation wave. Unexcited areas are transparent. The rotation axis f (filament) is shown by the broken line. White arrows indicate the direction of propagation. Approximately one-half of a rotation cycle is shown. Reentry was initiated using the cross-field stimulation method; the basic (S_1) and premature stimuli (S_2) were delivered from the front and left lateral surfaces, respectively (see text for further details).

Basic scroll wave filament shapes

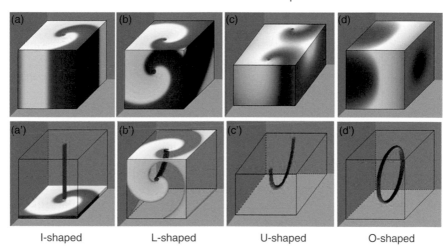

I-shaped   L-shaped   U-shaped   O-shaped

Figure 7.25 Basic configurations of vortex-like reentry in three dimensions. (a and a') Stable scroll wave organized by an I-shaped filament. The scroll rotates in the counterclockwise direction. Unstable scroll wave (b) rotating clockwise and organized by an L-shaped filament (b'). (c and c') Unstable figure-of-eight reentry organized by a U-shaped scroll filament. (d and d') O-shaped scroll wave and filament (see text for further details).

The rotation axis of the scroll wave is not rigid. Moreover, its rotation axis in space is not necessarily a straight line: it may curve and even form closed loops. This means that there are a variety of possible spatial configurations of 3-D vortices. Such different configurations may be described in terms of the filament, which is the line about which the excitation wave rotates. In Figure 7.25, we present four different examples of scroll wave filaments. Panel (a) shows a stable linear scroll wave (top) with its I-shaped filament (bottom) that spans the cube from top to bottom (bottom) in this simplistic cubic model of homogeneous cardiac tissue. In panel (b), a scroll wave with an L-shaped filament is shown. One end of the filament is on the top face of the cube; however, instead of running all the way down to the bottom, the filament turns toward the front and comes out on the frontal face of the cube, causing a spiral wave on this face. Panel (c) shows a scroll wave with a U-shaped filament. After making a loop (the turning point of the filament is close to the center of the cube), the filament comes back to the top surface. On the top of the cube, one may see therefore two counter-rotating spirals that in fact belong to the same scroll wave. At the same time on the bottom surface, one observes a breakthrough that initiates circular waves. Panel (d) shows a scroll wave with a filament forming a ring (O-shaped filament). In the literature this is known as a "scroll ring" or "vortex ring." From the outside, the excitation waves generated by the scroll ring look like spherical waves (top). However, the activity is clearly caused by an O-shaped rotor in 3-D space. Despite having the same nature and similar properties, the appearance on the surface of the four vortices shown in Figure 7.25 is quite different in each case. For example, on the top surface of the cube the vortex with the L-shaped filament (Figure 7.25b) appears as a single reentrant loop. The vortex with U-shaped filament (Figure 7.25c) generates a double reentrant loop or figure-of-8 reentry. Finally, the vortex with O-shaped filament (Figure 7.25d) appears on the top as a focal source of excitation. For the last case no reentrant activity can be seen from any surface of the cube.

Figure 7.26 depicts a more realistic simulation of a steady-state scroll wave with an I-shaped filament. In this simulation, the shell-like structure is a snapshot of the electrical activity in the heart. It surrounds the unexcited filament, shown as a tube extending between the two anchor points (epicardium on top, endocardium at the bottom), which help ensure filament stability. The complexity of the filament shape, as seen in Figure 7.26, is due to the changing directions of maximum propagation speed as a result of that gradual change in fiber orientation from the epicardial to endocardial surfaces, pretty much as in ventricular heart muscle; we refer to this configuration as "twisted anisotropy." Generally speaking, a rotating scroll, and especially its filament, is shaped by the geometry of the medium.

These 3-D simulations illustrate how the variability of the excitation patterns generated by 3-D vortices and manifested on one or another surface and their dependence on the cardiac tissue structure makes the characterization of a 3-D reentry based on surface recordings extremely difficult. A case in point is provided by the even more realistic simulation presented in Figure 7.27, which shows in panel (a) the intramural activity at 1990 milliseconds (10 cycles) after the onset of sustained reentry in a geometrically accurate model of the dog right (RV) and left (LV) ventricles. At that time, the repetitive generation of 3-D scroll waves (red) had become relatively stable. The scroll wave filament seen in panel (b) had curled such that one of its ends was located

(Transmural scroll wave)

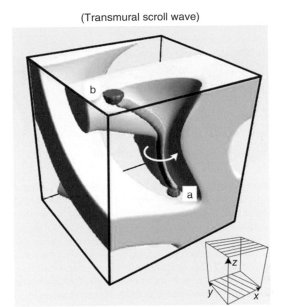

Figure 7.26 A steady-state scroll and filament under uniform left-handed twisted anisotropy. Near the top boundary, the fibers are parallel to the x-axis; near the bottom they are rotated by 120° (although still parallel to the xy plane). The twist and anisotropy are comparable to observations in the human ventricular wall. The propagating potential is displayed here as a snapshot of the region (yellow) where it is above a cutoff value equal to 50% of maximum. The filament (green) is the tubular surface described over time by the locus of two independent propagating variables with fixed assigned values; the scroll rotates in the direction of the small elliptical arrow. The filament is anchored to a pair of small boundary protrusions (red) "a" and "b." Note how the local anisotropy flattens the filament's cross section into approximately a small ellipse. The scroll results from the use of FitzHugh–Nagumo-type model. The choice of this model, as well as of a cubic enclosure, is for illustrative purposes only and does not reflect in any way on the generality of the work. (Reproduced with permission from Wellner *et al.*, *Proc Natl Acad Sci* 2002; 99:8015–8.)

near the center of the endocardium of the LV free wall. Toward its center, the filament aligned vertically downward, and then it bent steeply to form a horizontal loop around the LV apex and climbed upward to reattach its other end to the endocardium at the bottom of the LV free wall. Despite its complicated shape, the filament shown is topologically equivalent to a U-type filament and is therefore consistent with endocardial figure-of-8 reentry giving rise to a single epicardial breakthrough. Once again the complex shape of the filament results in great measure on the twisted anisotropy of the ventricular fibers (panel c), which change ~120 degrees in orientation from endocardium to epicardium. Analysis at later stages (not shown) demonstrated that the shape of the filament was not significantly different from that seen at 1990 milliseconds in Figure 7.27.

The concept of filament not only simplifies the classification of all possible configurations of 3-D vortices but also allows the shape of the wave front,

Scroll wave in whole heart model

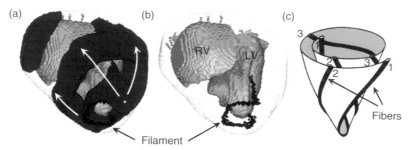

Figure 7.27 Three-dimensional visualization of scroll wave activity in a realistic geometrical model of the dog ventricles with twisted anisotropy. Simulations were carried out using FitzHugh–Nagumo kinetics. (a) An epicardial breakthrough (asterisk) emerged as a result of intramural reentry. Dark lines of points near the apex of the left ventricle (LV) outline the filament of the scroll wave, shown in panel (b) for clarity. Excited model elements are colored red, white arrows indicate the direction of propagation as seen on the epicardium, and the ventricular cavities are colored beige. Numbers indicate the time of activation in milliseconds. The U-type filament (left) is curled around the apex and results in the epicardial breakthrough. (c) Diagrammatic representation of twisted anisotropy in the left ventricle.

surface activation patterns, and dynamics to be predicted from the geometry of the filament.

Scroll waves with curved filaments and vortex rings can be formed by premature stimulation at the boundaries between zones of differing refractory periods, which are known to appear in damaged myocardium. Theory predicts that the geometry of filaments that emerge in this type of experiment should be determined by the geometry of the boundary between normal areas and areas with increased refractoriness and, thus, may be very complex.

Dynamics of Scroll Waves

The variety of 3-D configurations of scroll waves may develop a variety of dynamical behaviors even in homogeneous media. Any deformation of the filament and deviation from the rectilinear shape results in complex vortex dynamics. This motion involves not just drift but also evolution of the filament shape. Although the intrinsic motion of the filament is slow relative to the speed of excitation propagation, it may be responsible for the overall stability of the vortex and its lifetime. When applied to reentry in myocardium, such a motion (as well as the drift due to heterogeneities discussed previously) may account for the duration and stability of arrhythmia as well as formation of activation patterns similar to those of polymorphic tachycardia and torsades de pointes.

As a simple example of the intrinsic motion of the filament that might be applicable to reentry in the myocardium, consider the phenomenon of drift and shrinking of vortex rings. In contrast to simple scroll waves that are usually stationary and may rotate indefinitely in homogeneous media, a vortex with O-shaped filament is, as a rule, unstable (the same holds true for U- and L-shaped filaments). Its filament slowly shrinks and simultaneously drifts along the line perpendicular the filament plane. Both shrinking and drifting accelerate as the filament becomes smaller and its curvature increases. Eventually the filament shrinks to nothing or hits the border of the medium and the vortex disappears. This phenomenon was predicted in computer simulations of the FitzHugh–Nagumo model and later demonstrated experimentally in the B–Z reaction. It was hypothesized that vortices with shrinking O-shaped filaments underlie short-lasting paroxysms of tachycardia in myocardium. As already mentioned, the theory predicts that the speed of drift and shrinking is proportional to the curvature of the filament. The larger the initial size of the ring, the slower it drifts and shrinks and, thus, the longer it can exist.

It should be noted that we consider only the intrinsic motion of the vortices due to curvature of the filament. Heterogeneity and parameter gradients that cause drift of vortices in two dimensions are important in three dimensions as well. It is quite possible that the dynamics of 3-D vortices in myocardium is a combination of the intrinsic motion and drift due to parameter gradients. The study of 3-D vortices in heterogeneous media is still in its infancy. However, the significance of such combined effects was demonstrated in numerical experiments showing anchoring of drifting scroll waves to small localized inhomogeneities. Anchoring was thought of as one of the mechanisms responsible for the stabilization of high-frequency rhythms in the myocardium.

Experimental Detection of Three-Dimensional Vortex-like Reentry in Cardiac Muscle

The direct observation of 3-D vortex-like reentry would require highly sophisticated high-resolution intramural mapping techniques that remain elusive at the present time. However, certain inferences can be made on the basis of more readily available electrophysiological methods. For example, the question of what is happening in the thickness of the myocardium during spiral wave reentry may be readily inferred using simultaneous high-resolution recordings of electric activity from the endocardium and epicardium. In the top panel of Figure 7.28, we present seven consecutive snapshots of sustained, stationary reentrant activity recorded optically on the epicardium of the left ventricle of a Langendorff-perfused rabbit heart. The model in the bottom panel predicts that in this case, the activity must be the result of a transmural I-shaped filament whose two ends are anchored to the endocardium and epicardium. While no endocardial recordings were obtained in this particular case, the stability of the epicardial spiral wave pattern strongly suggests the presence of an I-shaped scroll filament. By contrast, Figure 7.29 shows another experimental example in which simultaneous epicardial and endocardial

(a) Surface spiral waves

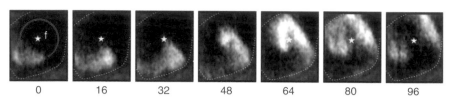

(b) Transmural scroll wave

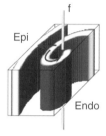

Figure 7.28 Deductive analysis of three-dimensional activity from surface optical recording of reentry in isolated Langendorff-perfused rabbit heart. (a) Seven consecutive snapshots of sustained, stationary stable spiral wave activity recorded from the epicardium. (b) Single three-dimensional scroll wave with I-shaped filament may explain the pattern of activity seen on the epicardium in this experiment.

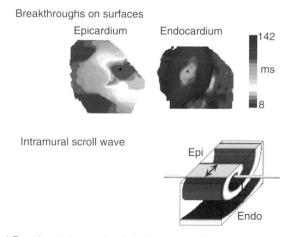

Figure 7.29 (top) Experimental example of simultaneous epicardial and endocardial recordings during sustained reentrant activity in a coronary perfused left ventricular wedge preparation. No spiral waves were observed on either surface. However, spatiotemporal periodic break-through patterns emerged on both surfaces in a coordinated manner from the mid-myocardium. Epicardial breakthroughs occurred always slightly ahead (see color bar) of the endocardial breakthroughs. (bottom) The experimental pattern may be explained by the presence of an intramural scroll whose filament lies parallel to both surfaces. (Reproduced with permission from Baxter *et al.*, *Biophys J* 2001; 80:516–30.)

recordings were obtained from the left ventricle in a wedge preparation during sustained tachycardia induced by rapid pacing. In this case, no spiraling activity was observed on either ventricular surface. Instead, spatiotemporal periodic patterns of breakthrough activity appeared on both surfaces in a coordinated manner, with epicardial breakthroughs occurring always slightly ahead (see color isochrones) of the endocardial breakthroughs. A reasonable interpretation for these results is that a scroll wave whose filament lies parallel to the surfaces was responsible for the activity. Alternatively, it is possible that this activity might have been produced by focal intramural ectopic pacemaker or triggered discharges. While the latter possibility may not be ruled out completely, the stability of the activity, and the experimental conditions in which such activity was initiated (rapid burst pacing) and maintained (healthy preparation, no calcium overload) lead one to favor the scroll wave hypothesis.

Summary

Reentrant arrhythmias occurring around functionally determined obstacles are analogous to spiral waves occurring in generic excitable media. Some of the clinical manifestations of these arrhythmias are poorly explained by more conventional electrophysiological models of reentry. The theory of spiral waves, on the other hand, offers a new approach for the study of arrhythmias. Spontaneously occurring complex patterns of activation, as well as various dynamics resulting from external stimulation, are clearly predicted by theoretical and experimental studies on spiral waves. In addition, this new approach offers new clues for the understanding of reentrant processes occurring in the complex three dimensionality of the heart.

8 Rotors and the Mechanisms of Atrial Fibrillation

Cardiac fibrillation is one of the most important causes of morbidity and mortality in the developed world, but its mechanisms are still far from being understood. For a number of years, investigators have focused on the role of certain ion channels and are also providing new fundamental knowledge about the dynamics and molecular mechanisms of both atrial (AF) and ventricular (VF) fibrillation in humans. In this and the following chapter, we make use of the fundamental knowledge outlined in Chapters 1–7 and in the relevant literature to provide a bird's eye view of the contemporary understanding of AF and VF mechanisms, evaluating the clinical relevance of such knowledge.

Approximately 2.3 million people in the United States are currently afflicted by AF, which makes it the most common sustained cardiac arrhythmia in humans. AF is also the most important cause of stroke. AF is an electrical derangement of cardiac excitation and propagation whose initiation depends on the presence of triggers and its maintenance requires an appropriate arrhythmogenic substrate. Yet, despite general awareness of the factors underlying normal and abnormal impulse initiation and propagation in the atria, the mechanisms of AF in humans have not been adequately explained and its therapy remains suboptimal. There appears to be the consensus, however, that most cases of sustained AF are initiated by abnormal electrical waves that emerge spontaneously from focal triggers, often localized in the great cardiac veins or the atria. The waves must propagate through an atrial tissue substrate that is conducive to AF maintenance. Although the precise nature of such foci is currently unknown, they are likely to generate rapid discharges secondary to the formation of EADs or DADs (see Chapter 6) at discrete sites as a result of local derangements of unknown etiology. Alternatively, AF may also be initiated by a wavebreak (see Chapter 7) formed by the interaction of a wave

Basic Cardiac Electrophysiology for the Clinician, 2nd edition. By J. Jalife, M. Delmar, J. Anumonwo, O. Berenfeld and J. Kalifa. Published 2009 by Blackwell Publishing, ISBN: 978-1-4501-8333-8.

front of any origin (e.g., an impulse generated by the sinus node) that encounters heterogeneously recovered atrial tissue in its path, leading to the initiation of reentrant activity. Regardless of its electrophysiological mechanism, the trigger does not act in isolation but AF initiation requires an appropriate substrate for its maintenance and for the formation of reentrant sources of sustained activity. Clearly, the normal atria may become such a substrate, at least transiently, as it occurs experimentally in animals and also in patients with paroxysmal AF. However, perpetuation of the arrhythmia, as in the case of chronic AF, requires a substantially altered substrate secondary to pathophysiologic changes in intercellular communication and in the intracellular and extracellular environments of the cardiac cells, which favor continuing formation and/or maintenance of the reentrant sources and abnormal impulse propagation.

The central objective of this chapter is to discuss recent experimental and clinical evidence supporting the hypothesis that sustained AF does not depend on a totally random propagation of electrical impulses. Rather, the data suggest that there is a high degree of determinism in AF whereby the fibrillatory waves organize both in space and time to generate measurable, yet complex patterns of atrial excitation and propagation. In other words, it has been shown in isolated hearts from sheep that maintenance of acute AF depends on localized high-frequency reentrant source(s) in the left atrium (LA) spawning fibrillatory conduction toward its periphery. On the other hand, in human patients, spectral analysis and measurements of the distribution of activation rates suggest that similar reentrant sources are localized for the most part at or near the pulmonary veins (PVs) in the case of paroxysmal AF, but elsewhere in the case of chronic AF. In this regard, the resulting high-frequency excitation patterns at the source and the complex dynamics of wave propagation underlying the fibrillatory activity are clearly predicted by theoretical and experimental studies on rotors and spiral waves.

Mechanism of Atrial Fibrillation: Multiple Wavelets versus Mother Rotor

In Chapter 7 we defined vortex-like reentry as a curved wave that rotates around an unexcited core and takes a spiral shape. The pivot point on the perimeter of the core is called the rotor and is the organizing center of the overall activity. Experimentally, optical mapping studies in atria and/or ventricles have shown a high degree of spatiotemporal organization during AF and rotors seem to be the drivers that maintain the activity, at least in some cases. Rotors may form when a wave breaks upon interacting with structural and/or electrophysiological heterogeneities in its path. In fact, it is now certain that wavebreak, leading to wavelet formation and rotor initiation (see Chapter 7), is the hallmark of any proposed explanation for AF or VF maintenance. When a rotor is formed, the rapidly succeeding wave fronts emanating from it propagate throughout the cardiac muscle and interact with

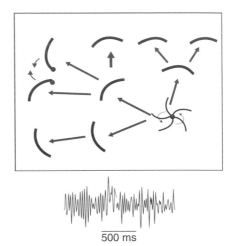

Figure 8.1 Schematic representation of a rotor generating rapidly succeeding wave fronts that propagate throughout the cardiac muscle and interact with anatomical and/or functional obstacles, causing fragmentation and new wavelet formation; i.e., fibrillatory conduction.

500 ms

anatomical and/or functional obstacles, causing fragmentation and new wavelet formation; i.e., fibrillatory conduction (Figure 8.1). Wavelets may undergo decremental conduction or may be annihilated by collision with another wavelet or a boundary, or may form new sustained rotors, resulting in a never-ending frequency-dependent fragmentation of wave fronts into what appears to be multiple independent wavelets. Accordingly, fibrillation is not totally unpredictable, but may be considered to have both deterministic and stochastic components; i.e., highly organized and periodic rotors as drivers, and randomly distributed fragmentation of the resulting wave fronts (fibrillatory conduction) leading to the formation of multiple wavelets. Thus, combining the rotor hypothesis with the multiple wavelet hypothesis offers a step closer to the understanding of the fibrillatory process. In other words, for multiple, randomly propagating wavelets to exist, there must be a source (e.g., a rotor) generating wave fronts at an exceedingly rapid rate. The interaction of those wave fronts with obstacles in their path results in the shedding of the wavelets. Therefore, irrespective of the underlying source, wavebreak and reentry account for the complex patterns of propagation, wavelet formation, and apparent aperiodic activity that characterize cardiac fibrillation. The manner in which different membrane ionic currents contribute to wavebreak, rotor stabilization, and wave fragmentation is now being successfully investigated at various levels of integration, from the molecule to the human patient. In the following sections we present some of the evidence supporting the idea that rotors are the sources that maintain AF.

The Sheep Model of Atrial Fibrillation

Since the late 1990s, extensive high-resolution mapping of the electrical activity during AF in the isolated Langendorff-perfused sheep heart has been an important source of information about AF dynamics and mechanisms. We selected the sheep heart because it resembles the human heart in overall size, morphology, and electrophysiological properties. Unless otherwise noted, the sheep were healthy and their hearts did not suffer from any disease. Hearts were excised and immediately connected to a Langendorff apparatus whereby oxygenated Tyrode's solution at body temperature and at pH of 7.4 was continuously perfused retrogradely against the aortic valve. The idea was to force the closure of the valve and direct the solution into the cardiac coronary arteries to keep the heart viable for the duration of the experiment. The Tyrode's solution contained a relatively low concentration of acetylcholine (ACh). Alternatively, the intra-atrial pressure was elevated to provide conditions for sustained AF for periods exceeding 20 minutes. Figure 8.2 is a diagram of the atria as seen from the head of the animal. It depicts the left atrial appendage (LAA), the right atrial appendage (RAA), the ostium of the PVs (in the sheep heart, the PVs often converge to a common ostium that opens into the posterior wall of the LA), the superior vena cava (SVC), the inferior vena cava (IVC), and the main bodies of the LA and RA. To study the patterns of activation during AF, we recorded potentiometric dye fluorescence simultaneously from about 20000 sites on either the RA free wall and on the LAA, or at the LAA and the LA posterior wall using two synchronized CCD cameras at a typical sampling interval of 8.33 milliseconds. The areas of each optically

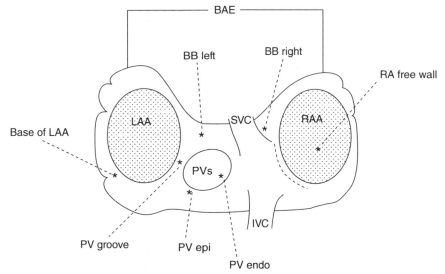

Figure 8.2 Schematic representation of the atria indicating the optical and electrode mapping locations. Hatched areas indicate optically mapped regions. BAE, biatrial electrogram; RAA, right atrial appendage; LAA, left atrial appendage; BB right, Bachmann's bundle right side; BB left, Bachmann's bundle left side; PVs, the region of the pulmonary veins (In the sheep, the four pulmonary veins often connect distally to the left atrium.); PV endo, endocardial surface of PV ostium; PV epi, epicardial surface of PV ostium; PV groove, groove between LAA and PV ostium; SVC, superior vena cava; IVC, inferior vena cava. (Reproduced with permission from Mandapati et al., *Circulation* 2000; 101:194–9.)

mapped region were usually 3×3-cm wide. In some cases, methoxyverapamil was added to the perfusion system to abolish motion artifacts; in others, the sole presence of ACh was sufficient to reduce contraction to a level that allowed optical recordings without such artifacts. Overall, when two synchronized cameras were focused simultaneously on the LAA and the RAA, the optical field comprised about 50% of the total epicardial surface of the atria. As shown in the figure, electrical bipoles were placed on other areas of the epicardium and endocardium to record the electrical activity at various selected sites. One electrode is located on the ventricle for evaluation of contamination of the atrial signals.

Wavebreak and Initiation of Reentry in the Atria

As discussed in Chapter 7, the essential step in the initiation of reentrant activity is the formation of a wavebreak. Wavebreaks may occur as a result of the interaction of the wave front with an anatomic or a functional obstacle. Phase mapping is a powerful method used in optical mapping to highlight the formation of wavebreaks and the resulting phase singularity points (PSs) that become the organizing centers (rotors) of reentry that pivot possibly at high frequencies. Briefly, the method consists of plotting the signal of any given camera pixel at an instant in time against the same signal at a time-delayed instance or by the use of the Hilbert transform. This mathematical transformation allows one to represent the action potential as a loop with time-variable phase value between $-\pi$ and π radians. The phase value at each pixel is then color-coded and phase maps for each instant are constructed for all pixels. Thus, during plane wave propagation, the wave front and its width are represented by one color (e.g., green), repolarization is represented by a sequence of different colors (e.g., yellow, blue, and purple), and rest is represented by yet another color (e.g., red). As discussed in Chapter 7, when a wave front encounters an obstacle of appropriate dimensions, it may break into two and result in phase singularities (PS) at the wavebreak points. In the phase map, a PS would be readily shown by a point where all colors (phases) converge and where the phase is not defined. Wavebreaks, as indicated by the presence of PSs, occur frequently during AF in the sheep heart. In Figure 8.3, we present data from an AF experiment in the sheep heart. At time 0 millisecond, a wave front propagates toward a functional obstacle at the center of the map and the wave front breaks. At 8 milliseconds, a pair of PSs is seen at the broken ends of the resulting wavelets. Eight milliseconds later, the PSs have drifted apart while at the same time rotating in opposite directions; full rotations will occur if there is enough "elbow room" between them. Thus, the PSs may become rotors and result in a long-lasting episode of figure-of-eight reentry. Measurements of the inter-PS distance in 15 cases of completed and 25 cases of incomplete figure-of-eight reentry showed that the two groups were uniformly distributed but in ranges that did not overlap; all inter-PS distances for incomplete reentry were found to be less than about 4 mm while

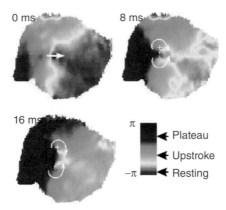

Figure 8.3 Wavebreak in the atrium. Consecutive phase maps show a wave front (green) moving from left to right at 0 millisecond. At 8 milliseconds, the wave front encounters a functional obstacle and breaks. Two PS (+ and –) are formed which begin to pivot in opposite directions. At 16 milliseconds, the phase singularities (PSs) have shifted apart and the convergence of all colors (phases) is clearly discernible at both. Note that if the two PSs have enough elbow room between them, full rotations will occur and two rotors (figure-of-eight reentry) will be formed. Color bar scale indicates phase value between –π and π radians with approximated action potential stages (see text for details). (Modified with permission from Chen *et al.*, *Cardiovasc Res* 2000; 48:220–32.)

all inter-PS distances for complete reentry were above that value. Thus, the minimal distance between two PSs that allows for the sustenance of a figure-of-eight reentry in the LA of the sheep heart is about 4 mm. It is therefore demonstrated that the interaction of wave fronts with obstacles in their path is a robust mechanism for the initiation of atrial reentry and AF.

A Single Reentrant Source may Drive Atrial Fibrillation

In Figure 8.4, we represent data from an optical mapping experiment in an isolated sheep heart during sustained AF in the presence of ACh. The biatrial electrogram at the bottom illustrates the overall fibrillatory behavior of the two atria. On top are snapshots of movies obtained simultaneously from the LAA and RAA and represented as phase maps. As shown by the inset, the phase maps allow visualization of the entire excitation–recovery cycle at each pixel location. Green represents depolarization during the upstroke of the local action potential while yellow, green, and purple represent consecutive phases of repolarization and blue represents rest. Each camera consisted of about 4000 pixels and the movies were obtained at 300 frames per second, which allowed determination of the dynamics of wave propagation with very high spatial and temporal resolution. The entire atrial activation was maintained by a sustained rotor anchored to the LAA, as revealed by the convergence of all phases of the action potential at the center of the map and the PS that pivots around the perimeter of a core. The rotor gyrated clockwise at more than 15 cycles per second, shedding spiral waves that propagated in all

LAA RAA

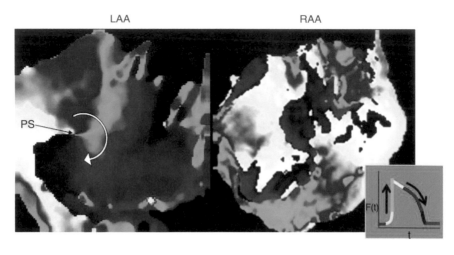

BAE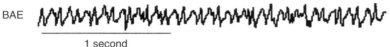

1 second

Figure 8.4 A single rotor in the LAA drives atrial fibrillation (AF). Optical mapping experiment in an isolated sheep heart during sustained AF in the presence of acetylcholine (ACh). Top: snapshots of phase movies obtained simultaneously from the LAA and RAA. Inset: color code for different phases of the excitation–recovery cycle at each pixel location. A rotor in the LAA generated spiral wave fronts that propagated to the RAA in complex patterns. A stable rotor in the LAA maintains AF. The phase map reveals the rotor as the pivot at the center of the rotating activity; i.e., where all colors converge and where the phase is not defined (i.e., the phase singularity point labeled as PS). On the RAA, the activity is slower and disorganized. Bottom: biatrial electrogram (BAE) shows fibrillatory behavior of both atria. LAA, left atrial appendage; RAA, right atrial appendage.

directions. Many of the generated waves moved across Bachmann's bundle (BB) and the coronary sinus and reached the RA and RAA appendage. However, as shown by the map on the left, the propagation patterns in the RAA were much more complex and the rate of activation at any pixel location was much slower than in the LAA. Thus, in this experiment, AF appeared to be maintained by a single high-frequency rotor in the left atrium with fibrillatory conduction toward the right atrium.

For reasons that will become evident later, it is convenient to characterize the optical or electrical signals not only as local electrical events in the time domain but also in the frequency domain using the fast Fourier transform (FFT). The latter allows generation of the power spectrum and determination of the frequency with the highest power as the dominant frequency (DF) at any pixel location. In Figure 8.5, we present data from another sheep heart experiment in which a site of high-frequency periodic activity that drove the atria during an entire AF episode was also localized. Time series are presented on the left with their corresponding power spectra on the right revealing that

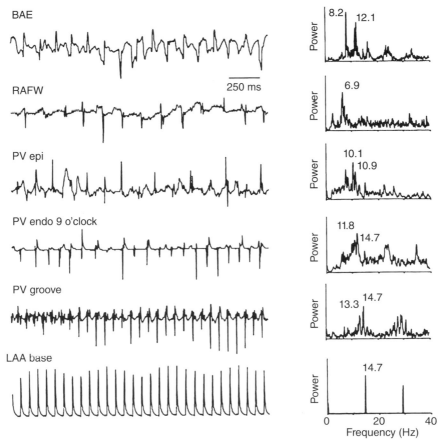

Figure 8.5 Simultaneously recorded electrograms and pseudo-electrograms and corresponding fast Fourier transforms during an atrial fibrillation (AF) episode. RAFW, right atrium free wall; PV endo 9 o'clock, PV endo at 9 o'clock position; BAE, biatrial electrogram; LAA, left atrial appendage. (Reproduced with permission from Mandapati *et al.*, *Circulation* 2000; 101:194–9.)

the biatrial and RA free wall electrograms were irregular, with DFs of 8.2 and 6.9 Hz, respectively. Signals from the epicardium and endocardium of the PVs and the common PV ostium were also irregular, with multiple peaks on their FFTs. Activity recorded from the groove between the PV ostium and LAA showed more rapid activity, with a DF at 14.7 Hz. The electrogram at the bottom, recorded from the base of the LAA, was rapid and regular, and its FFT showed a dominant peak at 14.7 Hz, suggesting that a stable source might have been present at that site. Examination of the LA optical movies established the mechanism underlying AF in this episode. In Figure 8.6a, an isochronal map (not a phase map as in Figures 8.3 and 8.4) of optical activity shows one cycle of a spiral wave that rotated clockwise and persisted for the entire duration of the arrhythmia episode of 25 minutes. A time series of the

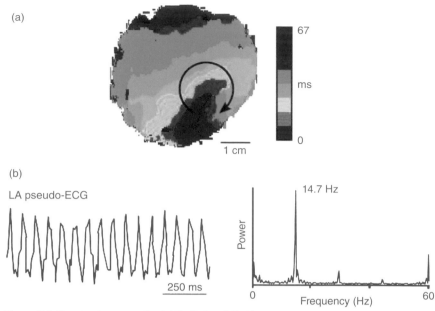

Figure 8.6 Reentrant source of atrial fibrillation (AF). (a) Isochrone map of optical activity from the free wall of the left atrium (LA) during sustained AF showing a clockwise reentry. (b) Optical pseudo-ECG of the LA during the same episode of AF with its corresponding power spectrum. (Reproduced with permission from Mandapati *et al.*, *Circulation* 2000; 101:194–9.)

summation of the optical activity throughout the field of view (representing a LA pseudo-electrogram in Figure 8.6b) demonstrated that the majority of the LA was being activated at a period of 69 milliseconds (left trace) which corresponded to the DF of 14.7 Hz. Notably, the electrode that recorded the periodic activity (bottom trace in Figure 8.5) was located at the base of the LAA ≈1 cm away from the rotor. The FFT of this signal showed a single peak at a frequency (14.7 Hz) that was identical to that of the rotor, indicating that the activity emanating from the rotor propagated to that site in a 1:1 manner. Thus, the results of the ACh-induced AF presented in Figures 8.3 to 8.6 supported the hypothesis that a single or a small number of sources of ongoing reentrant activity was the mechanism underlying AF in this particular isolated sheep heart model.

To assess more precisely the role of rotors and spiral wave activity in determining the global DF of an episode, we collected 14 identified LA vortices with completed rotations. A plot of the relationship between the rotation periods and the inverse of the global DFs obtained from the power spectrum of the corresponding LA pseudo-ECG (data not shown) yielded a linear fitted slope of 0.93 (R = 0.91). Measurements of the dimensions of the center of rotation (see Chapter 7) of these rotating waves revealed very small cores; the mean core perimeter and area were ~10 mm and ~4 mm^2, respectively, which correlated with the very high frequency of activation at those particular locations. Overall, the data strongly suggested that the periodicity of rotating spiral waves was the main contributor to the DF in the optically mapped region.

Left Atrium-to-Right Atrium Frequency Gradients

Further evidence in support of the idea that a small number of rotors maintain AF in the sheep heart model was sought by analyzing in detail dominant frequencies (DFs) in the power spectrum of multiple pixel locations and electrograms throughout both atria. We found the DFs to be organized in discrete domains in a pattern depicting a very reproducible hierarchy. Most notably, during the arrhythmia the activation frequencies in certain areas of the LA were consistently faster than any other areas. This is illustrated in panel (a) of Figure 8.7, which shows a dominant frequency map obtained

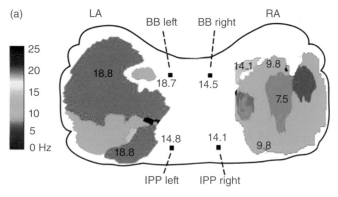

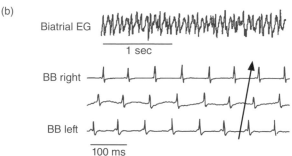

Figure 8.7 Relationship between activity in the left atrium (LA) and the right atrium (RA). (a) LA-to-RA gradient in dominant frequency (DF). DF maps of the epicardial surfaces of LA and RA, with values of DF along Bachmann's bundle (BB) and inferoposterior pathway (IPP). Numbers are expressed in Hertz. The areas of the color-coded frequency maps indicate the optical mapping field. (b) Left-to-right directionality of impulse propagation during AF. Recordings from a biatrial electrogram (EG, top trace) and three bipolar electrodes along BB, the tracing in the bottom being most leftward. (Reproduced with permission from Mansour *et al.*, *Circulation* 2001; 103:2631–6.)

during a 5-second episode of AF. In this representation, different colors indicate different frequencies in Hertz (Hz), as shown by the color bar.

The DF map was constructed from a 3-second episode of AF in the presence of ACh. It shows a high degree of organization with discrete frequency domains and an LA-to-RA frequency gradient. For the most part, the DF in the LA was highest at 18.8 Hz. The left side of BB shows a DF of 18.7 Hz whereas the inferoposterior pathway (IPP) on the same side was activated at 14.8 Hz. Moving further to the right, the DF at the right end of BB was 14.5 Hz; in the IPP it was 14.1 Hz. Finally, the RA shows a DF of 9.8 Hz. The same pattern of discrete DF domain distribution persisted for several minutes in all hearts, with less than ~20% temporal variability during sustained AF. Both the stability of the spatial distribution of DFs and the significant differences in activation frequency and organization between LA and RA strongly suggest that the underlying electrophysiologic properties of the former somehow enable it to support greater activation frequencies than the latter. Moreover, the results indicated that the largest decay in frequency occurred at the junction between BB and the RA, where significant pectinate muscle branching occurs.

Further support for the said hypothesis was sought by monitoring the direction of conduction along BB and IPP over a distance covered by a minimum of three consecutive bipolar electrodes located on each pathway—i.e., 2 cm over BB and 2.6 cm over IPP. Figure 8.6b illustrates an example of left-to-right propagation along BB during an episode of AF. The top trace is a biatrial electrogram (EG) of AF in a 3-second episode. The bottom three traces are EGs from the right, middle, and left of BB during the same episode. Propagation along the latter pathway was organized and occurred from left to right. Quantification of this finding revealed that wave fronts propagated from left to right in 81% and 80% of the analyzed activations along BB and IPP, respectively. Conversely, right-to-left propagation occurred in a significantly smaller percentage of cases. The finding that direction of propagation during AF occurs primarily from the areas of fast to areas of slow rate of activation has far-reaching implication. It suggests that the characterization of the spatial distribution of DFs may be used to localize a source of the arrhythmia by identifying the site with the highest DF. As will be demonstrated next, that insight has been utilized in AF patients where information on propagation patterns during AF is difficult to attain as a result of the low resolution of the electrode recordings available in the clinical electrophysiology lab.

It is important to note, however, that definite proof for the aforementioned mechanism is lacking for those AF episodes in which only electrograms were obtained or whose sources were outside the field of view of our imaging system. Nevertheless, one can infer the presence of high-frequency rotors and their crucial role in maintaining AF by the demonstration of increasing DF gradients in well-controlled experiments in which ACh is perfused at increasing concentrations while local DFs are measured simultaneously from multiple locations of both atria (see further discussion).

Dispersion of Activation Rate during Atrial Fibrillation

The data in Figures 8.5 and 8.6 suggested that waves emanating from a source during AF should be intermittently blocked and contribute to a spatial dispersion of DFs where notably, the activation frequencies in certain areas of the LA were always faster than any other region. Here we use computer simulation to gain some insight into the origin of such data. We start with the premise that the underlying mechanism of AF may be a highly periodic stationary source (e.g., a rotor or an automatic focus) located somewhere in the LA. In addition, we assume that, regardless of the nature of the periodic source, the complicated anatomy of the atria plays an integral role in the development of fibrillatory conduction. These assumptions are conveniently considered using a simplified mathematical model of a major pectinate muscle connected to a small area of the atrial wall. The three-dimensional model consisted therefore of a one-dimensional thin bundle attached to a two-dimensional sheet (see Figure 8.8). The kinetics assigned to each of the excitable elements (numerical cells) in the model were of a modified FitzHugh–Nagumo type, which roughly mimicked a cardiac action potential. Cells were connected to each other by low-resistance pathways. Periodic stimulation was applied to the top free edge of the thin (25 mm^2) bundle and the impulse was allowed to propagate downstream to invade the two-dimensional sheet. The traces on the right show the action potentials and corresponding power spectra of sites in the bundle and in the sheet. As shown by the top and bottom time series, stimulation at a constant period of 0.119

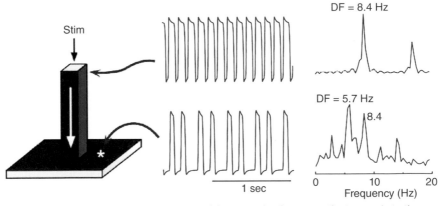

Figure 8.8 Computer model of action potential propagation from a pectinate muscle to the atrial wall. A 3-D (60 × 60 × 60 elements) model includes a 1-D bundle attached to a 2-D sheet (left panel). Periodic stimulation (Stim) was applied at the top edge of the bundle and the impulse was allowed to propagate downward with conduction velocity of ~0.29 m/s and to invade the 2-D sheet. The voltage time series and corresponding power spectra are shown for a site near the stimulation point and a site at the sheet. Comparison between the points indicates a 3:2 pattern of propagation into the sheet with a concomitant spectral transformation and a dominant frequency (DF) shift from 8.4 to 5.7 Hz. (Reproduced with permission from Jalife *et al.*, *J Cardiovasc Electrophysiol* 1998; 9:S2–12.)

second resulted in a 3:2 propagation pattern across the boundary between the thin bundle and the sheet. This is reflected also in the corresponding power spectra within the band between 0 and 20 Hz. While the source region (i.e., the thin bundle) displayed a DF of 8.4 Hz, the geometrical expansion into the sheet imposed a spectral transformation whereby the DF shifted to 5.7 Hz. The two power spectra display additional peaks originating from the combined effect of the sharp action potential deflections and the inter-beat cycle length variations. The constant cycle length at the thin bundle results in a narrow peak at a DF that is the exact inverse of the cycle length (CL, 1/0.119 = 8.4 Hz) with an additional smaller peak at about 16.8 Hz, which is an integer multiple of the DF (i.e., a harmonic). The CL of the activity in the sheet on the other hand is not constant and can be seen to alternate between short and long values. This in turn gives rise to a more complex profile. Several peaks are seen in the power spectrum, consequent of the combination of various intervals in the time series including not only the long and short CLs, but also their sum and difference. The Fourier algorithm, nevertheless, considers the most stationary combination of the CLs to be the DF at 5.7 Hz, which is the average number of local activations per second, corresponding to the 3:2 ratio of the input CL (frequency) of 0.119 second (8.4 Hz) represented by a smaller peak.

In general, the FFT provides a power spectrum that describes the stationary properties of the full-length signal. When the activation amplitude and CL are fixed during the full recording period T, then the electrophysiological meaning of the DF is simply 1/CL. However, beat-to-beat modulation in either the amplitude or CL complicates the relationship between each individual cycle and the resulted DF of the entire period T. Fischer *et al.* recently showed that a signal with a beat-to-beat CL variability that is up to about 30% of its mean CL would still render a good agreement between its DF and the mean activation rate. This similarity is very helpful as bipolar and unipolar recordings occasionally display power spectra with harmonic peaks that mask the peak corresponding to the activation rate, and that are erroneously labeled DF. To increase the likelihood of appropriately selecting the DF as the activation rate, its inverse value (i.e., 1/DF) is confirmed to match the approximate number of visual activations over a second. However, it appears that the greater the complexity of the electrograms in terms of inter-beat variation in morphology and CL, the less likely will the DF provide information about the activation rate. In that case, consideration of other activation characteristics, such as regularity and fractionation may be of significant help for the overall analysis of the arrhythmia.

Stretch and Activation in the Left Atrium during Atrial Fibrillation

As AF in humans is commonly associated with atrial dilation, we employed an experimental model of sustained AF under conditions of acutely increased intra-atrial pressure (IAP) to explore stretch-related AF dynamics. After perforation of the interatrial septum, all venous orifices were closed except for the left superior pulmonary vein (LSPV) (merged with the right superior pulmonary vein in eight of the nine animals) and inferior vena cava. Tubes connected to a digital IAP sensor were coupled to the inferior vena cava and LSPV at one edge and to an open-ended cannula, the height of which controlled hydrostatically the level of IAP. Our finding in the isolated sheep hearts, that the PV region is where the highest DFs are most likely to be located as well as selective PV angiography in patients with paroxysmal AF, suggested that AF triggers are most frequently located in dilated superior PVs. Therefore, we used this model of increased IAP-related AF to test the hypothesis that dilation induces arrhythmogenic LA sources emanating from the superior PVs. The persistence of the induced AF in this model was found to be highly dependent on the IAP; a pressure of 10 cm H_2O was found to be the lower limit to obtain sustained AF episodes while in comparison, below 10 cm H_2O, AF usually terminated after 10 to 20 minutes.

The studies presented show how frequency analysis can be used to characterize the organization of activity during AF and to establish the likelihood

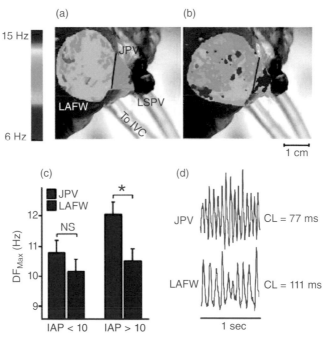

Figure 8.9 (a,b) Dominant frequency (DF) maps from one heart at intra-atrial pressures (IAPs) of 5 and 18 cm H_2O, respectively. DF maps are superimposed on color picture of a heart for illustrative purposes. Tubes connecting venous orifices to control IAP are seen at the bottom right of each panel. (c) Bar graph showing DF_{Max} (mean ± SEM) in the pulmonary vein junction (JPV, blue) and left atrium free wall (LAFW, red) at IAPs <10 and >10 cm H_2O (*P < 0.001). (d) Single-pixel recordings from JPV and LAFW at 30 cm H_2O. IVC, inferior vena cava; CL, cycle length. (Reproduced with permission from Kalifa et al., *Circulation* 2003; 108:668–71.)

of localizing sources maintaining the AF from which propagation is originating. In Figure 8.9, panels (a) and (b) are representative DF maps obtained simultaneously from the LA free wall (LAFW) and the LA superior PV junction (JPV) in one heart at IAPs of 5 and 18 cm H_2O, respectively. These maps clearly illustrate the strong dependence of frequency on IAP. Below 10 cm H_2O, the difference between the maximum dominant frequency (DF_{Max}) in the JPV and LAFW was not significant (10.8 ± 0.3 vs. 10.2 ± 0.3; $P = 0.6$; Figure 8.9c). However, at pressures >10 cm H_2O, DF_{Max} in the JPV was significantly higher than that in LAFW (12.0 ± 0.2 Hz and 10.5 ± 0.2 Hz, respectively; mean $\pm$ SEM; n = 9; $P < 0.001$; see also representative single-pixel recordings in panel d). At all pressures, DF_{Max} in both JPV and LAFW was significantly higher than the largest frequency recorded in the right atrial free wall (7.8 ± 0.3 Hz; $P < 0.001$).

Despite the general appearance of disorganized patterns of wave propagation during AF, optical mapping data reveal episodes where those waves are highly periodic, both spatially and temporally. Such spatiotemporal periodicities (STPs) may take various forms, including periodic waves emerging from the edge of the recording field, breakthroughs occurring at constant frequencies, and in some cases, stable rotors. We found similar STP waves in high IAP-associated AF. In Figure 8.10, we show quantification of directionality and STP of electrical activation as a function of the IAP during AF. Clearly, the direction of propagation from LSPV to LAFW (blue symbols) was very consistent. In all experiments, the directionality of local excitation in the JPV area (panel a) that corresponded to the highest frequencies correlated strongly with IAP ($r = 0.79$, $P = 0.02$; Figure 8.10b). In contrast, the directionality of LAFW to LSPV had a negative and statistically nonsignificant correlation with pressure ($r = -0.54$, $P = 0.09$). In Figure 8.10c, the number of STP wave fronts (normalized to the maximum number of STP wave fronts) in the JPV correlated strongly with IAP ($r = 0.92$, $P = 0.002$). Figure 8.10d shows an example of a rotor in the JPV, the cycle length of which (70 milliseconds) was equal to $1/DF_{Max}$ calculated from the same movie. Similar rotors were observed in three out of nine experiments. It was found that below 10 cm H_2O, AF terminates because its reentrant sources become slow and unstable. These data are particularly valuable when one considers that there is evidence that in patients with paroxysmal AF, the diameters of the superior PV ostia are markedly dilated compared with the inferior PV ostia, particularly when considered as arrhythmogenic PVs. However, the electrophysiological mechanisms linking PV and LA dilatation to maintenance of AF have not been established. Our data demonstrate that the sources of rapid atrial activation during stretch-related AF are located in the PV region and that their level of spatiotemporal organization correlates with pressure. The extent to which STP of excitation waves observed in the JPV are generated by microreentrant activity in the endocardial PV sleeves requires further investigation and those data only provide a partial mechanistic explanation for the precise role of the PVs in AF maintenance in the setting of atrial dilatation.

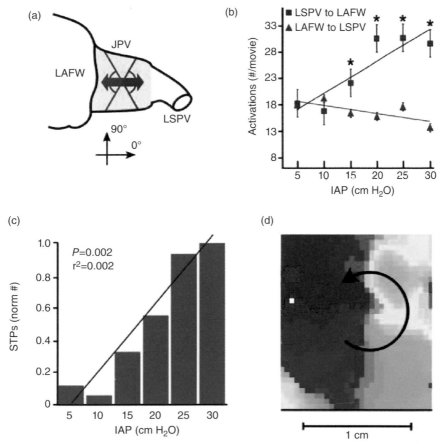

Figure 8.10 (a) Schematic directionality of activity from the pulmonary veins (PVs) to left atrium free wall (LAFW, blue arrow) and from the LAFW to left superior pulmonary vein (LSPV, red arrow) assessed at the pulmonary vein junction (JPV) region (shaded area). (b) Number of activations (mean ± SEM) moving from LSPV to LAFW and from LAFW to LSPV (*$P < 0.01$ compared with LAFW to LSPV). Colors are the same as in panel (a). (c) Relation between the normalized number of spatiotemporal periodicity (STP) wave fronts by episode and the level of pressure. (d) Phase map of a rotor recorded in the JPV at 15 cm H_2O. (Reproduced with permission from Kalifa *et al.*, *Circulation* 2003; 108:668–71.)

Vagal Effects on Rotors during Atrial Fibrillation

Both vagal stimulation and administration of ACh have been shown to result in AF. In experimental animal studies, vagal stimulation results in sustained AF as long as the vagus nerve is continuously stimulated and in dogs, catheter ablation of the cardiac parasympathetic nerves abolishes vagally mediated AF. It has also been demonstrated that AF cannot be induced in Kir3.4 (GIRK4) knockout mice. Thus, we have decided to study the role of $I_{K,ACh}$ in the mechanism of AF dynamics in our sheep model.

DF mapping is an excellent means of quantifying differences in activation frequency between the LA and RA during AF. However, power spectral analysis alone does not allow determination of mechanisms of propagation at the source area. On the other hand, phase mapping does provide direct demonstration of the underlying electrophysiologic mechanism of the arrhythmia. We therefore used the phase movies obtained from our optical mapping experiments to quantify mean rotor frequency as the inverse of cycle length (1/CL). Panel (a) of Figure 8.11 reproduces results obtained in six hearts in

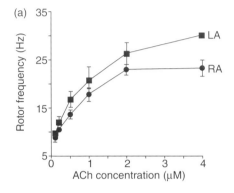

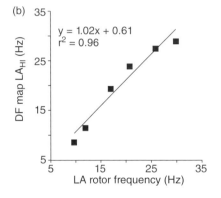

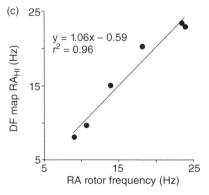

Figure 8.11 Relationship between acetylcholine (ACh) concentration and rotor frequency (1/CL). (a) ACh dose–response curves of left atrium (LA, squares) and right atrium (RA, circles) for the five longest living rotors for each of the six experiments. Rotor frequency is greater in LA than in RA at all concentrations. (b) LA rotor frequency vs. LA frequency measured by spectral analysis. (c) RA rotor frequency vs. RA frequency measured by spectral analysis. (Reproduced with permission from Sarmast et al., Cardiovasc Res 2003; 59:863–73.)

which the effects of varying concentrations of ACh on rotor frequency in both atria were investigated. The frequency was higher in the LA than in the RA at all concentrations. Similarly spectral analyses of optical and electrode data (see Figure 8.2) revealed that the LA-to-RA rotor frequency gradient increased with the ACh concentration (1.0 Hz at 0.1 μM vs. 6.2 Hz at 4.0 μM; $P < 0.05$). Furthermore, as shown in panels (b) and (c), the excitation frequencies of the longest living rotors in each atrium correlated well with the highest frequency domains of their respective DF maps.

Interestingly, while increasing the ACh concentration in the perfusate increased the rotor frequency and the frequency gradient, the same manipulation resulted in a progressive reduction in rotor life span. In addition, more wavebreaks were observed at the higher ACh concentration as demonstrated quantitatively as an increase in the PS density. The data suggested that the increase in the frequency gradient at the higher ACh concentration was a manifestation of increasing electrophysiologic heterogeneities in the tissue produced by a heterogeneous response to ACh. In other words, while at low ACh concentrations, the rotors remain relatively stable, at the unphysiologic ACh concentration of 4.0 μM, these faster spinning rotors encounter a substrate of augmented heterogeneity where there is a greater likelihood for wavelet production. In short, while it has long been known that elevated ACh concentrations are a recipe for more complex fibrillatory patterns, our results provided evidence that this is a direct result of the increased rotor frequency.

Ionic Mechanisms of Parasympathetic Modulation of Atrial Fibrillation

Left-to-right differences in AF frequency in the sheep heart may result from chamber specific differences in parasympathetic signaling at the level of ACh release from postganglionic vagal terminals, density of muscarinic receptors, inhibitory G-protein level, and/or density of the ACh-activated potassium Kir3.x (GIRKx) channel coupled to the muscarinic M_2 receptor. Obviously, differences in ACh release do not apply to the isolated heart. On the other hand, chamber-specific differences in muscarinic receptor density might play a role in establishing AF frequency gradients, as suggested by studies in rabbit hearts which have demonstrated that the density of muscarinic M_2 receptors is larger in the LA than in the RA. Whether such differences apply to the sheep heart is as yet unknown.

As an initial approach to determining the molecular mechanism underlying the different sensitivities of the LA and RA to the effects of ACh during AF, we measured the relative abundance of mRNA encoding Kir3.1 and Kir3.4 proteins. Figure 8.12 presents a ribonuclease protection assay (RPA) analysis for Kir3.1 and Kir3.4 using sheep DNA as a template. As shown in Figure 8.12b, quantifying the intensity of the RPA bands showed a differential expression of inwardly rectifying potassium channels, with the Kir3.1 and Kir3.4

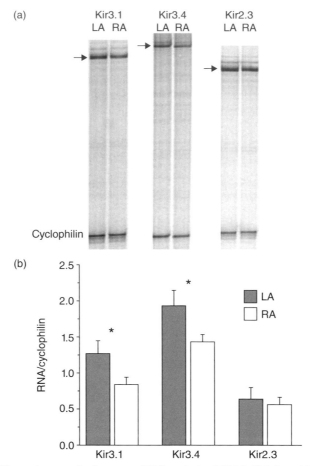

Figure 8.12 Ribonuclease protection assay (RPA) analysis of Kir3.1, Kir3.4, and Kir2.3 in the left (LA) and right atrium (RA). (a) Data from one sheep heart. Abundance of the isoform bands (arrows) was compared after scaling to the cyclophilin band in each lane. (b) mRNA concentrations from the LA and RA of five sheep are 1.28 ± 0.18 vs. 0.84 ± 0.1, 1.94 ± 0.21 vs. 1.44 ± 0.11, and 0.65 ± 0.16 vs. 0.57 ± 0.11 RNA/cyclophilin for Kir3.1, Kir3.4, and Kir2.3, respectively. Asterisks indicate $P < 0.05$. (Reproduced with permission from Sarmast *et al.*, *Cardiovasc Res* 2003; 59:863–73.)

mRNA being highly significantly greater in the LA than in the RA. Kir3.1 was ~45% more abundant in the LA than in the RA ($P = 0.008$) and Kir3.4 was ~34% more abundant in the LA compared with the RA ($P = 0.005$). Note that the Kir3.x channel complex responsible for $I_{K,ACh}$ is a heterotetramer of Kir3.1 and Kir3.4, although recently it has been shown in the bovine atrium that a significant proportion of channels exist as Kir3.4 homotetramers. Finally, as I_{K1} has been implicated in determining chamber-specific dynamics during fibrillation in a different species, we also measured the relative abundance of mRNA encoding its constituting channel proteins. Figure 8.12 shows also that the Kir2.3 channels, which have been suggested to be solely responsible for I_{K1} in the sheep atria, are about 12% more abundant in the LA compared with the RA but this difference is not statistically significant ($P = 0.178$). Thus, our measurements of the density of channels that may be implicated in the LA and RA different frequency of activity during AF suggest that the $I_{K,ACh}$ is more important than the I_{K1} in establishing that difference.

The data presented thus far suggest that the significantly different responses of the LA and RA to ACh during AF are somehow related to the dissimilar mRNA levels in the two atria of Kir3.1 and Kir3.4 channels responsible for $I_{K,ACh}$. To provide more definite proof for such a correlation, we examined the effects of three different concentrations of ACh (0.05, 0.1, and 0.5 µM) on $I_{K,ACh}$ current density of myocytes isolated from the LA and RA. We did not find any significant differences in ACh-activated potassium current ($I_{K,ACh}$) density between the LA and the RA at 0.05 µM (data not shown). However, as demonstrated in Figure 8.13, $I_{K,ACh}$ density was significantly higher in the LA than in the RA at 0.1 and 0.5 µM. Panel (a) shows the ramp-generated current in an LA myocyte in control and in the presence of 0.1- and 0.5-µM ACh showing

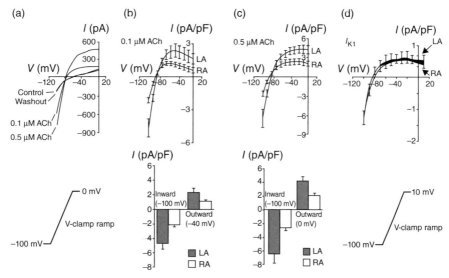

Figure 8.13 $I_{K,ACh}$ and I_{K1} densities in sheep atrial cells. (a) Top: voltage-clamp ramp generated currents in a sheep left atrium (LA) cell in control and in the presence of 0.1 and 0.5 µM acetylcholine (ACh). Note the reversibility of ACh effect upon washout. Bottom: voltage-clamp ramp protocol. (b) ACh = 0.1 µM. Top: $I_{K,ACh}$ density in left (n = 6) and right (n = 6) atrial cells. Bottom: peak inward (at −100 mV) and peak outward (at −40 mV) $I_{K,ACh}$ densities from top graph. (c) ACh = 0.5 µM. Top: $I_{K,ACh}$ densities in left (n = 7) and right (n = 6) atrial cells. Bottom, peak inward (at −100 mV) and peak outward (at 0 mV) current densities from top graph. LA $I_{K,ACh}$ density is higher than RA at both concentrations ($P < 0.05$). Note the apparent reduction in current rectification at the higher ACh concentration. (d) Top: I_{K1} density in LA (n = 5) and RA (n = 10) cells. Bottom: voltage-clamp ramp protocol. (Reproduced with permission from Sarmast et al., *Cardiovasc Res* 2003; 59:863–73.)

an increase in current with dose. The superimposed control and washout traces demonstrate the reversibility of the effects. The bottom of panel (a) is the ramp protocol used to generate the current traces. In panel (b), the top graph shows mean $I_{K,ACh}$ current density–voltage relations at 0.1 µM. The peak inward (at −100 mV) and peak outward (at −40 mV) current densities were significantly higher in the LA than in the RA, as shown by the bottom bar graph ($P < 0.05$). Panel (c) (top panel) shows mean $I_{K,ACh}$ current density–voltage relationships at 0.5 µM. Clearly, the LA has a higher $I_{K,ACh}$ density than the RA, as also demonstrated by the bottom graph, showing significant differences in both inward and outward currents ($P < 0.05$). Also, note that at the higher ACh concentration, there was an apparent reduction in current rectification. Therefore, peak outward current was measured at 0 mV (see top panel of Figure 8.13b). Panel (d) shows on top the I_{K1} density in the LA (n = 5) and the RA (n = 10) cells; the voltage-clamp ramp protocol is shown at the bottom. Clearly, I_{K1} density was similar in the RA and LA. Altogether, the results provide strong support to the idea that LA-to-RA gradients of excitation frequency and fibrillatory conduction in acute, cholinergically mediated AF are the result of significant differences in the functional expression of $I_{K,ACh}$ channels in RA and LA myocytes.

Remodeling of the Atrial Substrate in Chronic Atrial Fibrillation

There are at least two ways to classify AF in patients. One classification divides the arrhythmia into paroxysmal, persistent, and permanent, in reference to whether AF can terminate spontaneously, whether it can be terminated medically, or whether it cannot be terminated at all. Alternatively, AF may be classified based on its temporal patterns into acute or chronic, referring simply to its duration. Often the arrhythmia starts as paroxysmal AF but with time it frequently progresses to persistent and permanent AF. Thus, a somewhat different temporal classification of the patients can be used without reference to a clinical intervention as those patients with sustained AF at its initial stages and those at more advanced stages. In the former group, patients present AF of short duration and are referred to as paroxysmal AF (PAF) patients, regardless of whether their AF does or does not end spontaneously. Patients in the latter group present longer periods of AF that may be either persistent or permanent and are collectively referred to as chronic AF (CAF) patients.

Considerable work has been done using animal models to analyze the ionic currents of human atrial tissue and the basis of atrial action potential heterogeneity and rate dependence, two properties that are important determinants of AF. Regional variations in a variety of currents, including I_{Ca-L}, I_{to} and I_{K1} may play a role in action potential heterogeneity. Advances have been made in the understanding of atrial ion channels, membrane receptors, and gap junctions. High-resolution imaging tools are being applied to the monitoring of cellular events, including cell-to-cell propagation and the role of electrical sinks and sources in the establishment of frequency-dependent conduction block. Such tools are germane also to the elucidation of mechanisms of AF, particularly in regard to structure–function relationships in the atria, identification and localization of ischemic and/or fibrotic disease and atrial enlargement and its progression, and the role of such pathologic changes in the atria. Indeed, these advances are highly relevant to the understanding of the events leading to the substrate changes resulting in atrial electrical remodeling and to improvement of drug therapy for AF. In 1995, the group of Maurits Allessie described the electrophysiological changes induced by maintaining AF artificially in goats for a period of time that was longer than a day. Their main findings were that the artificially maintained AF led to a marked shortening of atrial effective refractory period, a reversion of its physiological rate adaptation, and an increase in rate, inducibility and stability of AF. Thereafter, the phenomenon of atrial tachycardia-induced remodeling, coined in that seminal publication as "AF begets AF," became well recognized. A variety of ionic current changes have now been described which likely account for the functional electrophysiological changes caused in experimental models by atrial tachycardia. Decreases are observed in I_{to}, I_{Ca-L} and I_{Na}. The decreases in I_{Ca-L} seem to be particularly important in explaining action potential abbreviation and loss of rate adaptation seen in AF. In the rapidly paced canine atrial model of AF, there is down-regulation of I_{Ca-L}, and several studies have reported that the electrophysiological remodeling accompanying AF could be prevented by pretreatment with calcium channel blockers, which implies that calcium overload is a key factor in the remodeling process. Thus, it has been suggested that calcium overload might trigger the intracellular signaling cascade which alters gene expression and eventually result in down-regulation of atrial K^+ and Ca^{2+} current densities. Indeed, recent studies in human have shown $I_{K,ACh}$ down-regulation following prolonged periods of AF; however, this decrease may be counteracted by an increase of I_{K1}, which is suggested to play an important role in stabilization and acceleration of functional reentry.

To determine the effect of the ionic remodeling and in particular the role of I_{K1} in the maintenance of rotors under simulated CAF conditions, we constructed a simplified 2-D model of human atrial cells which was devoid of any structural or electrophysiological heterogeneities, since adding these complexities can confound the interpretation regarding the ionic mechanisms underlying propagation dynamics. The CAF conditions were simulated by incorporating changes in a published model for human atrial myocytes. Two CAF conditions were simulated:

1. *CAF1 case*: This was simulated by incorporating a down-regulation in the densities of the transient outward K^+ current, I_{to} (by 50%), the ultrarapid delayed rectifier K^+ current, I_{Kur} (by 50%), and the L-type Ca^{2+} current, I_{Ca-L} (by 70%).

2. *CAF2 case*: The changes were similar to the CAF1 case. However, an additional increase in the density of the inward-rectifier K⁺ current, I_{K1} (by 100%) was also incorporated.

Figure 8.14a displays the simulated action potentials in single human atrial cells under control and chronic AF conditions; the APD was abbreviated in

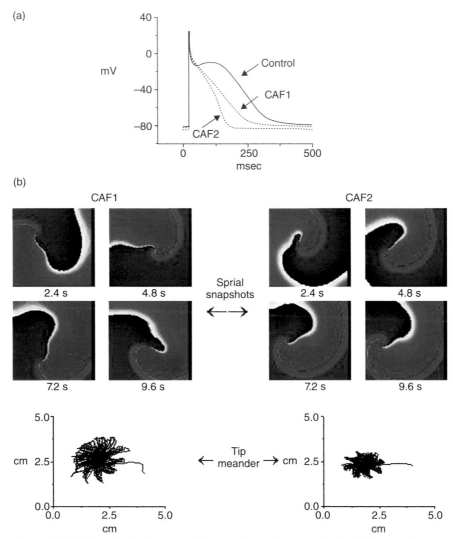

Figure 8.14 (a) Simulated action potentials in control and chronic atrial fibrillation conditions (CAF1, CAF2). (b) Spiral waves (phase movie snapshots) and tip meandering trajectories in chronic AF conditions (CAF1, CAF2). Phase movies are shown at four distinct times (2.4, 4.8, 7.2, and 9.6 seconds). The tip meander is plotted in a 5 × 5 cm, 2-D, atrial sheet. (Reproduced from Pandit *et al.*, *Biophys J* 2005; 88(6):3806–21.)

CAF1, and more so in CAF2. An increase in I_{K1} (CAF2) also caused a small hyperpolarization of the resting membrane potential (V_{rest}) by ~3.3 mV, compared with control and CAF1. This is in accordance with recent experimental results, which showed that the mean V_{rest} was hyperpolarized by 3.6 mV in chronic AF conditions when I_{K1} was increased. A sustained rotor was inducible only when the APD was shortened in CAF, and not under control, healthy, conditions. Figure 8.14b shows representative snapshots of phase movies of spiral waves in both CAF1 and CAF2 conditions at time intervals of 2.4 seconds. The spiral tip of those rotors was tracked by the location of their phase singularity points and displayed a quasiperiodic meander trajectory with a rosette-like pattern in both CAF1 and CAF2 cases. The tip meandering was ~2.6 cm wide in CAF1, and ~1.7 cm in CAF2. FFT analysis as in Figure 8.6 revealed that the DF (i.e., the rotation frequency) in the CAF1 case was ~5.7 Hz and it accelerated to ~8.4 Hz in the CAF2 case. Thus, we established that the up-regulation of I_{K1} at the CAF setting stabilizes and accelerates rotor activity. This finding is consistent with other studies from our laboratory which have suggested an important role for I_{K1} in sustaining rotor dynamics during ventricular fibrillation in the guinea pigs.

In addition to confirming a similar role for I_{K1} in the atrium, our simulations showed the mechanisms that are involved in rotor stabilization in CAF: namely, APD shortening and V_{rest} hyperpolarization. Normally, an increase in I_{K1} current will reduce cardiac excitability by opposing the stimulus current and preventing the approach toward threshold potentials. However, during reentry in CAF, the depolarizing wave front acts as a stimulus to drive a partially excitable/recovered tissue. An increase in I_{K1} hyperpolarizes V_{rest}, and causes a corresponding increase in the recovery of I_{Na} and subsequently the electrotonic current. The resultant enhancement of cardiac excitability causes faster spiral rotation. To confirm the role of V_{rest} hyperpolarization relative to the role of APD abbreviation in CAF, we also entirely blocked the I_{Ca-L} in the CAF1 case, without modulating V_{rest}. That causes indeed an abbreviation of the APD to be similar to the APD at CAF2; however, the spiral in this case accelerated only slightly to ~6.3 Hz and its meander slightly stabilized to ~2.0 cm. These results re-emphasize the fact that in addition to a shortening of the APD (which occurs when both I_{K1} is increased or I_{Ca-L} is blocked), increased availability of I_{Na} is an important factor in mediating rotor acceleration when I_{K1} is increased, due to hyperpolarization of diastolic membrane potential (which does not occur when I_{Ca-L} is blocked). Additionally, these results also show that I_{Ca-L} is an important determinant of spiral tip meander in this ionic model. The acceleration of the spirals in CAF2 vs. CAF1 is also in accordance with experimental results described earlier in which during ACh-mediated AF in sheep, higher activation frequencies in the LA were associated with a larger density of the ACh-activated K^+ current ($I_{K,ACh}$). Thus, even though an increased I_{K1} may have a protective effect against early or late afterdepolarizations at the cellular level, once AF is initiated, an increased I_{K1} will tend to stabilize rotor activity in the remodeled atrium.

Atrial Fibrillation in Humans: The Spatial Distribution of Dominant Frequencies

DF characterization in animal models has provided mechanistic insight into AF in animals. Not only did we find a clear difference between mean LA and RA DFs, but we also demonstrated that left-to-right impulse propagation was present in about 80% of cases along the BB and the IPP. Altogether, the data support the contention that AF, as seen on the ECG of normal hearts, results from rapidly successive wave fronts emanating from fast sources localized in the LA. The wave fronts propagating through both atria interact with anatomic and/or functional obstacles, leading to fragmentation and wavelet formation and reduction in activation rate.

A skeptical reader may begin to wonder at this point whether any of the foregoing is really applicable to human AF. After all, human AF is exceedingly complex and high-resolution optical mapping cannot be used in humans due to the phototoxicity of the voltage-sensitive dye. Yet, an important advantage of DF mapping is that it allows application of many of the tools used in the animal studies to generate new insight into AF in patient even when the resolution of the electrode generated maps is limited.

Several clinical studies have investigated how the cycle length of the atrial activity in patients during AF can contribute to its treatment. Recent studies employed Fourier methods to characterize rigorously the spatial distribution of DF during AF in patients. In 2005, Sanders *et al.* used the CARTO electroanatomic mapping system to acquire sequentially 5-second-long bipolar recordings from about 120 points throughout both atria and the coronary sinus (CS) in 32 patients during sustained AF in an electrophysiology study for an ablation procedure. The recorded signals were rectified and 3–15 Hz band-pass filtered, then FFT was used to determine the DF of each of 120 segments lasting 4.096 seconds with a resolution of 0.24 Hz. Patients with both paroxysmal and permanent AF demonstrated dominant frequency gradients from LA to RA to CS. However, compared with patients with paroxysmal AF, permanent AF patients demonstrated significantly higher average frequencies of activity.

Figure 8.15 shows four sample bipolar electrograms with their respective power spectra acquired from endocardial sites in the LA and RA of a patient with paroxysmal AF of spontaneous onset. On the left, typical AF recordings are seen with variable amplitudes and inter-beat intervals, which do not enable accurate cycle length analysis, particularly in the top recording. However, the spectra on the right show relatively narrow bands in the 3 to 15 Hz range with distinct peaks of DFs approximately corresponding to the activation rate and the inverse of the average cycle length in the electrograms.

In all 32 patients studied, electrograms were collected from multiple sites (typically 120 in both atria) and their corresponding DFs were superimposed on the atrial geometry created with the CARTO system to generate color DF maps, as illustrated in Figure 8.16. On each DF map, those sites that

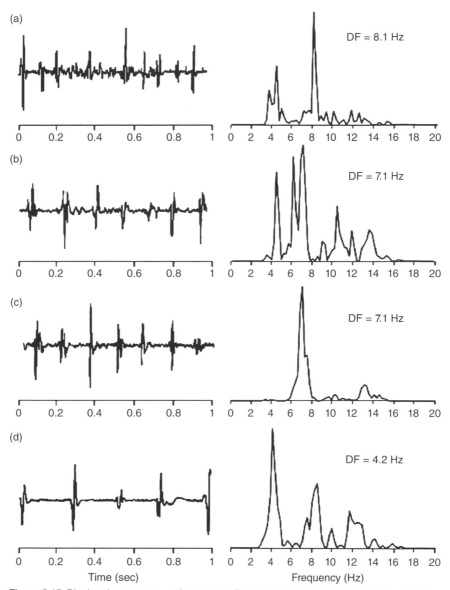

Figure 8.15 Bipolar electrograms and corresponding power spectra obtained from four points in a patient with spontaneous paroxysmal atrial fibrillation (AF). Each site shows a distinct dominant frequency (DF) value. Panel (a) clearly demonstrates the utility of spectral analysis. The bipolar recording shows low-amplitude complex signals that make accurate determination of frequency of activation difficult. The power spectrum clearly demonstrates the DF at 8.1 Hz. The DF map of this patient is shown in Figure 8.16a. Panel (a) is from the site of maximal DF at the right inferior pulmonary vein (RIPV). Panels (b) and (c) are from other high DF sites in the right (RSPV) and left superior pulmonary vein (LSPV). Panel (d) is from the posterior right atrium (RA). (Reproduced with permission from Sanders *et al.*, *Circulation* 2005; 112:789–97.)

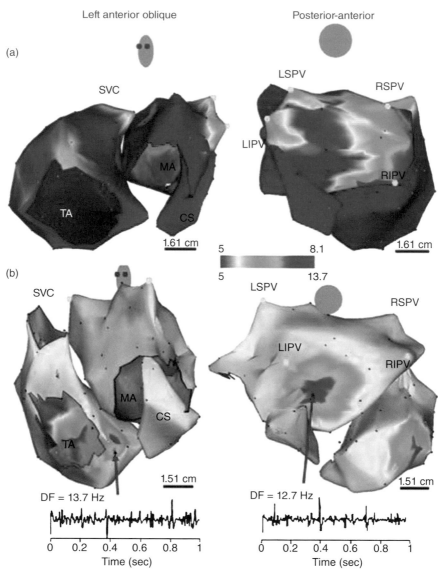

Figure 8.16 Dominant frequency (DF) maps of human atrial fibrillation (AF). (a) DF map in a patient with paroxysmal AF (6 hours). Note high DF sites in each of the pulmonary veins (PVs). Ablation sequence in this patient was LSPV, LIPV RSPV, and RIPV (site of AF termination); atrial fibrillation cycle length (AFCL) increased by 10, 25, 9, and 75 milliseconds, respectively, before termination. (b) DF map in a patient with permanent AF (24 months). The maximal DF and atrial frequency are higher than the patient in panel (a). In addition, many of the high DF sites are located outside the PVs. Ablation sequence in this patient was RIPV, RSPV, LSPV and LIPV; AFCL increased by 5, 2, 0, and 5 milliseconds, respectively. The electrogram of the site of maximal DF in the LA and RA is presented showing significant fractionation. SVC, superior vena cava; MA, mitral annulus; TA, tricuspid annulus; LSPV, left superior pulmonary vein; RSPV, right superior pulmonary vein; RIPV, right inferior pulmonary vein. Color bar, scale in Hz. (Reproduced with permission from Sanders *et al.*, *Circulation* 2005; 112:789–97.)

demonstrated high-frequency activity with a gradient of 20% or more relative to the surrounding atrial tissue were defined as high DF (HDF) sites. In this study, most HDF sites involved a single point, but in some the HDF site extended over two to three adjacent points. Figure 8.16a reproduces left anterior oblique (left) and postero-anterior (right) views of the same map showing fibrillatory activity at mean DF of ~4.8 Hz in the paroxysmal AF patient whose electrograms are shown in Figure 8.15. While frequency in the majority of the atria and CS was relatively slow (≤5 Hz), the posterior wall of the LA was activated at faster rates (7–8 Hz), with notable HDF sites at each of the PVs. In this patient, focal radio-frequency ablation applied to the HDF site near the right inferior PV (RIPV) effectively terminated AF. Figure 8.16b shows a DF map from a patient with permanent AF. Compared with the patient with paroxysmal AF, this patient not only had a higher frequency at the maximal HDF site (13.7 Hz), but also both atria demonstrated higher global frequency of activity and in addition, many of the HDF sites were located in the atria rather than in the PV region. We concluded that in the cohort of patients studied, paroxysmal AF was characterized by the hierarchical spatial distribution of DFs where the LA and PVs were always the fastest regions. By contrast, in persistent AF, a more uniform distribution of higher DF values was observed, where the highest DFs could not be found in the PV region.

Activation Frequency and Rotors as Atrial Fibrillation Drivers in Humans

The ability of RF ablation to terminate AF in some patients suggests that the arrhythmia depends on a focal small number of sources for its maintenance. However, whether those sources are of ectopic automaticity, triggers, or reentry-based drivers is not clear. Identifying rotors directly as drivers of AF in patients is not feasible with the existing mapping techniques. Yet, the results shown in Figure 8.11 offered an idea that led to the translation from the animal experiments to the patient and gave us an opportunity to obtain evidence, though indirect, for the presence of rotors as drivers through pharmacologic means. Translation was made possible also by the fact that adenosine, which is widely used in the clinic, is known to activate the same Kir3.x subfamily of inward-rectifier potassium channels as ACh, albeit through a different signaling pathway. By increasing K^+ conductance in the atrium, both ACh and adenosine hyperpolarize the cell membrane, abbreviate the action potential duration and the refractory period, and inhibit spontaneous pacemaker discharge as well as early and delayed depolarizations. On the other hand, as seen in Figure 8.11 for ACh, they both accelerate reentrant activity. Thus, in a study by Atienza et al. in 2006, adenosine was used to test the hypothesis that localized reentry maintains AF also in humans. We determined the effects of adenosine infusion on DF at varying locations of both atria to test the idea that adenosine-induced acceleration of HDF sites reveals reentry as the mechanism of AF maintenance and therefore rules out an

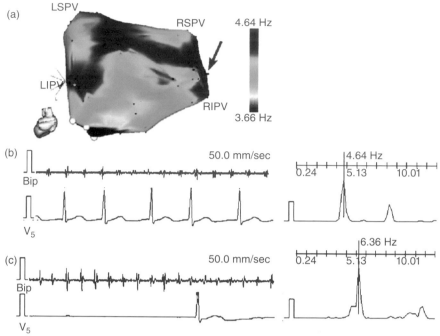

Figure 8.17 Accelerating effect of adenosine on a high dominant frequency (HDF) site. (a) Left atrium (LA) posterior view of a DF map from a paroxysmal atrial fibrillation (AF) patient. The DF map was produced by the real-time frequency-mapping CARTO system before infusion of adenosine. Red arrow indicates primary HDF site near the RIPV. (b) Baseline recording at the primary HDF site with its power spectrum and simultaneous V₅ reference. (c) Recording at the primary HDF site with power spectrum and simultaneous V₅ reference during peak adenosine effect showing increase of DF. LSPV, LIPV, RSPV, RIPV: left/right superior/inferior pulmonary veins (PVs); Bip, bipolar catheter. (Reproduced with permission from Atienza *et al.*, *Circulation* 2006; 114:2434–42.)

automatic or triggered mechanism. We generated baseline DF maps of the LA using real-time spectral analysis capabilities that allowed determination of the specific HDF site locations likely to harbor the AF drivers in four paroxysmal AF patients. Then the adenosine effect was measured at the highest and second-highest HDF sites in the LA. Figure 8.17 shows a representative example where the AF frequency at baseline was relatively slow (<5 Hz) and three HDF sites were identified with the highest HDF site being located near the RIPV (red arrow). Panels (b) and (c) show that while the adenosine infusion practically abolished the ventricular activity (through its effect on the atrioventricular node) as detected by V₅ on the surface ECG, the DF at the highest HDF site accelerated from 4.64 Hz at baseline to 6.35 Hz at the peak of the adenosine effect. An additional adenosine infusion performed while measuring activity at a secondary HDF site also showed an increase in DF, but to a lesser extent. Interestingly, in this patient, the arrhythmia terminated during post-mapping ablation at the primary HDF site, supporting again the critical role of such sites as AF driver locations. Compared with baseline, adenosine significantly accelerated the primary and secondary HDF sites in these four patients from about 5 to 6.7 Hz, demonstrating that the sites involved in the maintenance of AF are clearly affected by adenosine.

In a larger cohort of paroxysmal and persistent AF patients, Atienza *et al.* analyzed the effect of adenosine on the activation rate in specific regions at the junction of the PV and the LA (PV-LAJ), the roof of the RA (HRA), and the coronary sinus (CS). In general, patients with persistent AF demonstrated significantly higher maximal baseline DFs than paroxysmal AF patients ($P <$ 0.001). However, adenosine infusion in persistent AF patients increased local DFs only in the HRA. The increase in the PV-LAJ was not statistically significant and there was no change in the CS DF. In sum, adenosine infusion increased frequency primarily at sites that activated at the highest rate at baseline. In paroxysmal AF patients, adenosine increased activation frequency in the PV-LAJ. In persistent AF patients, the highest-frequency sources accelerated by adenosine were located in either atria but not at PV sites. Thus, the response to adenosine is consistent with reentrant drivers maintaining AF that have different locations in paroxysmal compared with persistent AF patients.

Summary

Experimental studies of cholinergic AF in the isolated sheep heart demonstrated that high-frequency reentrant sources in the left atrium can drive the fibrillatory activity throughout both atria. Following those results and based on a large body of work investigating how measurements of AF cycle length in patients can contribute to its treatment, we focused our analysis on the organization of DF of the activity during AF in humans. Using electroanatomic mapping and Fourier methods, we generated three-dimensional, whole-atrial DF maps in patients undergoing AF ablation procedures and identified relatively small areas where the DF was particularly higher than its surrounding. In patients with paroxysmal AF, those sites are often localized to the posterior left atrium near the ostia of the PVs. In contrast, patients with permanent AF demonstrate high DF sites that are more often localized to either atrium than the posterior left atrium–PV junction. The response of the arrhythmia to adenosine is consistent with the mechanistic hypothesis that reentry in those high DF sites maintains human AF, and that reentrant drivers have different locations in paroxysmal compared with persistent AF patients.

9 Molecular Mechanisms of Ventricular Fibrillation

Ventricular fibrillation (VF) is the leading immediate cause of sudden cardiac death in the industrialized world, accounting for an estimated 300 000 fatalities annually in the United States of America alone. On ECG, VF is characterized by the presence of an aperiodic and irregular rhythm, suggesting that the activation of the ventricles is highly complex and disorganized. Thus, according to conventional wisdom, VF is the result of totally random electrical excitation of the ventricles. However, as for AF (see Chapter 8), an old idea on the mechanism of fibrillation has reemerged from theoretical and experimental studies showing that wave propagation during VF is not totally random. The postulate is that "rotors" are the major organizing centers of fibrillation, and that certain specific molecular properties of the cardiac muscle at the ion channel level contribute to rotor stability and frequency, as well as to the overall complexity of the arrhythmia. This chapter has three major objectives: (1) to review the most significant literature on wave propagation dynamics and VF maintenance; (2) to discuss recently published data on the molecular mechanism of VF in the structurally and electrophysiologically normal heart; such mechanisms may be explained in part on the basis of chamber-specific differences in the level of expression of cardiac potassium channels; and (3) to summarize new evidence that strongly supports the idea that the fundamental concepts reviewed in the foregoing chapters, including the idea of rotor and wavebreaks, are applicable to the understanding of the mechanism of VF and sudden cardiac death in all mammals, including humans.

Wavebreaks and Rotors

About three decades ago, theoretical and experimental findings demonstrated that the heart could sustain a self-organized electrical activity that rotated about a functional obstacle. These "rotors" were thought to be the major

Basic Cardiac Electrophysiology for the Clinician, 2nd edition. By J. Jalife, M. Delmar, J. Anumonwo, O. Berenfeld and J. Kalifa. Published 2009 by Blackwell Publishing, ISBN: 978-1-4501-8333-8.

organizing centers of fibrillation. Since then, much work has focused on rotors as the underlying mechanism for VF in the heart. However, two schools of thought have emerged. First, many recently proposed mechanisms for VF have focused on the instability and breakup of rotors. Over the past two decades, substantial experimental and theoretical work has accumulated suggesting that "turbulence" in VF is associated with breakup of a single spiral wave or a pair of counter-rotating spiral waves into a multispiral disordered state. To explain this phenomenon, the restitution hypothesis suggests that the breakup of the rotor into a multispiral state ensues when the oscillations of the action potential duration (APD) are of sufficiently large amplitude to cause block of conduction along the wave front. This idea builds on previous work demonstrating that the slope of the electrical restitution relation determines certain dynamical behavior that may be conducive to the development of ventricular fibrillation. In particular, if the slope of the action potential restitution curve, in which duration of the action potential is plotted against the preceding diastolic interval, is >1, then APD alternans are possible. The initiation of APD alternans has been proposed to be the first step in period-doubling sequences that culminate in complex behavior. Subsequently, this process would result in the destabilization of the wave fronts and the formation of a multispiral state. Another mechanism for breakup focuses on the fact that propagation within the 3-D myocardium is highly anisotropic due the intramural rotation of the fibers, thus producing twisting and instability of the organizing center (filament), which results in its multiplication following repeated collisions with boundaries in the heart. Second, work from our laboratory has also focused on rotors as the primary engines of fibrillation. However, in contrast to the breakup mechanism, we have proposed that under appropriate conditions, rotors may be long lasting even in the structurally normal heart and result in a high degree of spatial and temporal organization, although during VF there may be a wide spectrum of rotor behaviors. On one end, it has been demonstrated that a single drifting rotor can give rise to a complex pattern of excitation that is reminiscent of torsades de pointes or even VF, depending on rotation frequency. On the other end, it has been suggested that VF is the result of a high-frequency rotor stabilized somewhere in a small area of myocardium and the complex patterns of activation that are observed throughout the ventricles are the result of the fragmentation of emanating electrical activity from that rotor, i.e., fibrillatory conduction.

Fibrillatory Conduction

Gray *et al.* demonstrated unequivocally in 1995 that, in the rabbit heart, even a single drifting rotor could produce an ECG that is indistinguishable from VF. However, it has been demonstrated also that in other hearts, a more complex spatiotemporal organization may prevail. This has led us to suggest that some forms of fibrillation depend on the uninterrupted periodic activity of discrete reentrant circuits. The faster rotors act as dominant frequency (DF) sources that maintain the overall activity. The rapidly succeeding wave fronts emanating from these sources propagate throughout the ventricles and interact with functional and anatomical tissue heterogeneities, leading to fragmentation and wavelet formation (see Chapter 5). The newly formed wavelets may undergo decremental conduction or they may be annihilated by collision with another wavelet or a boundary, and still others may form new sustained rotors. Thus, the result would be fibrillatory conduction or the frequency-dependent fragmentation of wave fronts, emanating from high-frequency reentrant circuits, into multiple independent wavelets. Spectral analysis of optical epicardial and endocardial signals for sheep ventricular slabs has provided additional evidence in favor of the idea that fibrillatory conduction may be the underlying mechanism of VF. Data were presented showing that the DFs of excitation (i.e., peak with maximal power) do not change continuously on the ventricular surfaces of slabs. Rather, the frequencies are constant over regions termed "domains." Moreover, there are only a small number of discrete domains found on the ventricular surfaces. They also demonstrated that the DFs of excitation in the adjacent domains were often 1:2, 3:4, or 4:5 ratios of the fastest DF domain and this was suggested to be the result of intermittent Wenckebach-like conduction blocks at the boundaries between domains. Thus, the conclusion was drawn that, in the ventricular slab model, VF may be the result of a sustained high-frequency 3-D intramural scroll wave, which creates a highly complex pattern of activation when wave fronts emanating from it fragment as the result of interaction with the heterogeneities present in the cardiac tissue.

The Guinea Pig Heart Model of Ventricular Fibrillation

In 2001, Samie *et al.* from our laboratory presented new evidence in the isolated Langendorff-perfused guinea pig heart that strongly supported the hypothesis that fibrillatory conduction from a stable high-frequency reentrant source is the underlying mechanism of VF in this species. Optical recordings of potentiometric dye fluorescence from the epicardial ventricular surface were obtained along with a volume-conducted "global" ECG. Spectral analysis of optical signals (pixel by pixel) was performed and the DF from each pixel was used to generate a DF map, which revealed that DFs were distributed throughout the ventricles in clearly demarcated domains (see Figure 9.1). The highest DF domains were always found on the anterior wall of the left ventricle (LV). Moreover, optical data showed that wavebreaks and intermittent conduction block occur at the boundaries between high- and low-frequency domains.

Nature of the Fastest Dominant Frequencies

In Figure 9.2a, we present the ECG from another heart during VF. In Figure 9.2b, the DF map of that VF episode shows the LV-to-RV gradient of DFs.

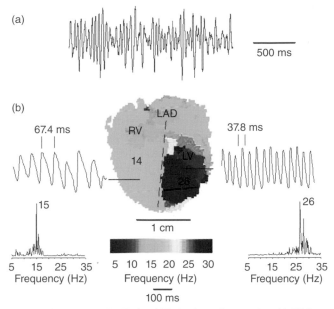

Figure 9.1 Analysis of ventricular fibrillation (VF) dominant frequencies. (a) ECG trace.
(b) Dominant frequency map with single-pixel recordings (top tracings) and respective power
spectra (bottom tracings) from the right ventricle (RV, left) and left ventricle (LV, right). LAD, left
anterior descending artery. (Reproduced with permission from Samie *et al.*, *Circ Res* 2001;
89:1216–23.)

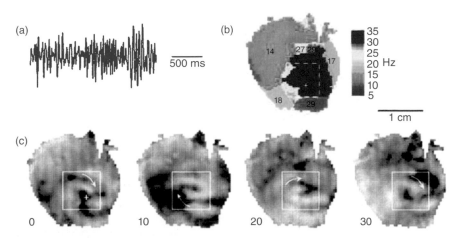

Figure 9.2 High-frequency rotor. (a) ECG trace of ventricular fibrillation (VF). (b) Dominant
frequency (DF) map showing the left to right ventricle (LV-RV) gradient in frequencies.
(c) Snapshots of a long-lasting rotor on the anterior LV wall at four different times during one
rotation. Numbers in panel (b) are in Hz; numbers in panel (c) are in milliseconds. (Reproduced
with permission from Samie *et al.*, *Circ Res* 2001; 89:1216–23.)

Further observation in the optical recordings demonstrated that, in fact, a relatively stable high-frequency rotor was responsible for the fastest DF domain in the LV. Figure 9.2c shows snapshots of the rotor at four different times during one rotation. In this example, the rotor was on the epicardial surface for ≈150 rotations at 32 Hz. Thus, the activity of a high-frequency rotor gave rise to the fastest DF domain in this heart. To establish the contribution of rotor activity to the fast frequency domain in other eight hearts, 11 rotors were identified. We calculated the frequency of each rotor and correlated it with the fastest DF. A strong correlation ($R = 0.95$) existed between the two parameters, suggesting that the rotor was the main contributor to the frequency of the fastest domain. However, despite the stability of the highest frequency domain in the LV, and the excellent correlation between the rotation frequencies and the highest DFs, inspection of the LV epicardium revealed rotors of variable persistence (ranging 4 to 150 rotations). Thus, while it is likely that all dominant rotors remained in the anterior LV wall, some probably took an intramural position and thus were hidden from view.

Action Potential Abbreviation and Rapid Rotation Frequency

During VF, the activation rate is significantly faster than that achievable by either pacemaker activity or rapid pacing. Similarly in our experiments, rotors achieve cycle lengths (CLs ~30–40 milliseconds) that are significantly briefer than expected from the guinea pig heart whose APD is ~200 milliseconds, at 1 Hz. Recent computer simulations suggest that the activation at extremely fast rates by stationary rotors may be the result of the strong repolarizing influence exerted by their core, which abbreviates the APD in its proximity. This is explained by the fact that the core contains excitable but unexcited cells that remain near the resting potential. Thus, during reentry there is a sink-to-source mismatch, which results in the flow of electrotonic currents between cells in the core and cells in the immediate vicinity of the core. Such electrotonic currents drive neighboring cells toward repolarized potentials, and hence, shorten APD. However, with increasing distance from the core, this influence weakens and the APD progressively increases. Consequently, the tissue close to the core achieves very fast CLs, whereas far from the core, the myocardium cannot conduct at the rate of the rotor and nonuniform (i.e., other than 1:1) conduction develops. In theory, this effect may provide a basis for the gradient in DFs observed in the guinea pig ventricles during VF. As illustrated in the paper by Samie *et al.* published in 2001, propagation near the rotor is usually 1:1; however, at a certain distance from the rotor, intermittent conduction block and wavebreaks develop and slower DF domains are formed. Nevertheless, while this mechanism may account for the shortening of the APD and the formation of DF domains, it does not explain the consistent localization of the fastest DF domain to the anterior free wall of the LV.

Background Current in Left Ventricle versus Right Ventricle

Numerical simulations have demonstrated the importance of the background inward-rectifier potassium current (I_{K1}) in the establishment of a fast and stable reentry. As discussed in the previous chapters, the prediction is that I_{K1} helps to abbreviate the APD near the core; in addition, I_{K1} is also essential in maintaining the stability of rotors. Therefore, we decided to use the whole-cell voltage-clamp technique to characterize the background current in the RV and the LV, and relate its spatial distribution to differences in excitation frequencies. Panel (a) of Figure 9.3 shows the current density–voltage ($I–V$) relations of the background current of two different cells from the LV and the RV in the same heart. As seen, the outward conductance is clearly larger in the LV cell than in the RV cell. Similar results were obtained for 19 LV cells and 18 RV cells isolated from 10 guinea pig hearts. Panel (b) shows the mean $I–V$ relations of those cells, indicating that the magnitude of the outward conductance is significantly higher in the LV than in the RV (−50 mV: RV 5.3 ± 0.4; LV 7.4 ± 0.6 pA/pF, $P = 0.009$). In additional experiments using a standard subtraction procedure after measuring the current density in the presence and the absence of 1-mM Ba^{2+} to obtain the Ba^{2+}-sensitive current, we confirmed that the density of the outward component of I_{K1} is indeed greater in the LV than in the RV myocytes. A number of mechanisms may underlie this

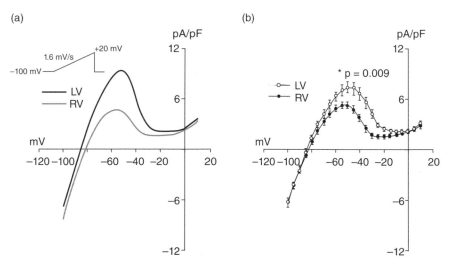

Figure 9.3 Current–voltage relations for background current (I_B). (a) Current–density voltage relation of I_B for sample cells from the right ventricle (RV) and left ventricle (LV) of the same heart. Inset: voltage-clamp protocol. A slow ramp of 1.6 mV/s was applied from a holding potential of −100 to +20 mV. (b) Mean $I–V$ relation for I_B (nRV = 18 and nLV = 19). Currents were normalized to cell capacitance and averaged. Mean RV and LV capacitances, 165 and 167 pF, respectively. (Reproduced with permission from Samie *et al.*, *Circ Res* 2001; 89: 1216–23.)

difference in the outward component of I_{K1} density observed in the right and left ventricles. Two possibilities, based on differences in specific genes expressed between the LV and the RV, are (1) the genes for specific ion channels or (2) the genes for proteins that directly, or indirectly, regulate the function of these channels. Notably, however, we found that the density of the inward component is essentially the same in both ventricles (see Figure 9.3), which may be due to the contribution of other conductances to the inward background current in the myocytes, particularly, the Na+ background current. An alternative explanation is that the inward-rectifier channel complex responsible for I_{K1} actually is formed by heteromultimers of protein isoforms encoded by two or more different but closely related genes.

An Ionic Mechanism of Stable Ventricular Fibrillation

Our studies strongly suggested that the stabilization of the rotor in the LV was related to a difference in the I_{K1} density of cells in the RV and the LV. The single-channel conductance and mean open time of I_{K1} are 40 pS and 100 milliseconds, respectively. Furthermore, the time independency of I_{K1} guaranties that its $I–V$ relationship is maintained similar at different activation rates; particularly at the high activation rates that characterize reentrant sources of ventricular fibrillation. I_{K1} contributes a large inward conductance at membrane potentials below the potassium equilibrium potential (E_K), which together with the relatively large outward conductance at potentials just above E_K, helps maintain the resting membrane potential close to E_K. In addition, I_{K1} is an important determinant of the duration and shape of the normal cardiac action potential; it also helps I_{Kr} and I_{Ks} to end the plateau and is responsible for the terminal phase of rapid repolarization. During functional reentry, however, APD is significantly abbreviated near the center of rotation. Under these conditions, premature repolarization near the core is speculated to depend less on I_{Kr} or I_{Ks} and to be mediated via the combined influence of I_{K1} and the electrotonic repolarizing current provided by the core. Computer simulations show that in addition to controlling the APD, the large I_{K1} stabilizes reentry by reducing the wave front–wave tail interaction. As shown in Figure 9.3, subsequent experiments showed that the outward component in $I–V$ relation of I_{K1} is different in the cells of the RV and the LV. With such data in hand, we carried out numerical studies to determine the consequences that a significant difference outward current density may have on the dynamics of rotors and the waves emanating from them. As illustrated in panel (a) of Figure 9.4, upon incorporation of the experimental current–voltage relations corresponding to the RV and LV into a single-cell computer model, the action potential of the cell with the higher outward current component from the LV showed an abbreviated action potential. Further incorporation of those current–voltage relations data into a 2-D model of reentrant cardiac excitation shown in panel (b), the model with small outward conductance of I_{K1}, simulating the RV, was unable to sustain a rotor because the wave front and wave

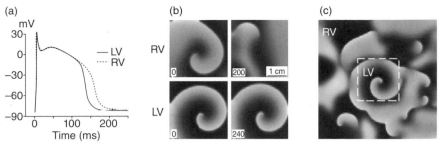

Figure 9.4 Computer simulations of functional reentry using experimentally obtained I_{K1} current–voltage relations in the modified Luo and Rudy model. (a) Simulated action potentials in single cells incorporating the left and right ventricle (LV and RV) I_{K1} current–voltage relations. Notably, the increased outward component of I_{K1} in the LV results in an abbreviation of its action potential. (b) Two snapshots of numerical data obtained in a 3×3 cm^2 sheet simulating the RV and LV models. (c) Snapshot of numerical data in the combined RV-LV model of 6×6 cm^2. Values in all panels are in milliseconds. Broken lines in panel (b) show the perimeter of the LV model (area, 2×2 cm^2). (Modified with permission from Samie et al., Circ Res 2001; 89:1216–23.)

tail collided, trapped the tip of the rotor, and thus terminated the activity. In contrast, simulating the LV activity, we observed that the large outward conductance of I_{K1} produced the necessary abbreviation of the APD for the establishment of a stable high-frequency rotor. Moreover, as shown in panel (c), when LV and RV models were coupled in a 2-D sheet, the numerical results accurately reproduced the experimental VF data. Under these conditions, the high-frequency rotor in the LV (center) became the engine that maintained the overall activity in both ventricles, with the RV (periphery) producing multiple short-lived wavebreaks and non-sustained reentry whose intrinsic frequency was much slower than in the LV. Thus, our simulations predict that, by reducing APD near the core and preventing wave front–wave tail interactions, the larger amplitude of the outward component of I_{K1} in LV myocytes stabilizes the high-frequency rotor in the LV.

The Kir Family of Channel Proteins

A very large number of genes encoding potassium channels have been cloned over the last several years and excellent reviews have appeared on this subject (see also Chapter 2). As illustrated in Figure 9.5, members of the family of channels known as the inwardly rectifying potassium (Kir) channels are composed of four subunits, but there is conflicting evidence whether these channels existed as homo- or heterotetramers in vivo. As shown in panel (a), each subunit has cytoplasmic N- and C-termini, two transmembrane domains (M1 and M2). As shown in panel (b), the loop structure (P or H5) between M1 and M2 is responsible for the formation of the pore. The P loop contains the characteristic GYG/GFG stretch that determines K+ selectivity in all potassium channels. The first Kir proteins to be cloned were Kir1.1 and Kir2.1

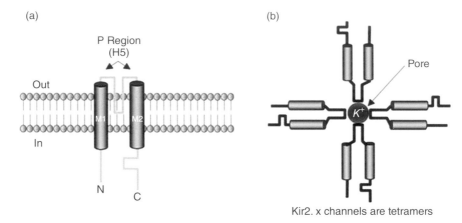

Figure 9.5 (a) Schematic diagram of the deduced topology of a Kir channel protein. (b) Four subunits form a Kir channel with the P region lining the pore.

(originally named ROMK1 and IRK1). Since then, many other Kir channels have been discovered that are now classified into seven subfamilies with diverse properties and expression patterns. Only the Kir2.x and 3.x subfamilies are functional in the heart under normal conditions. The Kir2.x subfamily members are strong inward rectifiers whose time and voltage-dependent rectification properties are almost identical to native I_{K1} in the heart. The Kir3.x subfamily members, found mostly in pacemaker and atrial cells, are G-protein activated and are responsible for the negative chronotropic and inotropic effects observed after vagal stimulation. Kir6.x channels activate only during periods of ischemia by sensing low ATP/ADP ratios during intracellular metabolic stress. Other Kir subfamilies, including Kir1.x, 4.x, 5.x, and 7.x, do not seem to be expressed in cardiac tissue.

Inward Rectification and Kir2.x Channels

Rectification is described as a non-ohmic current–voltage relationship such that a channel's conductance changes with voltage. Inward-rectifier potassium channels of the Kir2.x subfamily pass inward currents at potentials more negative than the reversal potential of K+, but much less current at potentials positive to the reversal potential. Thus, Kir2.x proteins are the strongly rectifying potassium channels that carry I_{K1} and whose main function is to stabilize the resting membrane potential and the excitation threshold; lower I_{K1} conductance through these channels at more depolarized voltages prevents short-circuiting the action potential. However, the Kir channels do pass small but critical amounts of outward current contributing to final repolarization of the action potential. As such, the Kir2.x channels are crucially important for heart function. Katz first described inward rectification in 1949 and Armstrong suggested that inward rectification might be due to an intracellular positively charged molecule blocking the channel pore. Later work in cardiac myocytes showed that intracellular Mg^{2+} blocked Kir channels in a voltage-dependent manner. Once the Kir proteins were cloned in the early 1990s, the more critical role of intracellular polyamines as the "rectifier molecules" for inward-rectifying potassium channels was established. Polyamines block outward currents through Kir channels in a steeper voltage-dependent fashion than Mg^{2+}. Interestingly, although all Kir channels are blocked by intracellular polyamines, the sensitivity of block is different among Kir subfamilies. A weak inward rectifier would permit more outward current as compared with a strong rectifier, which would permit less current. To date, there has not been a comprehensive characterization of the extent of rectification, the Mg^{2+} and polyamine sensitivity, and current–voltage relationship of the Kir2.x subfamily uniformly in a mammalian expression system. Work by Liu *et al.* in 2001 has studied the current–voltage relationship of the guinea pig Kir2.x series using single-channel recordings, but only the inward current was described. This group did not study outward currents and thus, differences in the extent of rectification among the Kir2.x subfamily were not explored. Also, although some basic electrophysiology study has been done in *Xenopus* oocytes and mammalian cells in culture, since ionic conditions of the bath and pipette solutions have been different from one lab to the next, there are no unifying data comparing all Kir2.x isoforms together. Characterization of the Kir2.x channels in a mammalian cell line is urgently needed to allow us to determine if a difference in whole-cell I_{K1} is due to the unique properties of the Kir2.x isoforms and how they are expressed in the heart.

Kir2.x Channels in the Right and Left Ventricle

To establish an underlying mechanism for the different outward components of the background current in LV and RV myocytes, we investigated chamber-specific differences in the level of expression of Kir2.x channels. In panel (a) of Figure 9.6 are shown RNAse protection assay (RPA) data for Kir2.1 and Kir2.3 mRNAs from a single experiment demonstrating denser bands for both genes in the LV. Figure 9.6b clearly demonstrates that mRNAs for both protein isoforms are significantly larger in the LV than in the RV (LV/RV for Kir2.1: 1.97 ± 0.45; Kir2.3: 1.43 ± 0.08; $P < 0.05$ vs. 1). Interestingly, neither Kir2.2 nor Kir2.4 was present at significant levels in the ventricular tissue of either chamber (data not shown). Thus, the difference in the expression of the Kir2.1 and 2.3 transcripts in the guinea pig heart, the levels of both messages being significantly greater in the LV than in the RV, helps explain the significant differences in the outward component of I_{K1} observed in the two ventricles.

Why the Kir2.x Channels?

Compelling evidence for I_{K1} and Kir2.x channel involvement in the mechanism of VF maintenance was the demonstration that pharmacologic

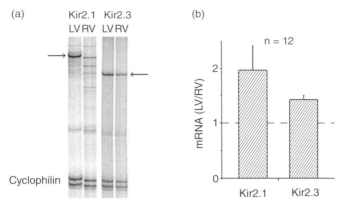

Figure 9.6 (a) Representative RPA showing bands corresponding to Kir2.1, Kir2.3, and cyclophilin (internal loading control) mRNA in the left ventricle (LV) and right ventricle (RV). (b) mRNA levels of Kir2.1 (1.97 ± 0.45) and Kir2.3 (1.43 ± 0.08) in LV normalized with respect to RV (n = 12). Horizontal dashed line at "1" indicates equal mRNA level in the LV and RV. (Reproduced with permission from Warren et al., J Cardiovasc Electrophysiol 2003; 14:621–31.)

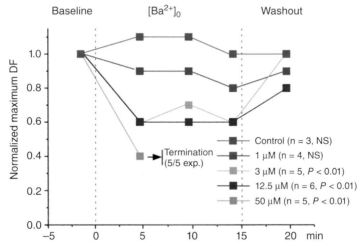

Figure 9.7 Time course of Ba^{2+}-induced changes in left ventricular dominant frequency (DF; normalized to the maximum during baseline) and after washout. All Ba^{2+} concentrations produced significant changes ($P < 0.05$) at 5 minutes, except 1 µmol/L. (Reproduced with permission from Warren et al., J Cardiovasc Electrophysiol 2003; 14:621–31.)

blockade of this current could terminate reentry and fibrillation. It was found that the relative effect of selective blockade by micromolar concentrations of Ba^{2+} on the outward component of I_{K1} is greater in LV than in RV myocytes. Importantly, at the range of concentrations known to selectively block I_{K1}, Ba^{2+} perfusion terminated VF in the Langendorff-perfused guinea pig heart in a dose-dependent manner. Figure 9.7 shows the evolution of the normalized average maximum DF frequency in each dosage group. Clearly, whereas maximum DF was not significantly altered in three control hearts, 3, 12.5, and 50 μmol/L Ba^{2+} produced the largest effect with very rapid (maximum effect ≤5 minutes) and significant decreases in DF ($P < 0.01$). Washout with normal Tyrode's solution partially restored the DF. The most striking effect of Ba^{2+} was termination of VF in a concentration-dependent manner. Specifically, 50 μmol/L Ba^{2+} terminated VF in five out of five experiments within 10 minutes; 1 μmol/L Ba^{2+} did not terminate any of the episodes. Although 50 μmol/L Ba^{2+} terminated VF reproducibly, usually sinus rhythm was not restored. Instead, slow polymorphic arrhythmias ensued with beat-to-beat change of epicardial breakthrough site, indicating that Ba^{2+} may have induced slow spontaneous discharges at subepicardial locations, perhaps at varying sites within the His-Purkinje network.

The rectification properties of Kir2.x channels mirror whole-cell I_{K1} very closely, but there is also a significant difference in the outward component of rectification between the cloned Kir2.1 and 2.3 channels when expressed in mammalian cells. These channels do not require modulation by intracellular factors (e.g., G-proteins) to pass current as is seen in the Kir3.x and 6.x subfamilies. To our knowledge, no one has yet studied how individual properties of the Kir2.x subfamily members contribute to differences in I_{K1} in different regions of the heart and used this information to understand ventricular fibrillation. It is of interest that it has been proposed that dominant negative mutations of Kir2.1 function are responsible for dysmorphic features, periodic paralysis, and cardiac arrhythmias in patients with Andersen-Tawil (AT) syndrome, also known as LQT7. Studies by Preisig-Müller *et al.* in 2001 have presented strong evidence that the mutant allele of Kir2.1 responsible for AT syndrome may combine with wild-type Kir2.1, Kir2.2, and Kir2.3 proteins to form heterotetrameric channels of Kir2.x potassium channels which may contribute to the great variability in the phenotype of these patients. It has been established that AT syndrome is caused by mutations in KCNJ2, which encodes Kir2.1. In a recent study by Tristani-Firouzi *et al.* in 2002, it was shown that in mutation carriers, long QT syndrome is usually the primary cardiac manifestation and about 64% of these patients present cardiac arrhythmias. However, none of the subjects studied by this group suffered sudden cardiac death. In numerical studies in which the effects of Kir2.1 reduction were studied in a model of single ventricular myocytes, the same investigators showed that the terminal phase of the cardiac action potential was prolonged. When a reduced extracellular K$^+$ was simulated, Na$^+$/Ca^{2+} exchanger-dependent delayed afterdepolarizations and spontaneous arrhythmias developed. While these observations suggest that the substrate for arrhythmia susceptibility in AT syndrome was somewhat different from the other forms of inherited long QT syndrome, it did not provide any insight into the absent incidence of sudden death in these patients. We speculate that the reduced I_{K1} in AT syndrome patients conveys an important degree of protection against initiation of reentrant arrhythmias by premature excitation associated with delayed repolarization. As demonstrated by the 2-D computer simulations presented in Figure 9.4a, it is likely that APD and wavelength prolongation induced by I_{K1} reduction renders the ventricles of these patients unable to sustain any stable rotors because the wave front and wave tail interactions lead to spontaneous termination of the activity.

I_{K1} Up-Regulation in the Mouse Heart

Genetically engineered mice represent invaluable tools in which the electro-physiological consequences of manipulating ion channels at the molecular level can be directly determined. Li *et al.* in 2004 generated a transgenic (TG) mouse in which I_{K1} was up-regulated by overexpressing the Kir2.1 protein in the heart under control of the α-myosin heavy chain promoter. Two viable lines (lines 1 and 2) that overexpressed the Kir2.1–GFP fusion protein were generated. Surface ECG recordings from anaesthetized line 2 mice revealed dramatic abnormalities of excitability expected from increased I_{K1}, including short corrected QT interval (QTc), slowed heart rate, junctional escape, atrio-ventricular block, atrial flutter, and sudden death. Line 1 mice survived longer than line 2 mice, and had a prolonged QRS interval and shortened QTc interval compared with wild-type (WT) mice. The effective refractory period in isolated hearts was reduced in both lines. Figure 9.8 shows volume-conducted

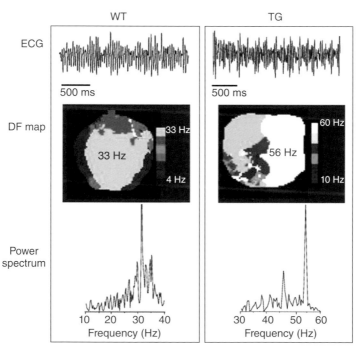

Figure 9.8 Ventricular fibrillation in wild-type (WT, left) and transgenic (TG; up-regulation of I_{K1}; right) isolated mouse hearts. Top: ECGs; middle: dominant frequency (DF) maps; bottom: corresponding power spectra of the ECG traces. Color scales: WT, 4–33 Hz; TG, 10–60 Hz. (Reproduced with permission from Noujaim *et al.*, *J Physiol* 2007; 578:315–26.)

ECGs, DF maps, and power spectral plots from representative WT and TG hearts from line 1 in VF. In both cases, the ECGs (top) are compound, with polymorphic wave shapes characteristic of VF, but the complexes are narrower in the TG compared with the WT heart. In both cases, the arrhythmias were complex. In the WT heart, the DF map (middle left) reveals a 33-Hz frequency domain (yellow) in addition to other slower domains, consistent with the power spectrum of the ECG trace (bottom left), which displays a DF of 34 Hz along with additional small peaks in an overall pattern that is typical of VF. The DF map of the TG heart (middle right) shows a domain (white) of 56 Hz, coexisting with other slower frequency domains. The power spectrum of the ECG (bottom right) displays a large peak at 56 Hz coexisting with multiple other smaller peaks. Again, this pattern is indistinguishable from VF. Altogether, the data from those WT and TG mice, as well as those from the guinea pigs, optical mapping experiments demonstrate that I_{K1} has a crucial role in controlling frequency and stability of rotors responsible for VT/VF.

I_{Ks} and Fibrillatory Conduction

The data presented earlier and in the preceding chapters clearly support the idea that VF is characterized by the presence of electrical rotors that spin at exceedingly high frequencies, generating wave fronts that block intermittently in a spatially distributed manner, with consequent wave front fragmentation (wavebreak), and wavelet formation. This suggests that at least some forms of VF are highly organized and depend on the uninterrupted periodic activity of a small number of high-frequency reentrant sources. The rapidly succeeding wave fronts emanating from such sources propagate throughout the ventricles and interact with tissue heterogeneities, both functional and anatomical, leading to fragmentation and wavelet formation, the end result being fibrillatory conduction (see Chapter 5). The following question remains, however: what are the molecular mechanisms of wavebreaks and how do they lead to fibrillatory conduction?

As discussed in Chapter 5, the gating kinetics of the delayed-rectifier K+ current (I_K) contribute to post-repolarization refractoriness leading to frequency-dependent intermittent excitation failure in isolated cardiomyocytes. However, until recently, the impact of such kinetics on arrhythmogenesis, particularly VF, was unknown. Recently, we used neonatal cardiomyocyte monolayers as a 2-D biological excitable medium to investigate the consequences of the overexpression of the slow component of I_K, I_{Ks}, on excitation, propagation, and the dynamics of reentrant activation. We hypothesized that expression of I_{Ks} in rat cardiomyocyte monolayers contributes to wavebreak formation and facilitates fibrillatory conduction by promoting postrepolarization refractoriness. Consequently we performed optical mapping experiments using rat ventricular myocyte monolayers infected with an adenovirus carrying the genomic sequences of KvLQT1 and minK (molecular correlates of I_{Ks}) and littermate controls infected with a GFP adenovirus. APD

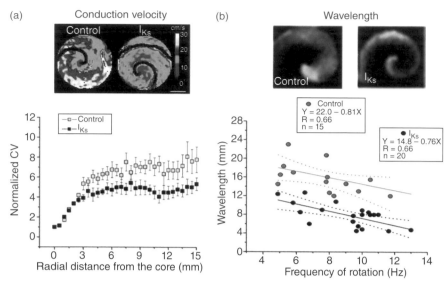

Figure 9.9 Conduction velocity (CV) and wavelength during reentry in cardiomyocyte monolayers. (a) Top: CV maps. Note greater velocities in the core periphery of control (left) than I_{Ks} (right) monolayer; bottom: normalized CV as a function of radial distance from the core. (b) Top: snapshots of electrical spirals in control (8.3 Hz; left) and I_{Ks} (10.1 Hz; right) monolayers. Wavelength, defined as the spatial extension of the excited state, was greater in control than I_{Ks}; bottom: wavelength, measured 5 mm from the core was significantly larger in control than I_{Ks} at all rotation frequencies. (Modified with permission from Muñoz *et al.*, *Circ Res* 2007; 101:475–83.)

was significantly shorter in I_{Ks} than in control monolayers at all rotation frequencies. Moreover, as shown in Figure 9.9a during reentry, conduction velocity (CV) as a function of distance from the core had a significantly less pronounced increase in the I_{Ks} monolayers, consistent with a less excitable preparation. As a result, wavelengths in the latter were significantly shorter than in littermate controls at all rotation frequencies (Figure 9.9b). Consequently, stable rotors occurred in both groups, with significantly higher rotation frequencies, lower conduction velocities, and shorter action potentials in the I_{Ks} group.

Another important difference was that unlike control monolayers, the waves emanating from rotors in the I_{Ks} preparations frequently underwent wavebreak, fibrillatory conduction, and formation of new, short-lived rotors in a time-dependent fashion. Figure 9.10 illustrates the contrasting evolution of the two groups. In panel (a), the top frames show individual phase maps of a control monolayer obtained at 0, 120, 240, and 360 seconds of the onset of the experiment. The bottom frames show similar phase maps of littermate monolayers infected with I_{Ks} at 0, 90, 180, and 270 seconds after the onset of the experiment. In both cases, waves were generated by a single reentrant source rotating at 8.2 Hz (control) and 9.4 Hz (I_{Ks}). It is clear from these examples that while in the control there was a single rotor giving rise to

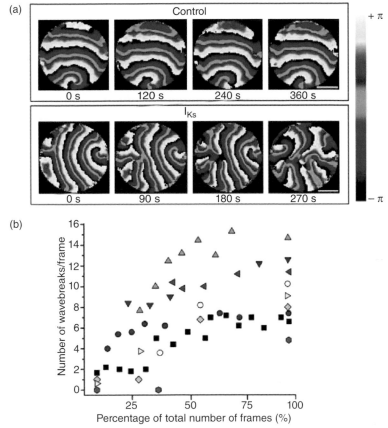

Figure 9.10 I_{Ks} overexpression results in fibrillatory conduction. (a) Top: sequential phase maps of a control monolayer; bottom: phase maps of littermate monolayers infected with I_{Ks}. Waves are generated by a single reentrant source rotating at 8.2 and 9.4 Hz for top and bottom, respectively. Scale bars = 10 mm; numbers, time in seconds. (b) As indicated by the various colored symbols, the number of wavebreaks increased progressively in the nine I_{Ks} monolayers that developed fibrillatory conduction. Different symbols indicate different experiments. (Reproduced with permission from Muñoz *et al.*, *Circ Res* 2007; 101:475–83.)

well-organized wave fronts at all times, I_{Ks} overexpression resulted in a time-dependent increase in the density of wavebreaks and the complexity of the fibrillatory conduction pattern. As shown in panel (b), the number of wave-breaks increased progressively. Moreover, the density of wavebreaks increased with time as long as a stable source sustained the fibrillatory activity. None of the controls showed any wavebreaks other than the original rotor giving rise to sustained reentrant activity.

It is important to note at this point that apparently chaotic waves often recorded optically during VF in intact hearts and attributed to fibrillatory conduction may be generated by sources outside the field of view. In mono-layers, however, the area recorded corresponded to the entire preparation, allowing the strong conclusion that all the episodes of fibrillatory conduction were sustained by at least one stable rotor. In summary, during sustained reentry, I_{Ks} overexpression decreases APD, CV, and wavelength (WL) at frequencies ranging between 4.9 and 13 Hz. However, despite inducing such a significant WL shortening, I_{Ks} overexpression results in "history-dependent" sink/source mismatch during diastole that leads to wavebreak and fibrillatory conduction particularly at high frequencies of reentry.

The Universal Law of Ventricular Fibrillation Frequency Scaling Across Species

During VF, the ventricular activation sequence is profoundly abnormal and electrical wave fronts no longer follow the usual paths. Yet, it has been hypothesized that the perpetuation of the abnormal excitation depends on a driver in the form of a self-sustaining reentrant activation across species. Such common mechanism maintaining the fibrillatory behavior is illustrated by the data in Figure 9.11, which was obtained by high-resolution optical mapping of Langendorff-perfused hearts from four different mammals. Fluorescent voltage-sensitive dye and a CCD camera that was focused on the anterior ventricular surface of those hearts recorded the electrical activity. Snapshots taken from phase movies of wave-propagation dynamics during stable VF

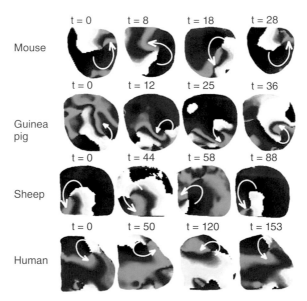

Figure 9.11 Stable ventricular fibrillation in the hearts of four different mammals, from mouse to humans. Four action potential phase snapshots depict a rotation of spirals in mouse, guinea pig, sheep, and human hearts. Vortex-like reentry is apparent in all hearts. The white circular arrows mark the location of the center and the direction of rotation. Numbers above each map represent time in milliseconds after an arbitrary zero. (Reproduced with permission from Noujaim *et al.*, *Proc Natl Acad Sci U S A* 2007; 104:20985–9.)

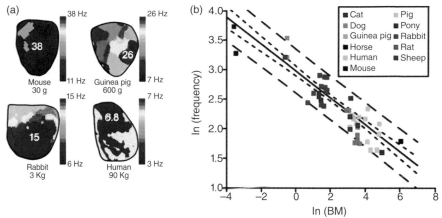

Figure 9.12 Scaling of ventricular fibrillation (VF) frequency in mammalian hearts. (a) Dominant frequency (DF) maps of epicardial electrical activity of mouse, guinea pig, rabbit, and human hearts during VF. The frequencies of excitation are distributed in clearly demarcated domains. The fastest domain in the mouse heart is 38 Hz, in the guinea pig heart is 26 Hz, in the rabbit heart is 15 Hz, and in the human heart is 6.8 Hz. (b) Double logarithmic plot of frequency vs. body mass (BM) covering 11 species, from mouse to horse. Best fit line: y = 2.94 ± 0.04 − 0.23x ± 0.014; R = −0.93; P < 0.01. Solid black line indicates best fit, short dashed lines indicate 95% confidence limits, and long dashed lines indicate 95% prediction limits. (Reproduced with permission from Noujaim et al., Proc Natl Acad Sci U S A 2007; 104: 20985–9.)

reveal sustained vortices (rotors) whose rotation frequency depends on the species (mouse, 38 Hz; guinea pig, 26 Hz; sheep, 12 Hz; human, 6.8 Hz).

Figure 9.12a shows DF maps of VF obtained by fast Fourier transform (FFT) analysis of the high-resolution optical signals in the examples taken from those four different species (mouse, guinea pig, rabbit, and human) spanning three orders of magnitude in their body mass (BM). Altogether, these data demonstrate that during VF, the ventricles do not activate in synchrony. Some areas excite at higher rates than others and the DFs organize in clearly demarcated domains. As demonstrated in hearts from guinea pigs and mice, the frequency of the vortices, or their rotation period (1/frequency), closely matched the frequency of fibrillation or cycle length calculated from the DF maps or the ECG. Notable, however, is the fact that the highest DF domain decreases with increasing body size (mouse, 38 Hz; guinea pig, 26 Hz; rabbit, 15 Hz; human, 6.8 Hz).

Scaling of Ventricular Fibrillation Frequency

In the late 1990s, West et al. demonstrated how biological processes such as metabolic rate, life span, and respiratory rate scale with BM according to the universal law of allometric scaling: $Y = aBM^b$, where Y is the biological process, and b is the scaling exponent, which often is a multiple of 1/4. It has been proposed, using metabolic rate (MR) scaling (MR $\propto$ BM$^{3/4}$), that the underlying mechanism of the 1/4 power law is an evolutionary means to optimize biological systems brought about by the maximization of exchange surface areas and the minimization of transport distances and times. Following a similar reasoning, cardiovascular variables have been predicted and shown to scale with BM as well. For example, in the ECG of the mammalian heart, the time intervals that define the normal inter-beat interval (RR), atrioventricular conduction (PR), duration of ventricular activation (QRS), and duration of the excited state (QT) are all proportional to BM$^{1/4}$. It was recently proposed that the PR interval is $\propto$BM$^{1/4}$ because of the delivery of the action potential from the sinoatrial node, to the ventricles, and through a branching self-similar network (the specialized conduction system). Consequently, it is established that the propagation of the electrical impulse from the atria to the ventricles in the mammalian heart depends on body size. Of note is the left ventricular ejection time, which is $\propto$BM$^{1/4}$, suggesting that, across mammalian species, the normal electrical makeup of the heart is tightly coupled to its pumping function. However, it remained unknown until very recently whether the abnormal electrical wave propagation that characterizes VF holds a relation of dependence on BM.

To establish whether VF frequency actually scales with BM, we obtained data from 11 species, ranging from the 30-g mouse to the 400-kg horse in 40 different published studies, as well as in additional studies we performed in mouse, pig, and sheep hearts. When the frequency of fibrillation is plotted against BM on a double logarithmic scale, the best linear fit yields an intercept of 2.95 $\pm$ 0.04 and a slope of -0.23 ± 0.014 ($R = -0.93$, $P < 0.01$; Figure 9.12b). It follows that the frequency of VF $\approx$ 18.9$\cdot$BM$^{-1/4}$, and that the inter-beat interval of VF equals about 53$\cdot$BM$^{1/4}$. The plot in Figure 9.12b shows that there is variability in the frequency of VF in relation to BM$^{1/4}$. Because most of these values were collected from the literature, inherent differences in the experimental conditions are likely to be present. Also, fundamental chamber-specific differences in gene expression may contribute to such deviations. For example, in the mouse heart, there are regional differences in the distribution of the Kv1.4 gene responsible for the transient outward potassium current, which is known to be more pronounced in mouse than in guinea pig heart. However, expression of the inwardly rectifying potassium current is chamber-specific in the guinea pig heart. The delayed-rectifier potassium current is negligible in the rabbit and rat, but not in the guinea pig and human hearts. Such differences in ion channel expression and/or distribution may significantly affect the frequency and organization of VF. Then again, frequency itself is likely to control VF organization: the higher the frequency, the lower the degree of organization, which helps to explain why VF in human, being slower, seems more organized than in species like pigs and dogs, as suggested by numerical simulations by Ten Tusscher *et al.* The scaling of the inter-beat interval of VF with BM$^{1/4}$ is consistent with the scaling of many physiological time intervals in normal biology, including cardiac cycle, respiratory cycle, life span, total blood circulation time, gestation time, all of which have been shown to be $\propto BM^{1/4}$. However, here we demonstrate that the inter-beat interval of VF, a timescale incompatible with life and a cause of death also follows the same trend, spanning four orders of magnitude in BM.

Mechanism of Ventricular Fibrillation Scaling

The question remains as to the mechanism(s) underlying the scaling of the VF frequency as $BM^{1/4}$. Under normal conditions, in order for the mouse heart to beat much faster than the elephant heart, not only its energetic demand must be met but also the entire electrical excitation–recovery cycle; i.e., the APD must accommodate appropriately to allow fast beating rates. If the APD is too long, then when the next impulse arrives, it will find the tissue ahead of it refractory, and thus unexcitable, leading to failure of propagation. If the APD is too short, then the excitation–contraction coupling phenomenon will be compromised, jeopardizing cardiac function. On ECG, the QT interval measures the global electrical activation–recovery cycle of the ventricles. QT scales in proportion to $BM^{1/4}$. It therefore follows that the APD of the ventricular cells is also $\propto BM^{1/4}$. It is important to stress that although this energetic demand argument does not hold for VF, during which ventricular contraction is asynchronous and force generated is negligible after each excitation, it is clear that APD does change with body size and VF frequency.

Given the constant CV of action potential propagation in mammalian hearts and the scaling of the QT interval during sinus rhythm and VF cycle length to $BM^{1/4}$, we propose that the rotors that maintain VF from small to large animals spin at periods that are strongly dependent on APD. Our premise here is that as the APD increases, the frequency of VF decreases. To validate such a premise, and to authenticate the postulate that the scaling exponent of VF frequency vs. BM is $-1/4$, we carried out computer simulations of vortex-like reentry in five imaginary species with characteristic heart sizes, $L = 1, 2, 4, 8,$ and 16 cm, covering three orders of magnitude in body size (i.e., BM = 0.017–68 kg). We assumed that the density of these hearts is equal to that of water (1 g/cm^3) and that their total mass represents 0.6% of the BM; consequently, BM = $L^3/0.006$. The cell size was assumed to be invariant across species along with the universal formalism of their simple excitation and recovery, for which we used FitzHugh–Nagumo-type membrane kinetics. The membrane model parameters, however, were adjusted for each species; the time constant and repolarization parameters were scaled such that the APD of each model was close to the realistic values of the species and scale precisely as $BM^{1/4}$ (Figure 9.13a), while maintaining a fixed plane wave CV across all species. This operation yielded vortices whose frequency of rotation was $\propto BM^{-1/4}$ (Figure 9.13b) and $\propto APD^{-1}$ (Figure 9.13c). Although somewhat simplistic, these simulations demonstrate that, in general, one can obtain rotors whose frequencies scale like the VF frequencies with a $-1/4$ exponent by scaling the APD similarly to the QT interval, which in turn is proportional to

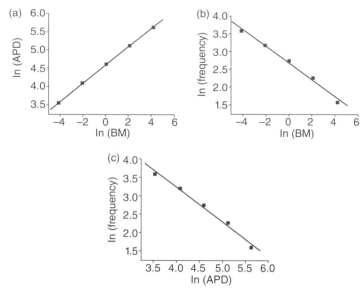

Figure 9.13 Action potential duration (APD) and rotor frequency in computer simulations of imaginary species' hearts. (a) ln(APD) vs. ln(BM): y = 4.58 ± 0.008 + 0.25x ± 0.003; R = 1; P < 0.01. (b) ln(frequency) vs. ln(BM): y = 2.7 ± 0.05 − 0.24x ± 0.02; R = −0.99; P < 0.01. (c) ln(frequency) vs. ln(APD): y = 7 ± 0.3 − 0.94x ± 0.7; R = −0.99; P < 0.01. Gray lines indicate best fit. (Reproduced with permission from Noujaim *et al.*, *Proc Natl Acad Sci U S A* 2007; 104:20985–9.)

the BM with a 1/4 exponent. The experimentally determined best fit for ln (DF) vs. ln (BM) (2.94 − 0.23x) is very close to that determined theoretically from the computer model (2.7 − 0.24x).

What Is the Significance of Ventricular Fibrillation Frequency Scaling?

Despite more than a century of conjecture and experimentation, the mechanisms that initiate and maintain VF remain far from being understood. As such, the ability to identify patients at risk as well as preventing VF remains awfully inadequate. The mechanisms of initiation and maintenance of cardiac fibrillation have traditionally been studied using large animal models and numerical simulations. Work from many laboratories has led to the conviction that the onset of fibrillation occurs when an electrical wave first breaks and begins to rotate at an exceedingly high frequency; it escalates into full fibrillation as the wave fronts generated by rotors encounter tissue that is not ready for excitation, and more wavebreaks occur, leading to completely irregular excitation. Yet, what are the electrical conditions leading to that wavebreak, and how can it be prevented? We simply do not know. In recent years, transgenic and knockout mouse models have become essential for the elucidation and establishment of general principles underlying cardiac channel diseases and their electrophysiologic and arrhythmogenic consequences. This makes allometric scaling relationships essential when it comes to translating the findings to the clinical setting. Mice and other small mammals are used in research due to their size, short life spans, and affordability, with a supposed correlation between their metabolic and organ function to that of humans. Mouse models have become particularly important as newer inroads into cardiac genomics, proteomics, and phenomics hold the promise of defining, at the molecular, cellular, and systemic levels, the functional roles of ion channels and their regulation in the mechanisms of VF and sudden cardiac death. Thus, although the appropriate rendition of the molecular underpinnings of fatal arrhythmias from small mammals to humans is still incomplete, our demonstration that the inter-beat interval of VF scales as $BM^{1/4}$ suggests that there might be a strong similarity in the underlying mechanisms of VF in most, if not all, mammalian species, which may be of considerable fundamental and practical significance.

Summary

In this chapter, we have reviewed the most significant literature on wave propagation dynamics and VF maintenance. We have also discussed recently published data that strongly support the hypothesis that the molecular mechanism of VF in the structurally and electrophysiologically normal heart may be explained in part on the basis of chamber-specific differences in the level of expression of cardiac potassium channels, particularly the inward-rectifier potassium channels responsible for I_{K1}. In addition, we have reviewed some recent experiments in 2-D rat cardiomyocyte monolayers strongly suggesting that the slow component of the delayed-rectifier current, I_{Ks}, plays an important role in the mechanism of fibrillatory conduction. Finally, we summarized recent exciting data demonstrating that the inter-beat interval of VF scales as a function of body mass, according to a universal allometric scaling law ($VF_{Cycle\ length} = 53*BM^{1/4}$), spanning over four orders of magnitude in BM, from mouse to horse. Overall, a clearer picture of VF dynamics and its molecular mechanisms is emerging, which might eventually lead to more effective prevention of sudden cardiac death.

10 Inheritable Arrhythmogenic Diseases

In this chapter, we briefly address some salient features of the clinical manifestations, genetic bases, and cellular mechanisms of the arrhythmias seen in some of the most widely studied heritable arrhythmogenic diseases, including long QT syndrome (LQTS), Brugada syndrome, short QT syndrome (SQTS), catecholaminergic polymorphic ventricular tachycardia (CPVT), and arrhythmogenic right ventricular cardiomyopathy (ARVC).

In recent years, the identification of the disease loci underlying the currently known mutations in proteins that form sarcolemmal ion channels, particularly the LQTS, has greatly contributed to the understanding of the substrate for life-threatening arrhythmias. In addition, studies in large numbers of patients with ischemic heart disease and heart failure have brought attention to a possible genetic foundation in the vulnerability to sudden cardiac death (SCD). However, the underlying molecular and electrophysiological mechanisms of SCD in common acquired heart diseases remain elusive. On the other hand, the study of arrhythmogenic mechanisms in familial diseases shows potential for revealing more common arrhythmogenic disorders in which the genetic background makes possible the initiation of ventricular arrhythmias and SCD.

Congenital Long QT Syndrome

An important characteristic of many inheritable ion channel diseases is an abnormal, inhomogeneous ventricular repolarization. Individuals affected by the most widely studied of such diseases, the long QT syndrome, are predisposed to ventricular tachyarrhythmias caused by prolonged and unstable repolarization, which often leads to SCD as the first manifestation of the disease. LQTS can be heritable or acquired. The heritable form, better known

Basic Cardiac Electrophysiology for the Clinician, 2nd edition. By J. Jalife, M. Delmar, J. Anumonwo, O. Berenfeld and J. Kalifa. Published 2009 by Blackwell Publishing, ISBN: 978-1-4501-8333-8.

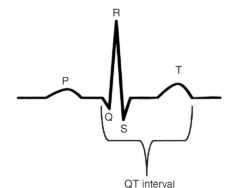

Figure 10.1 On ECG, the QT interval reflects the activation–recovery cycle of the ventricular myocardium, measured from the beginning of the QRS complex to the end of the T-wave.

as congenital LQTS, is caused by mutations in genes that encode ion channels, either the sodium channel gene *SCN5A*, or one of several genes that code for potassium or calcium channels, or even non-ion channel proteins that result in a LQTS phenotype. On ECG, the most salient feature of congenital LQTS is prolongation of the QT interval, reflecting abnormal myocardial repolarization. Clinically, LQTS is characterized by a propensity to potentially fatal ventricular arrhythmias, particularly torsades de pointes, which may lead to syncope, cardiac arrest, or sudden death in otherwise healthy young adults and children. The syndrome is most often transmitted in families as an autosomal dominant trait (Romano–Ward syndrome).

As illustrated in Figure 10.1, on ECG, the QT interval reflects the activation–recovery cycle of the ventricular myocardium, measured from the beginning of the QRS complex to the end of the T-wave. Since the duration of the ventricular action potential and thus of cardiac repolarization depends on the rate of ventricular activation, more accurate assessment of the QT interval requires correction for the heart rate. Although not universally accepted, the Bazett equation is used for this purpose, as follows: $QTc = QT/\sqrt{R\text{-}R}$ interval. When the QT interval is corrected for heart rate (QTc) and remains longer than 0.44 second (for convenience, QTc is measured also in seconds similar to the QT), it is generally considered abnormal, though a normal QTc can be slightly prolonged in women (up to 0.46 second). The longest QT interval is usually observed in the right precordial leads. An abnormally prolonged QTc reflects an abnormally prolonged myocardial repolarization, which increases the likelihood of dispersion of refractoriness, when some part of myocardium might be refractory to subsequent depolarization. In LQTS, QT prolongation can lead to polymorphic ventricular tachycardia (VT), or torsades de pointes, ventricular fibrillation (VF), and SCD (see Figure 10.2). As discussed in Chapter 6, at the cellular level, the mechanisms of initiation of these often-fatal arrhythmias are thought to be the formation of early afterdepolarizations (EADs). Prolongation of the ventricular action potential duration (APD) prolongs the time window during which calcium channels remain open and facilitates the formation of EADs (Figure 10.3). Any other condition that

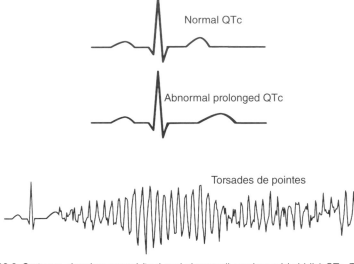

Figure 10.2 Cartoons showing normal (top) and abnormally prolonged (middle) QTc. The latter reflects an abnormally prolonged myocardial repolarization, which increases the likelihood of polymorphic ventricular tachycardia, or torsades de pointes (bottom), ventricular fibrillation (VF) and sudden cardiac death (SCD).

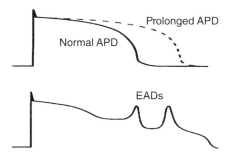

Figure 10.3 Prolongation of the ventricular action potential duration (APD) prolongs the time window during which calcium channels remain open and facilitates the formation of early afterdepolarizations (EADs).

accelerates the reactivation of calcium channels (e.g., increased sympathetic tone) increases the risk of EAD, which in the presence of dispersion of repolarization may result in wavebreak and initiation of functional reentry in the form of torsades de pointes (Figure 10.4). In patients with LQTS, a variety of adrenergic stimuli, including exercise, emotional stress, loud noise, and swimming may precipitate an arrhythmic response. However, it also may occur without such preceding conditions.

Genetic Types in Long QT Syndrome
LQTS has long been recognized as mainly Romano–Ward syndrome (i.e., familial occurrence with autosomal dominant inheritance, QT prolongation, and ventricular tachyarrhythmias) or as Jervell and Lang–Nielsen (JLN) syndrome; i.e., familial occurrence with autosomal recessive inheritance,

Conditions that promote
reactivation of calcium channels and EADs:

Autonomic	- Increased sympathetic tone
	- increased catecholamines
	- Decreases vagal tone
Metabolic	- Hypoxia
	- Acidosis
	- Cesium
	- Hypokalemia
Drugs	- Potassium channel blocking agents
	(e.g., sotalol, quinidine, and n-acetylprocainamide)
Intrinsic	- Bradycardia

Figure 10.4 Conditions that accelerate the reactivation of calcium channels increase the risk of early afterdepolarizations (EADs).

Table 10.1 Genetic background of inherited forms of long QT syndrome (LQTS)

Type of LQTS	Chromosomal locus	Mutated gene	Protein	Ion current affected
LQT1	11p15.5	KVLQT1 or KCNQ1 (heterozygotes)	KvLQT1	Potassium (I_{Ks})↓
LQT2	7q35–36	KCNH2	HERG,	Potassium (I_{Kr})↓
LQT3	3p21–24	SCN5A	Nav1.5	Sodium (I_{Na})↑
LQT4	4q25–27	ANK2	Ankyrin-B	$I_{Na,K}$↓ I_{NCX}↓
LQT5	21q22.1–22.2	KCNE1 (heterozygotes)	minK	Potassium (I_{Ks})↓
LQT6, SIDS	21q22.1–22.2	KNCE2	MiRP1	Potassium (I_{Kr})↓
LQT7 (Andersen-Tawil syndrome)	17q23	KCNJ2	Kir2.1	Potassium (I_{K1})↓
LQT8 (Timothy syndrome)	12q13.3	CACNA1C	Cav1.2	Calcium (I_{Ca-L})↑
LQT9, SIDS	3p25	CAV3	caveolin-3	Sodium (I_{Na})↑
LQT10	11q23	SCN4B	$Na_{vβ}4$	Sodium (I_{Na})↑
Jervelle and Lange Nielsen1	11p15.5	KCNQ1	KvLQT1	Potassium (I_{Ks})↓
Jervelle and Lange Nielsen2	21q22.1	KCNE1	minK	Potassium (I_{Ks})↓

congenital deafness, QT prolongation, and ventricular arrhythmias. As summarized in Table 10.1, LQTS is most commonly caused by mutations of the genes for cardiac potassium or sodium ion channels. Long-QT-associated gene mutations in sodium or even calcium channels lead to gain of function with increased Na$^+$ or Ca$^+$ influx, whereas those in the K$^+$ channels lead to loss of function with reduced K$^+$ efflux. Mechanistically, the end result that is common to all changes in channel function is sustained depolarization secondary to the perturbation of the balance between inward and outward currents during the plateau of the action potential.

To date, 10 different LQTS subtypes have been identified (see Table 10.1). LQT1, LQT2, and LQT3 account for most cases, with estimated prevalence of 45%, 45%, and 7%, respectively. LQT1 and LQT2 result from mutations in genes *KCNQ1* and *KCNH2*, respectively, encoding two distinct delayed-rectifier potassium channel proteins, KvLQT1 and HERG, respectively, which are important in the termination of the action potential plateau. LQT5, LQT6, and LQT7, which are more rare, also result from gene mutations in potassium channel (α or β) subunits (*KCNE1*, *KCNE2*, and *KCNJ2*, respectively). LQT3 is a sodium channel disease that results from gain-of-function mutations in *SCN5A*. LQT4 results from mutations in ankyrin-B, a binding protein that associates with other proteins implicated in cardiac electrophysiology and intracellular calcium homeostasis. LQT8, also known as Timothy syndrome, is based on mutations in the α-subunit of the slow calcium channel (*CACNA1C*). Finally, LQT9 and LQT10 are both quite rare; LQT9 is based on mutations in the *CAV3* gene that encodes caveolin-3, the most abundant protein in membrane caveolae of striated muscle. On the other hand, LQT10 is the result of mutations in *SCN4B*, which encodes $Na_{v\beta}4$, a β_4-subunit that is thought to co-assemble with the α-subunit to form the fully functional cardiac sodium channel.

In general terms, QT prolongation in LQTS is attributed to positive charge overload in the intracellular space of the cardiac cell during repolarization. In LQT1, LQT2, LQT5, LQT6, and LQT7, potassium currents are reduced, increase with a larger than normal delay, or they deactivate much more rapidly than when they are in normally functioning channels. These changes decrease the potassium outward current and prolong repolarization. QTc prolongation in LQT4, LQT9, and LQT10 is the result of mutations in proteins other than ion channels. For example, ankyrin-B mutants result in the disruption of calcium homeostasis and formation of EADs, whereas *CAV3* or *SCN4B* mutants underlie an increase in the persistent sodium current and thus APD prolongation.

Pathophysiology of Long QT Syndrome Types

In most LQTS patients, there is autosomal dominant inheritance of mutations in either *KCNQ1* (LQT1) or *KCNH2* (LQT2). In these patients, ventricular tachyarrhythmias and sudden death are often triggered by emotional stress or physical exercise. The only available therapeutic approaches are symptomatic treatment with beta-blockers, which reduces the frequency of arrhythmias, and the implantation of an automated cardioverter defibrillator.

The LQT1 gene is *KCNQ1*. It encodes for the protein KvLQT1, which upon co-assembling with an ancillary protein (minK) forms the channel that carries the slowly activating and deactivating, delayed-rectifier potassium current, I_{Ks} (see Chapter 2). More than 170 mostly missense mutations have been reported for this gene (Figure 10.5). Their net effect is decreased outward

KvLQT1

(a)

(b)

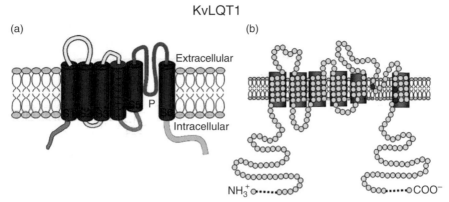

Figure 10.5 Two different models of the deduced sequence of the KvLQT1 protein, which forms the α-subunit of the slow delayed-rectifier I_{Ks} channel. (a) Tube model shows that the protein consists of intracellular amino and carboxyl terminals and six putative membrane-embedded homologous domains (S1 to S6), S4 being the voltage sensor. P, P-loop (see Chapter 2 for further details). (b) A different representation of KvLQT1 illustrates in red the approximate location of three of the more than 170 mostly missense amino acid mutations that have been reported for the *KCNQ1* gene.

HERG

(a)

(b)

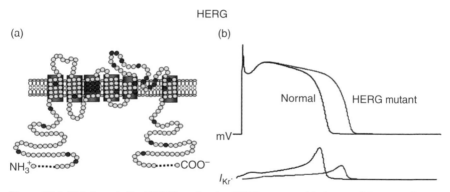

Figure 10.6 Mutations in the *KCNH2* coding for HERG cause rapid closure of the potassium channels and decrease the normal rise in I_{Kr}. (a) Cartoon of the deduced sequence of HERG illustrating the approximate locations (in red) of amino acid mutations leading to loss of function in I_{Kr}. (b) Action potentials (top) and I_{Kr} current (bottom) in a normal (black) and a hypothetical cell expressing mutant HERG channels (red).

potassium current during the plateau, which allows inward plateau currents to predominate with a consequent delay in ventricular repolarization and QTc prolongation.

The LQT2 gene (*KCNH2*) encodes for HERG which forms the rapidly activating, rapidly deactivating, delayed-rectifier potassium channel that carries I_{Kr}. As shown in Figure 10.6, mutations in this gene cause rapid closure of the potassium channels and decrease the normal rise in I_{Kr}. They also result in delayed ventricular repolarization and QT prolongation. About 200 mutations in this gene have been reported to date.

Studies using genetically engineered mouse models of the LQTS have demonstrated that expression of dominant negative mutations in either *KCNQ1* or *KCNH2* leads to prolongation of the APD, EADs, regional electrical heterogeneities, and ventricular arrhythmias. In addition, in the mouse, the down-regulation of one potassium current is often associated with compensatory up-regulation of other K$^+$ currents. In contrast, in a recently developed transgenic LQTS rabbit model, elimination of I_{Ks} in ventricular cardiomyocytes was associated with the elimination of I_{Kr}, and vice versa, which suggested an interaction between the rabbit ERG and KvLQT1. In both cases, there was prolongation of APD and the QT intervals, as well as increased dispersion of ventricular repolarization. Interestingly, however, unlike LQT1 rabbits, LQT2 rabbits showed a high incidence of spontaneous SCD secondary to polymorphic VT (Figure 10.7). This seems to correlate well with the fact that LQT2 patients with a pore mutation have the highest risk of arrhythmic events. Moreover, adult LQT2 patients have a higher risk of sudden death than LQT1 patients, and the risk is increased in those with a longer QT interval and in women.

LQT3 results from gain-of-function mutations in the gene *SCN5A* which encodes for the protein forming the cardiac voltage-gated sodium channel (Na$_V$1.5). Studies using genetic linkage analysis first localized an LQTS gene to a region on chromosome 3p (LQT3 locus) in a small number of families. This mutation in *SCN5A* resulted in the deletion of three amino acid residues (delKPQ 1505–1507) from the cytoplasmic loop that connects transmembrane domains 3 and 4 of Na$_V$1.5. The mutation led reduced sodium current inactivation, which manifested as a persistent residual sodium current during the plateau phase of the cardiac action potential with consequent QTc prolongation (Figure 10.8). Since then more than 70 distinct mutations have been identified in families with LQT3. Studies using functional expression of specific mutant proteins in heterologous systems such as human embryonic kidney (HEK) cells or Chinese hamster ovary (CHO) cells, or in genetically engineered mouse or rabbits, have helped to better understand the pathophysiological mechanisms of LQT3, and have demonstrated how one abnormal allele is sufficient to result in prolonged depolarization and arrhythmias. *SCN5A* mutations typically yield incompletely inactivating Na$^+$ channels and residual sodium depolarizing current (see Figure 10.8), leading to unbalanced depolarizing oscillations throughout the action potential plateau.

As illustrated in Figure 10.9, mutations are found throughout the Na$_V$1.5 channel sequence, though multiple mutations tend to cluster in a small number of regions of the channel structure, particularly the S4 segment of domain 4, which is critical for sensing the transmembrane voltage and in the control of channel inactivation. Another interesting cluster of mutations can be found in the proximal carboxyl-terminus, which is also implicated in channel inactivation. Overall, approximately 10% of autosomal dominant

(a)

(b)

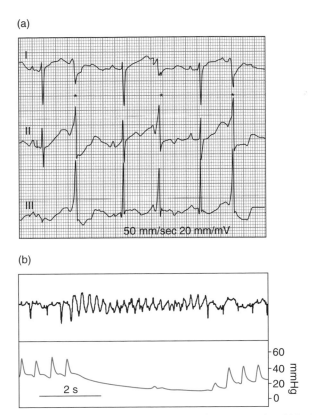

Figure 10.7 Sudden death and spontaneous arrhythmias in a transgenic rabbit of LQT2. (a) Simultaneous 3-lead (I to III) ECG strip showing prolonged QTc, ventricular extrasystoles (bigeminy) with R-on-T phenomenon in the LQT2 founder rabbit under midazolam sedation. Asterisks denote ventricular extrasystoles. This rabbit died suddenly approximately 2 weeks after this recording. (b) Spontaneous polymorphic tachycardia in a ketamine/xylazine-anesthetized rabbit. Top panel shows ECG lead II. Bottom panel shows simultaneous arterial pressure recorded from the ear artery. (Adapted from Brunner *et al.*, *J Clin Invest* 2008; 118:2246–59.)

LQTS can be attributed to mutations at LQT3, Some loss-of-function mutations in the same gene may lead to Brugada syndrome.

LQT4 is of interest in that it demonstrates that mutations in proteins other than ion channels, in this case the binding protein ankyrin-B, can also be involved in the pathogenesis of LQTS. Ankyrin-B is an intracellular binding protein that associates with proteins involved in the control of cardiac electrical activity. It may bind to several membrane ion pumps and channel proteins, such as the anion exchanger (chloride-bicarbonate exchanger), sodium-potassium adenosine triphosphatase (ATPase), the sodium channel, and the sodium-calcium exchanger (NCX), and calcium-release channels (including those mediated by the receptors for inositol triphosphate [IP$_3$] or ryanodine).

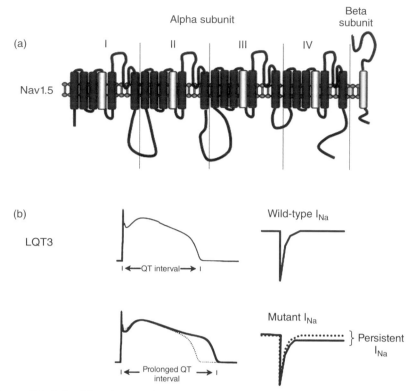

Figure 10.8 Gain-of-function mutations in the *SCN5A* gene coding for the voltage-dependent sodium channel result in LQT3. (a) Deduced sequence of the alpha- and beta-subunits of Na$_v$1.5 showing the location (in blue) of the ΔKPQ mutation, which includes an in-frame deletion of three amino acids (Lys-1505, Pro-1506, and Gln-1507). (b) Top: normal action potential and sodium current (wild type); bottom: prolonged action potential duration (APD) and mutant Na$^+$ channel current showing residual I_{Na}. SCN5A mutations typically yield incompletely inactivating Na$^+$ channels and residual sodium depolarizing current, leading to prolongation of APD and thus QT prolongation, unbalanced depolarizing oscillations throughout the action potential plateau, early afterdepolarizations (EADs), and polymorphic ventricular tachycardia (VT).

Five different mutations in the ankyrin-B gene have been shown to result in LQT4. Ankyrin-B mutations result in interference with the function of several of these pumps and channels, resulting in increased intracellular calcium concentration and fatal arrhythmia.

LQT5 is a relatively uncommon autosomal dominant form of LQTS. It involves mutations in the gene *KCNE1* which encodes for minK. As discussed earlier, co-assembly of minK with KvLQT1 forms the slowly activating delayed-rectifier channel responsible for I_{Ks}. Similar to LQT1, LQT5 results in a decreased outward current of potassium and in QT prolongation. In its rare homozygous forms, LQT5 can lead to Jervell and Lange–Nielsen syndrome.

LQT3 –Na channel gain-of-function
mutations

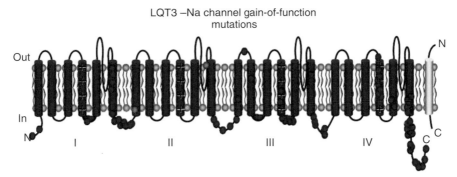

Figure 10.9 Mutations, shown in blue, are found throughout the alpha-subunit of the Na$_V$1.5 channel sequence, though multiple mutations tend to cluster in a small number of regions of the channel structure, particularly the S4 segment of domain 4, which is critical for sensing the transmembrane voltage and in the control of channel inactivation.

LQT6 involves mutations in the gene *MiRP1*, or *KCNE2*, which encodes for the potassium channel, β-subunit, minK-related protein 1 (MiRP1). *KCNE2* encodes for β-subunits of potassium channels that carry I_{Kr}.

LQT7 is also known as Andersen–Tawil syndrome. It results from mutations in *KCNJ2* which encodes for the strong inward-rectifier potassium channel protein, Kir2.1, responsible for the I_{K1} current. I_{K1} is the main background potassium current maintaining resting membrane potential of the ventricular myocyte. I_{K1} is also involved in the control of cardiac cell excitability and plays an important role in ensuring the return to the resting membrane potential during the final phase of repolarization (see Chapter 2); i.e., during phase 3 of the action potential. In LQT7, QT prolongation is less prominent than in other types, and the QT interval is sometimes in the normal range. Since in addition to the heart, Kir2.1 is expressed in other organs such as skeletal muscle, Andersen–Tawil syndrome is associated with periodic paralysis and skeletal developmental abnormalities, including clinodactyly, low-set ears mandibular hypoplasia, short stature, and scoliosis. Although Andersen syndrome patients develop ventricular tachyarrhythmias, including torsades de pointes, SCD is rare in these patients.

Mutations in the LQT8 gene (*CACNA1C*) cause loss of L-type calcium current. So far, a limited number of cases of Timothy syndrome have been reported. They have been associated with abnormalities such as congenital heart disease, cognitive and behavioral problems, musculoskeletal diseases, and immune dysfunction.

LQT9 is caused by mutations in the membrane structural protein, caveolin-3, which forms specific membrane invaginations called caveolae that contain voltage-gated sodium channels. This LQTS type was discovered in 2006 in an analysis of the *CAV3* gene in 905 unrelated patients with long QT syndrome who had previously been tested for mutations in known LQT genes. In six such patients, four heterozygous missense mutations were identified that were not found in more than 1000 controls. Functional expression studies showed that the mutant caveolin-3 resulted in a two- to threefold increase in the late sodium current of the cardiac sodium channel. Subsequently, three missense mutations were identified in an analysis of the *CAV3* gene in necropsy tissue from 134 unrelated cases of sudden infant death syndrome (SIDS). Voltage-clamp studies demonstrated a fivefold increase in late sodium current for all three mutations compared with controls. Thus, similar to LQT3, these particular mutations increase the persistent sodium current which delays repolarization and prolongs the QT interval (see Figure 10.8).

LQT10, a recently discovered gene for LQTS, is *SCN4B* encoding the protein $Na_V\beta4$, which is an auxiliary subunit to the pore-forming voltage-gated sodium channel of the heart ($Na_V1.5$). Only one mutation has been found in a 5-year-old girl, who at 21 months had asymptomatic bradycardia (<60 bpm), profound QT prolongation with a QTc of 712 milliseconds, intermittent 2:1 AV block and macroscopic T-wave alternans during 1:1 conduction. Her medical history included fetal bradycardia noted at 24 weeks of gestation and a ventricular septal defect that spontaneously closed by 6 months of age. She remained asymptomatic after placement of an epicardial pacemaker. She had two paternal great aunts who had SCD, one at age 35 and the other at age 8 years. The patient's ECG features were similar to those seen in *SCN5A*-mediated LQT3.

Acquired Long QT Syndrome

Drug-induced QT prolongation may also increase the risk of ventricular tachyarrhythmias (e.g., torsades de pointes) and SCD. The ionic mechanism is similar to that observed in congenital LQTS, i.e., mainly intrinsic blockade of cardiac potassium efflux. Hence, a long list of drugs known as potassium channel blockers, including some antiarrhythmic drugs in class 1A (e.g., quinidine) or class 3 (e.g., sotalol) can induce long QT syndrome because of their effects in delaying repolarization. It is generally accepted that these drugs induce prolonged QT only in individuals who are susceptible. However, the mechanism(s) underlying such susceptibility has not been elucidated and its genetic basis is the subject of scrutiny in the fields of pharmacogenetics and pharmacogenomics. It is possible that susceptible individuals have a mutation in one of the channel proteins that is unmasked by potassium channel blockers, which is very difficult to ascertain because screening for familial mutations is a tedious and highly time-consuming endeavor. Nevertheless, it has been suggested that as many as 10–15% of patients who develop drug-induced LQTS present single nucleotide polymorphisms (SNPs) primarily in genes coding for cardiac potassium channels.

In addition to medications, several other factors can prolong the QT interval. Important risk factors for drug-induced QT prolongation are female sex, electrolyte disturbances (hypokalemia and hypomagnesemia), structural heart disease, and bradycardia. Some have also suggested that affected individuals have mutations that affect cardiac ion channels, altering repolarization reserve. Polymorphic VTs occurring in patients with the congenital form of the disease are indistinguishable from those observed in the acquired form of the syndrome. However, the precipitating factors are different. Arrhythmias occurring in the congenital form of long QT syndrome are induced by stress, fright, and arousal, indicating that they are mediated by sympathetic stimulation. Arrhythmias can be suppressed or prevented by Q blockers or ablation of the left stellate ganglion and, in selected patients with congenital long QT syndrome, by Na channel blocking agents, such as lidocaine. In this group of patients, sympathomimetic maneuvers (treadmill exercise, cold pressor, valsalva), rapid pacing, or infusion of epinephrine, norepinephrine, or isoproterenol may lead to an increase in the amplitude of the QT-U interval and facilitate the onset of ventricular arrhythmias. In addition, exercise-related tachycardia is associated with T-wave alternans, which seems to herald the onset of VT.

Arrhythmia Mechanisms and the Long QT Syndrome

Three major mechanisms have been implicated in the mechanisms of VT associated with the long QT syndrome:

1. *Delayed afterdepolarization (DAD)-induced triggered activity* was implicated in the mechanisms of onset of ventricular arrhythmias observed in the congenital form of the syndrome. As discussed previously, DADS are enhanced by rapid pacing as well as by catecholamines and other maneuvers that lead to intracellular Ca overload.
2. *Early afterdepolarization (EAD)-induced triggered activity* is probably associated with both congenital and acquired form of the syndrome, in which the arrhythmias are facilitated by long pauses or bradycardia. The relation between EAD and torsades de pointes was suggested by the experiments by Brachmann *et al.* in the early 1980s, which showed that the combination of Cs, a K channel blocking agent, and bradycardia resulting from chemical ablation of the AV node, led to the occurrence of long QT interval and torsades de pointes type of VT in dogs, whereas the same combination resulted in EADs in isolated canine Purkinje fibers. More recent experimental work as well as simulations also supports the participation of EAD and triggered activity in the arrhythmias observed in the congenital long QT. EAD-induced triggered arrhythmias (TAs) were demonstrated in monophasic action potential recordings from patients with the long QT syndrome. Polymorphic QRS patterns were observed simultaneously with monophasic action potential recordings showing EAD-type of activity in the endocardial surface of the ventricles in the isolated Langendorff-perfused rabbit heart. Yet there were some concerns regarding the association between EAD and polymorphic tachycardia. Early experiments indicated that EADs were only possible in the specialized Purkinje system. Although

in vitro experiments showed that EAD-induced TA arising in Purkinje fibers may indeed propagate to the muscle, the relatively low mass of Purkinje cells in relation to that of the ventricular cells casts some doubt upon such a hypothesis. EADs and TAs were observed in cells of the mid-myocardial wall (i.e., M cells). Because the relative mass of M cells seems to be significantly larger than that of Purkinje fibers, EAD, and TA arising from M cells, these cells were suggested to contribute to the genesis of this type of arrhythmias. However, this idea remains controversial as well.

The following are some of the facts that support the idea that EADs are involved as a trigger in torsades de pointes: (1) the arrhythmia occurs in the setting of a prolonged QT interval, which is analogous to the APD prolongation necessary for the occurrence of EADs; (2) the ectopic activity occurs exclusively or is favored by either bradycardia or long pauses and is prevented by rapid pacing; (3) the coupling interval of the first ectopic beat is relatively long; and (4) low K is a predisposing factor. The administration of K is expected to reduce the incidence of the arrhythmia or totally abolish it. The higher the concentration of K, the lower is the incidence of ectopic activity and the lower is the heart rate at which EADs are expected to occur. (5) Low Mg is a predisposing factor. Even in the presence of normal Mg, administration of Mg may abolish the arrhythmia without altering the duration of the QT interval. (6) There is a clear overlap between the lists of agents known to give rise to EADs in the experimental setting (Chapter 6) and the agents known to induce torsades de pointes (Table 10.2). (7) Finally, patients with the congenital form of long QT syndrome may improve after left stellate gangliectomy, thus supporting the contribution of changes in the sympathetic innervation (e.g., the imbalance between left and right sympathetic effects) to the development of ventricular arrhythmias. This observation is consistent with the fact that DADs and EADs may be enhanced by catecholamines.

3. Functional *reentry* may be associated with both congenital and acquired forms of the syndrome. Long QT syndrome patients may have greater-than-normal dispersion of refractoriness, which may favor the occurrence

Table 10.2 Some agents associated with torsades de pointes

1. Class IA antiarrhythmic drugs (quinidine, disopyramide, procainamide)
2. Class IB antiarrhythmic drugs (lidocaine, tocainide, mexiletine)
3. Class IC antiarrhythmic drugs (flecainide, encainide, indecainide)
4. Class III antiarrhythmic drugs (amiodarone, sotalol, clofidium, bretylium)
5. Phenothiazine
6. Tricyclic and tetracyclic antidepressants
7. Erythromycin
8. Antihistaminics
9. Amiloride

of unidirectional block and reentrant activation. Even though there is multiple evidence indicating that triggered activity is indeed responsible for at least the initiation of torsades de pointes in patients with long QT interval, it is still unclear how such ectopic activity may result in the characteristic ECG presentation of torsades de pointes. Experiments using a voltage-sensitive dye and a video camera to map the epicardial surface of the isolated ventricles, together with computer simulations, suggest that non-stationary vortex-like reentry (spiral waves) may explain the polymorphic ECG appearance of torsades de pointes (see Chapter 7). Similar studies demonstrated that, in the isolated rabbit heart exposed to low K and quinidine or a class III antiarrhythmic drug, EADs may originate at multiple sites throughout the endocardium and give rise to excitation waves that spread across both ventricles. Because the site of origin of EADs may change over large distances on a beat-to-beat basis, EADs can give rise to polymorphic patterns of arrhythmias. However, it seems likely that the typical pattern of torsades de pointes can only be achieved if at least two EAD-induced wave fronts interact in such a way as to initiate nonstationary reentrant activity. In other words, it appears that, in the setting of bradycardia and long QT, polytopic EADs may be the trigger whereas vortex-like reentry may be the mechanism that maintains classical torsades de pointes. The relationship between torsades de pointes and reentry is discussed in more detail in Chapter 7.

Brugada Syndrome

Brugada syndrome is an inheritable form of idiopathic ventricular arrhythmia that is associated with ECG abnormalities and with mutations in the *SCN5A* gene, which encodes for the α-subunit of the sodium channel. Brugada syndrome patients typically have a family history of unexplained sudden death and an increased risk for potentially lethal polymorphic VT or fibrillation, particularly during sleep, even in the absence of structural heart disease. Brugada syndrome occurs predominantly in males and inheritance is autosomal dominant. Most Brugada syndrome patients that are positive for *SCN5A* mutation are heterozygous (i.e., only one allele carries the mutation) but there have been a few reports of individuals who carry two different mutations inherited from each parent (homozygous). However, in most families that carry a mutation, there is a low concordance between the genotype and the clinical manifestation of the disease (i.e., there is incomplete or low penetrance).

Prevalence and Clinical Manifestations

It has been difficult to estimate the true prevalence of Brugada syndrome in the general population. Some investigators suggest that it occurs in 1–5 per 10 000 inhabitants worldwide. Prevalence is highest in Southeast Asia, especially in Thailand and the Philippines where Brugada syndrome is often

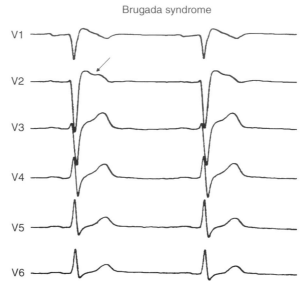

Brugada syndrome

Figure 10.10 The ECG of Brugada syndrome patients is characterized by a coved-type ST-segment elevation in the right precordial leads (arrow), apparent right bundle branch block in the absence of myocardial ischemia or electrolyte abnormalities, and normal T interval duration.

referred to as sudden unexplained nocturnal death syndrome (SUNDS) and is considered to be the major cause of sudden death in young individuals. *SCN5A* mutations make up 18–30% of Brugada syndrome cases. The mean age at the time of first diagnosis or sudden death is approximately 40 years but the range is very wide; i.e., between 2 days and 84 years of age.

As illustrated in Figure 10.10, on ECG, Brugada syndrome is characterized by a coved-type ST-segment elevation in the right precordial leads, apparent right bundle branch block in the absence of myocardial ischemia or electrolyte abnormalities, and normal T interval duration. In a few cases, the characteristic ECG abnormalities are concealed, but may be unmasked by the administration of sodium channel blocking agents (i.e., procainamide, flecainide, and ajmaline), vagotonic agents, tricyclic antidepressants, cocaine, and propranolol intoxication, as well as fever. Patients may be at increased risk for atrial fibrillation and intraventricular conduction abnormalities.

Three types of ECG pattern in the right precordial leads may be recognized in Brugada syndrome (Figure 10.11). Type 1 is characterized by a coved 0.2-mV ST-segment elevation followed by a negative T-wave. This pattern elevation is diagnostic of Brugada syndrome. In type 2, the elevated ST-segment has a saddleback configuration with an initial elevation of ~0.1 mV followed by a trough and then either a positive or biphasic T-wave. Type 3 ST-segment elevation has either a saddleback or coved appearance with an ST-segment elevation of less than 0.1 mV. All three patterns may appear spontaneously

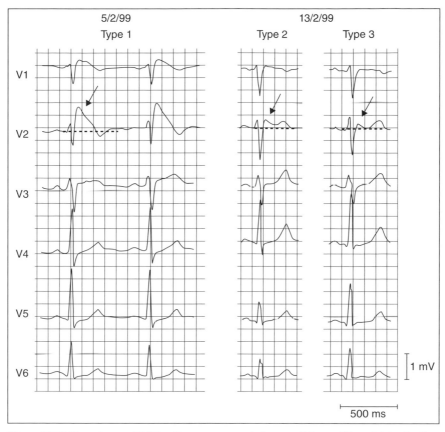

Figure 10.11 Three types of ECG pattern were recorded sequentially on different dates by the right precordial leads in the same patient with Brugada syndrome. Type 1 is manifested as a coved 0.2-mV ST-segment elevation followed by a negative T-wave. In type 2, the elevated ST-segment has a saddleback configuration with an initial elevation of ~0.1 mV followed by a trough and then either a positive or biphasic T-wave. Type 3 ST-segment elevation has either a saddleback or coved appearance with an ST-segment elevation of less than 0.1 mV. (Adapted from Wilde *et al.*, *Circulation* 2002; 106:2514.)

and sequentially in the same patient or may be induced upon the administration of a sodium channel blocking agent (e.g., ajmaline or flecainide) While types 2 and 3 ECG are suggestive of the Brugada syndrome, only type 1 should be considered diagnostic and a definite diagnosis is established when the type 1 pattern is seen in more than one right precordial lead in association with one or more of the following: documented VF, polymorphic VT; a family history of SCD in patients who are less than 45 years old; coved-type ECGs in family members; inducible VT with programmed electrical stimulation; syncope; or nocturnal agonal respiration.

The ECG is often used to distinguish between *SCN5A* mutation-positive and mutation-negative subjects. In addition to ST-segment elevation, a prolonged PQ interval and a correspondingly longer HV time are more common in Brugada syndrome patients with *SCN5A* mutations than in subjects that do not have a mutation. The QRS duration may also be prolonged in Brugada syndrome caused by *SCN5A* mutations, and the intraventricular conduction defects may worsen with age in some of these patients.

The sudden unexplained death syndrome (SUDS) is clinically similar to Brugada syndrome and causes sudden death, typically during sleep, in young and middle-aged males in Southeast Asian countries. *SCN5A* mutations have also been identified in subjects with SUDS. For example, while the basal ECG of a 19-day-old infant who was successfully resuscitated from VF did not show features of Brugada syndrome, DNA analysis revealed a missense mutation (R1193Q) in *SCN5A*, previously linked with the Brugada syndrome.

Genetic Bases and Pathophysiology of Brugada Syndrome
The first report of SCN5A mutations in Brugada syndrome was followed by many publications reporting an increasing number of mutations. SCN5A mutations have also been identified in subjects with SUDS. In contrast with LQT3, which results primarily from missense mutations leading to gain of function in the sodium channel, many mutations in Brugada syndrome are predicted to cause truncated proteins by either introduction of a frameshift, premature stop codon (nonsense mutations), or predicted splicing errors, all of which has suggested that the disorder results from loss of function. Moreover, some missense mutations in *SCN5A* have also been demonstrated to result in impaired protein trafficking from their site of production inside the cell to the cell membrane, or in disruption of ion conductance, and thus in nonfunctional channels. Therefore, at the cellular level, reduced sodium current (see Figure 10.12) is the primary pathophysiological consequence in Brugada syndrome and this is consistent with *SCN5A* mutations predicted to encode nonfunctional channels.

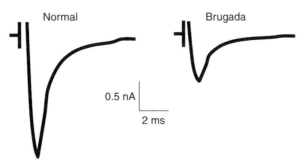

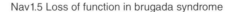

Figure 10.12 Schematic representation of voltage-clamp data to illustrate the sodium current changes produced by an *SCN5A* loss-of-function mutation. Reduced sodium current is the primary pathophysiological consequence in Brugada syndrome and this is consistent with *SCN5A* mutations predicted to encode nonfunctional channels.

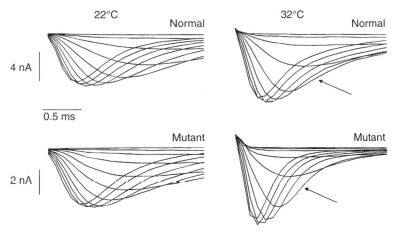

Figure 10.13 Effect of temperature on sodium current inactivation in normal and Brugada syndrome mutant Na$_v$1.5 channels transfected in mammalian cells. Whole-cell currents obtained at test potentials between −70 and −20 mV, in increments of 5 mV, demonstrated accelerated I_{Na} inactivation (faster decay of current) at 32°C but not at 22°C. (Adapted from Dumaine *et al.*, *Circ Res* 1999; 85:803–9.)

Of the nearly 100 mutations in *SCN5A* that have been linked to Brugada syndrome, only a small fraction have been studied in heterologous expression systems and shown to result in loss of function of the sodium channel in the form of: (1) lack of functional expression; (2) shift in the voltage- and time dependence of I_{Na} activation, inactivation, or reactivation; (3) persistence of the channel in a state of inactivation from which it recovers more slowly than normal; or (4) premature inactivation of the current. As shown in Figure 10.13, the accelerated inactivation of the sodium current is sometimes observed at physiological temperatures, but not at room temperature. Accelerated I_{Na} inactivation was further increased at higher-than-normal temperatures, providing a basis for the increased risk of arrhythmias in Brugada syndrome patients who develop fever.

A number of studies have led to the conclusion that repolarization abnormalities at the right ventricular outflow tract (RVOT) are the cause of the characteristic type 1 electrocardiogram in Brugada syndrome patients. In addition, magnetic resonance imaging studies have shown that the RVOT is selectively dilated in these patients, reflecting the presence of structural changes that contribute to the development of an arrhythmogenic substrate. It has been speculated that connexin43 defects in the RVOT may contribute to the development of the Brugada syndrome phenotype by impairing electrotonic communication and augmenting repolarization heterogeneities that contribute to slowing of conduction and arrhythmia development.

From the cellular electrophysiology point of view, two alternative mechanisms have been proposed to explain the arrhythmias in the Brugada syndrome. Proponents of the first mechanism suggest that a reduction in myocardial sodium current amplifies differences in APD between endocardium and epicardium that are brought about by unequal distribution of transient outward current (I_{TO}). I_{To} is a repolarizing current that contributes to the characteristic spike and dome shape of the epicardial action potential. In this scheme, reduced myocardial sodium current causes disproportionate shortening of epicardial action potentials because of unopposed I_{TO} leading to an increased transmural voltage gradient, dispersion of repolarization, and a substrate promoting so-called transmural phase 2 reentrant arrhythmias (Figure 10.14). The second hypothesis postulates that the main effect of reduced myocardial sodium current is conduction slowing and delayed activation on the epicardium of the right ventricle and RVOT (Figure 10.15). Thus, a steep repolarization gradient that develops in the epicardium, but not the endocardium, leads to phase 2 repolarization-extrasystoles, which might degenerate into VF as a result of further depolarization and repolarization

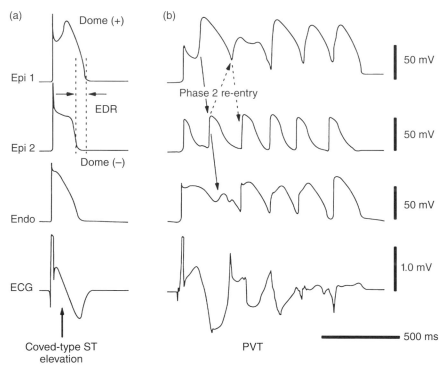

Figure 10.14 Proposed mechanism of arrhythmogenesis in Brugada syndrome. Coved-type ST-segment elevation and subsequent non-sustained polymorphic ventricular tachycardia (VT) caused by premature beats induced by phase 2 reentry in a Brugada model, employing an arterially perfused canine right-ventricular wedge preparation. (a) Reduced myocardial sodium current associated with the loss-of-function mutation of the sodium channel protein causes disproportionate shortening of epicardial action potentials because of unopposed I_{TO}. (b) This ultimately leads to an increased transmural voltage gradient, dispersion of repolarization, and a substrate promoting so-called "phase 2 reentry" from epicardium to endocardium. (Reproduced with permission from Shimizu *et al.*, *Nat Clin Pract Cardiovasc Med* 2005; 2:408–14.)

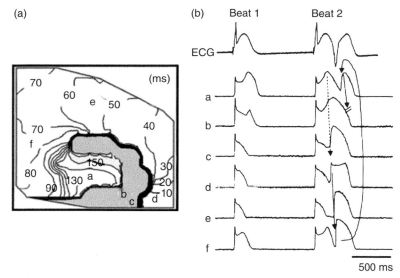

Figure 10.15 Alternative hypothesis for reentry initiation in Brugada syndrome. (a) Isochrone map of an extrasystole obtained by epicardial optical mapping of the canine wedge preparation. (b) Transmural electrogram and optical action potentials at each site ("a–f") demonstrate epicardial phase 2 reentry from "a" through "f." (Modified with permission from Aiba *et al.*, *JACC* 2006; 47:2074–85.)

abnormalities. Additional studies have suggested that the negative T-wave in the ECG of type 1 Brugada syndrome patients is the result of preferential prolongation of the epicardial action potential secondary to accentuation of the notch during phase 1 of the action potential in the region of the right ventricular outflow tract. Further studies are needed to decide which of the two hypotheses prevails.

Short QT Syndrome

The SQTS is an inherited disorder that occurs in individuals with a structurally intact heart and an increased susceptibility to arrhythmias and sudden death. The disease is characterized by a remarkably accelerated repolarization that is reflected in a shorter-than-normal QTc (Figure 10.16). Clinical manifestations of SQTS overlap with those of other genetic arrhythmic syndromes caused by ion channel abnormalities, including LQTS, Brugada syndrome, and CPVT, and range from syncopal events to cardiac arrest; affected and asymptomatic individuals have also been identified.

Although few families with SQTS have been described, three genetic loci, responsible for SQT1, SQT2, and SQT3 have already been linked to the disease, demonstrating that SQTS is a genetically heterogeneous disease, allelic to LQTS. As illustrated in Figure 10.17a, SQT1 is caused by a gain-of-function substitution **(N588K)** in the *KCNH2* gene encoding the α-subunit of the HERG (I_{Kr}) channel. As discussed earlier, loss-of-function mutations in this gene

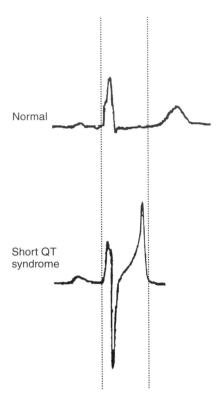

Normal

Short QT
syndrome

Figure 10.16 Short QT syndrome (SQTS). ECG recordings from a normal individual (top) and a patient with SQTS, which is manifest as a shorter-than-normal QT interval.

cause LQT2. As shown in Figure 10.17b, SQT2 is caused by a gain-of-function mutation **(V307L)** in the *KCNQ1* gene encoding the α-subunit of the KvLQT1 (I_{Ks}) channel. Again, loss-of-function mutations in this gene cause LQT1. We recently reported a novel locus associated with SQTS and demonstrated that a gain-of-function mutation (D172N) in the *KCNJ2* gene encoding for the strong inwardly rectifying channel protein Kir2.1 is associated with an accelerated repolarization process. We classified it as type 3 short QT syndrome or SQT3 (Figure 10.17c).

The mutations linked to the three forms of SQTS shorten the APD. However, a variation in the T-wave phenotype distinguishes the different mutations because of the dissimilar time dependence and voltage ranges at which I_{Kr}, I_{Ks}, and I_{K1} operate. As illustrated in Figure 10.18, computer simulations of human ventricular cells incorporating one of the three different mutations suggested that, in SQTS1 and SQTS2, significant APD abbreviation starts at the level of the plateau, but the overall morphology of the action potential remains unchanged. In contrast, the I_{K1} mutant is characterized by an abrupt increase in the rate of final repolarization of the action potential and a significant change in the action potential shape. Additional simulations using a 2-D model in which a precordial ECG lead recorded the changes in the QT duration and T-wave morphology of the simulated cardiac sheet showed that

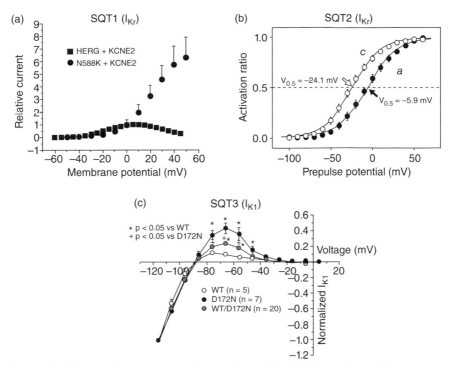

Figure 10.17 Ionic basis and current–voltage relations of the three types of short QT syndrome. (a) SQTS1, characterized by gain of function of I_{Kr}. Normalized current–voltage relationships for wild-type (WT) (i.e., HERG+KCNE2) and mutant (N588K + KCNE2) channels expressed in mammalian cells. Mutation N588K abolishes rectification of HERG. Current amplitudes were normalized to their respective values at 0 mV (maximum for HERG). (Modified with permission from Brugada et al., Circulation 2004; 109:30–35.) (b) SQT2 results in gain-of-function of I_{Ks}. Current–voltage relation for the tail current of wild-type (closed circles, n = 9) and V307L (open circles; n = 14) mutant of KCNQ1 gene coding for KvLQT1 (I_{Ks}). Mutant V307L shifted the voltage at half maximum activation (V0.5) to the left. (Modified with permission from Bellocq et al., Circulation 2004; 109:2394–7.) (c) SQTS3 is characterized by gain-of-function in I_{K1}. Voltage-clamp data CHO cells. Currents were elicited by 400-millisecond depolarizing voltage steps from –120 to +20 mV and from a holding potential of –60 mV. Current–voltage relationships were plotted as the current normalized to the current recorded at –100 mV. At each voltage from –75 to –45 mV, the current amplitude of the D172N channel is significantly larger than the WT ($P < 0.05$). For the WT/D172N current, amplitude is larger than WT at voltages between –75 and –50 mV. (Adapted with permission from Priori et al., Circ Res 2005; 96:800–7.)

all three gain-of-function mutations shortened the QT interval. However, as illustrated in Figure 10.19, only the D172N mutation in Kir2.1 accounted for the tall and asymmetrical T-wave morphology that characterizes SQTS3. Therefore, in the setting of the SQT, there seems to be an apparent genotype–phenotype correlation between the specific mutation and the resulting shape of the T-wave.

The arrhythmogenic potential of the Kir2.1 mutation may be attributable to the larger-than-normal I_{K1} outward current that shortens the APD and allows

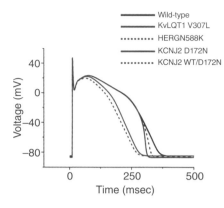

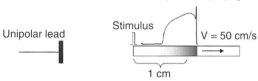

Figure 10.18 Computer simulations of human ventricular cells incorporating the gain-of-function mutation in each of the three different SQTS types. In SQTS1 and SQTS2, significant action potential duration (APD) abbreviation starts at the level of the plateau, but the overall morphology of the action potential remains unchanged. In contrast, the I_{K1} mutant is characterized by an abrupt increase in the rate of final repolarization of the action potential and a significant change in the action potential shape. (Modified with permission from Priori et al., Circ Res 2005; 96:800–7.)

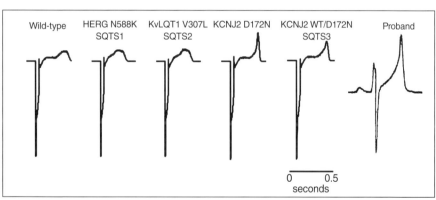

Figure 10.19 ECG morphologies of short QT syndrome (SQTS) in computer simulations of action potential propagation using a two-dimensional model. A precordial ECG lead (red) recording the changes in the QT duration and T-wave morphology of the simulated cardiac sheet showed that all three gain-of-function mutations shortened of QT interval. Only the D172N mutation in Kir2.1 accounted for the tall and asymmetrical T-wave morphology that characterizes SQTS3. Therefore, in the setting of the SQT, there seems to be an apparent genotype–phenotype correlation between the specific mutation and the resulting shape of the T-wave. (Reproduced with permission from Priori et al., Circ Res 2005; 96:800–7.)

for stabilization of rotors. I_{K1} plays an important role in stabilizing the resting membrane potential, in modulating excitability, and in causing the final repolarization phase of the action potential in both atria and ventricles. The current shows strong rectification between −50 and 0 mV, which means that the channels remain closed during the action potential plateau; they only open when

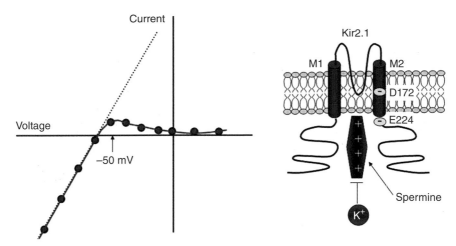

Figure 10.20 I_{K1} shows strong rectification between –50 and 0 mV, which means that the channels remain closed during the action potential plateau; they only open when the membrane potential returns to levels between –30 and –80 mV, which in the normal action potential occurs during the last phase of repolarization. Rectification is achieved by a voltage-dependent blockade by one of the positively charged intracellular polyamines (putrescine, spermine, and spermidine), which are known to interact with at least two negatively charged amino acid residues (D172 and E224) located in the M2 region inside the pore of the Kir2.1 channel complex.

the membrane potential returns to levels between –30 and –80 mV, which in the normal action potential occurs during the last phase of repolarization (Figure 10.20). Rectification is achieved by a voltage-dependent blockade by intracellular magnesium and/or one of the polyamines (putrescine, spermine, and spermidine), which are known to interact with at least three amino acid residues located inside the pore of the channel complex. SQTS3, which is characterized by asymmetrical T-waves, and a genetic defect in the *KCNJ2* gene cardiac inward-rectifier Kir2.1 channel cause a significant increase in the outward component of the *I–V* relation of I_{K1}. Moreover, genomic screening of the *KCNJ2* gene disclosed the presence of a single base pair mutation resulting in a D172N substitution located in the second transmembrane region of the channel, which has been shown to be important in rectification (Figure 10.21). The proband of the study in which the SQTS3 was discovered had no history of cardiac arrhythmias. During exercise stress testing, she developed isolated premature ventricular complexes with left bundle branch block morphology that were asymptomatic. The father of the proband and carrier of the D172N mutation had experienced repeated episodes of nocturnal palpitation and a syncopal event; however, no documentation of arrhythmias was available. Overall, in analogy with other patients with the electrocardiographic diagnosis of SQTS, these patients did not present clinically documented tachyarrhythmias. Computer simulations, however, supported the view that, by increasing the outward component of I_{K1}, the D172N mutation creates a

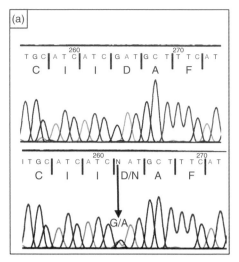

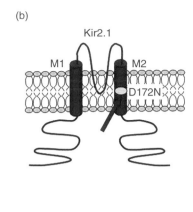

Figure 10.21 SQTS3 mutation. (a) Genomic screening of the *KCNJ2* gene disclosed the presence of a single base pair mutation resulting in a D172N substitution. (b) The substation of N for D at position 172 (blue arrow) is in the second transmembrane region of the channel, which has been shown to be important in rectification (see Figure 10.2) because of its interaction with intracellular polyamines upon membrane depolarization. (Modified with permission from Priori *et al.*, *Circ Res* 2005; 96:800–7.)

vulnerable substrate that may facilitate development of atrial and ventricular tachyarrhythmias even in a heterozygote substrate. To be sure, whereas the increased outward current resulting from the D172N mutation is expected to reduce the likelihood of EADs or DADs, it is reasonable to surmise that the steeper restitution associated with such a mutation would enhance the possibility of T-wave alternans, thereby increasing vulnerability to fibrillation when the heart rate is high. By analogy, transgenic overexpression of I_{K1} in the mouse heart has been demonstrated to shorten repolarization, as evidenced by shortening of the ventricular action potential and the QT interval (Figure 10.22). Consequently, this provided the basis for a possible VF stabilizing effect. However, the direct involvement of I_{K1} in arrhythmia mechanisms was not demonstrated. Therefore, as described in detail in Chapter 9, the mouse model of I_{K1} overexpression was used subsequently to study the effect of I_{K1} increase on VF at the molecular level. The results show that there is significant correlation between the stability and frequency of rotors responsible for VF and the magnitude of the outward component of I_{K1}. Hence, at the range of frequencies of VF, a larger outward current should result in shorter APD to allow higher frequency rotors to stabilize. By inference, SQT3 patients with demonstrated D172N mutation are expected to have an increased vulnerability to sustained VF.

As discussed earlier, loss-of-function mutations in the *KCNJ2* gene have been identified in patients affected by Andersen-Tawil syndrome, which is also

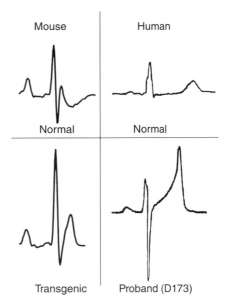

Figure 10.22 ECG pattern of Kir2.1 overexpression in mouse. Analogous to patients with SQTS3, transgenic overexpression of I_{K1} in the mouse heart shortens repolarization, as evidenced by shortening of the ventricular action potential and the QT interval.

referred to as LQT7 and is characterized by prolonged repolarization and by periodic hypokalemic paralysis. In the Andersen-Tawil syndrome, reduction of I_{K1} leads to prolongation of the QT interval and predisposes to cardiac arrhythmias. In contrast, an increase of I_{K1} has been demonstrated to shorten repolarization, evidenced by shortening of the monophasic action potential and the QT interval, and to exert a proarrhythmic effect both in the atria and the ventricles in a transgenic mouse model of up-regulation of Kir2.1, although changes in rectification characteristics need not be similar to up-regulation of I_{K1}.

Catecholaminergic Polymorphic Ventricular Tachycardia

CPVT is a highly lethal familial disease that usually manifests in childhood and adolescence. It is characterized by stress or exercise-induced bidirectional ventricular tachycardia (biVT) or PVT leading to syncope and/or SCD. CPVT is caused by enhanced Ca^{2+} release through defective sarcoplasmic reticulum release (ryanodine receptor or RyR2) channels in the cardiac myocyte. CPVT patients have a structurally intact heart and do not have ECG abnormalities that would allow establishment of the diagnosis upon evaluation of the resting ECG. Induction of VT during exercise stress test or during Holter monitoring is therefore pivotal for diagnosis. The prevalence of the disease is not yet defined. Since mortality among untreated patients is up to 30% by the age of 40 and since SCD may be the first manifestation of the disease, it is essential to identify these patients early in life and implement appropriate therapeutic strategies. Beta-blockers are the preferred therapy in CPVT patients even though these agents seem more effective in slowing VT and increasing the

Bidirectional tachycardia

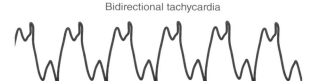

Figure 10.23 Diagrammatic representation of the ECG appearance of bidirectional VT in a patient with catecholaminergic polymorphic ventricular tachycardia (CPVT).

threshold for the appearance of catecholamine-related arrhythmias rather than in preventing sudden death. Implantation of an implantable cardioverter defibrillator (ICD) is the treatment of choice for patients who are not adequately protected by beta-blockers. CPVT patients commonly present with biVT, which manifests on ECG as an alternating axis of the QRS complexes during VT (Figure 10.23). Interestingly, biVT is considered to be a distinctive feature of digitalis intoxication, which led investigators to speculate that calcium overload-mediated DADs could represent the cellular mechanism of initiation of arrhythmias in CPVT patients, even before the genetic basis of the disease was elucidated.

The Ryanodine Receptor and Its Function

The sarcoplasmic reticulum (SR) is an intracellular-membrane demarcated structure that plays an essential role in contraction and relaxation of the cardiac muscle (Figure 10.24). Its function is mediated by two primary transport proteins, the Ca^{2+} release channel (RyR2) and the Ca^{2+} pump, which are responsible, respectively, for the rapid release and reuptake of SR Ca^{2+} and thus for the control of muscle contraction and relaxation. RyR2 is vital to excitation–contraction (EC) coupling in the heart. In ventricular myocytes, the large amount of calcium that is needed to elicit the contraction of the cardiac cell is released from the junctional SR by the RyR2 in response to an influx of a small amount of Ca^{2+} through the L-type voltage-dependent calcium channels (LTCC). A spatiotemporal coordination exists between Ca^{2+} influx through LTCCs located within the t-tubules of the sarcolemma and Ca^{2+} release from functionally coupled RyR2 channels located in near proximity at discrete areas in the junctional SR membrane (Figure 10.24). Thus, the process of Ca^{2+}-induced Ca^{2+} release results from a relatively small Ca^{2+} influx current that triggers an approximately 1000-fold greater intracellular Ca^{2+} efflux through the sum of all RyR2 activations during systole. These synchronous Ca^{2+} release events known as Ca^{2+} "sparks" allow binding of Ca^{2+} to troponin C, which promotes myofilament contraction. Interestingly, in Purkinje fibers, the function of RyR2 is not confined to junctional complexes between SR and the sarcolemma. Ultrastructural studies have demonstrated that Purkinje cells lack t-tubules and have at least two different but continuous SR regions, namely the junctional SR and the corbular, or non-junctional SR. Similar to atrial myocytes, in Purkinje cells, RyR2 is localized to junctional, as well as corbular SR which is densely distributed in interfibrillar spaces of the I-band

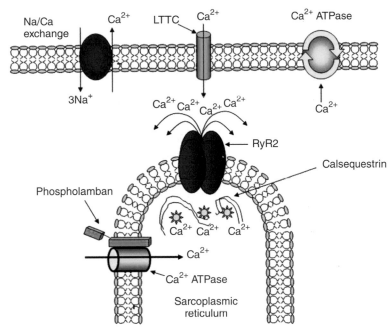

Figure 10.24 The cardiac ryanodine receptor (RyR2) of the sarcoplasmic reticulum (SR) and its role in intracellular calcium homeostasis and excitation–contraction (EC) coupling. SR function is mediated by two primary transport proteins, the Ca^{2+} release channel (RyR2) and the Ca^{2+} pump (Ca2+ ATPase, regulated by phospholamban), which are responsible, respectively, for the rapid release and reuptake of SR Ca^{2+} and thus for the control of muscle contraction and relaxation. RyR2 is vital to EC coupling. In the lumen of the SR, calcium binds to calsequestrin. In ventricular myocytes, the large amount of calcium that is needed to elicit the contraction of the cardiac cell is released from the junctional SR by the RyR2 in response to an influx of a small amount of Ca^{2+} through the L-type voltage-dependent calcium channels (LTCC). A spatiotemporal coordination exists between Ca^{2+} influx through LTCCs located within the t-tubules of the sarcolemma and Ca^{2+} release from functionally coupled RyR2 channels located in near proximity at discrete areas in the junctional SR membrane. Calcium is extruded from the cell through sodium-calcium exchange or pumped actively by the sarcolemmal calcium ATPase.

regions, suggesting that corbular SR is a site of calcium-induced calcium release via RyR2.

RyR2 is regulated by several physiological mediators and may also release calcium in response to SR calcium overload, which may occur under pathological conditions such as physical and emotional stress, or digitalis toxicity, and may be arrhythmogenic. A high load of Ca^{2+} in the SR directly increases the amount of Ca^{2+} available for release through the RyR2, but also greatly enhances the fraction of SR Ca^{2+} that is released for a given I_{Ca} trigger. This has been explained in part by the stimulatory effect of high intra-SR free Ca^{2+} concentration on the RyR2 channel, which is thought to be the mechanism that triggers spontaneous SR Ca^{2+} release and is the basis of "aftercontractions," transient inward current and DADs that may lead to arrhythmias.

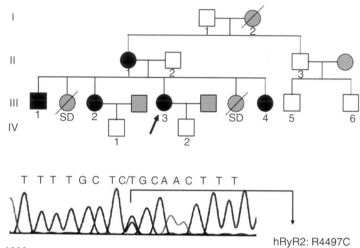

TTTTGC TC/TGCAACTTT

hRyR2: R4497C

Figure 10.25 Family tree (top) and DNA sequencing (bottom) in a kindred with R4497C mutation. Filled symbols represent clinically and genetically affected patients. Open symbols represent clinically and genetically unaffected individuals. Gray symbols represent individuals who were not tested. Arrow represents proband. SD, unexplained sudden death at young age. The presence of a hRyR2R4497C mutation was identified in the proband and in clinically affected family members by DNA sequence analysis (bottom). (Adapted from Priori SG, et al. *Circulation* 2001;103:196.)

RyR2 Mutations and Catecholaminergic Polymorphic Ventricular Tachycardia

Dr. Silvia Priori from the University of Pavia in Italy reported the first RyR2 mutation in a family (Figure 10.25) affected by a highly malignant form of CPVT that was resistant to beta-blockers. The mutation (R4497C) was subsequently identified in other CPVT families. After that initial report, other groups identified novel hRyR2 mutations in patients affected by CPVT. To date, as many as 40 point mutations in the human RyR2 (hRyR2) linked to defective RyR Ca^{2+} channel function have been reported in individuals affected by CPVT. In general, inheritance of the mutation is of the autosomal dominant form. A recessively inherited CPVT phenotype was reported for a family that presented a missense mutation in a highly conserved region of the calsequestrin2 gene (CASQ2). The CASQ2 protein serves as the major Ca^{2+} reservoir in the SR of cardiac myocytes and is part of a protein complex that contains the ryanodine receptor. Studies in rat cardiomyocytes using adenoviral transfer techniques have suggested that the CASQ2 mutation impairs the SR Ca^{2+} storing and release functions and destabilizes the Ca^{2+}-induced Ca^{2+} release mechanism. Finally, similar to missense mutations of the highly homologous hRyR1 gene underlying the skeletal muscle disorders malignant hyperthermia (MH) and central core disease (CCD), the RyR2 missense mutations seem to cluster in the N-terminal, central, and C-terminal regions of the hRyR2 gene. This suggests that RyR1 and RyR2 may have similar structural and functional abnormalities.

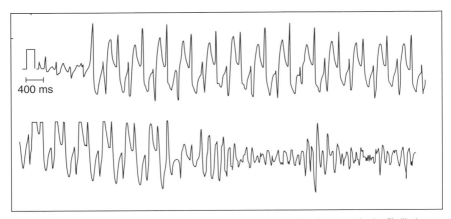

Figure 10.26 An example of bidirectional tachycardia deteriorating into ventricular fibrillation (VF) in a patient with catecholaminergic polymorphic ventricular tachycardia (CPVT).

The RyR2$^+$/RyR2^{R4496C} Mouse

The R4497C mutation seems to be highly life-threatening in humans. As shown by Dr. Priori and her associates (see also Figure 10.26), cardiac arrest occurred in 53% of carriers of the mutation and in four of those it was lethal. Furthermore VT or VF also occurred in five patients during beta-blocker therapy, suggesting that these agents provide insufficient protection against life-threatening events in CPVT. In an effort to better understand the molecular bases of the CPVT phenotype, the Priori lab undertook the development of a unique genetically engineered ("knock-in") mouse model (RyR2$^+$/ RyR^{R4496C}) that carries the murine equivalent of the human R4497C mutation in RyR2 that results in CPVT. Their data proved that PVT and even biVT may be elicited in the RyR2$^+$/RyR2^{R4496C} mice under conditions that closely resemble those eliciting cardiac arrhythmias in CPVT patients (Figure 10.27). In fact, not all RyR2$^+$/RyR2^{R4496C} mice developed arrhythmias, which is also consistent with the incomplete penetrance of the CPVT phenotype in humans. Similar to patients, treatment with propranolol also was ineffective in preventing arrhythmias in RyR2$^+$/RyR2^{R4496C} mice. However, experimental evidence linking this mutation to the bidirectional and polymorphic VTs that characterize the disease was still lacking.

Mechanisms of Arrhythmogenesis in Catecholaminergic Polymorphic Ventricular Tachycardia

BiVT occurs mainly as a result of digitalis intoxication and is a common ECG finding in about 30–50% of CPVT patients. Cardiac glycosides are known to lead to intracellular Ca^{2+} overload and to DAD generation in cardiomyocytes, and evidence from electrophysiological studies during arrhythmia induction with isoproterenol infusion in CPVT points toward DAD generation as the mechanism of biVT. From these observations, it was inferred that biVT is a triggered arrhythmia resulting from DADs, secondary to spontaneous SR Ca^{2+}

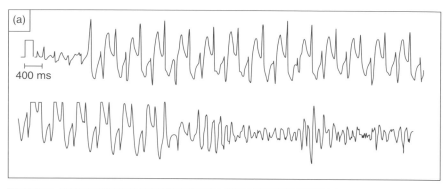

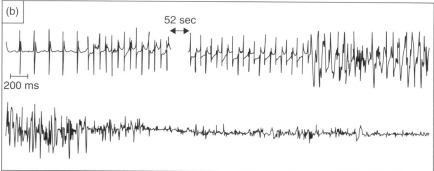

Figure 10.27 (a) Bidirectional tachycardia (BiVT) and ventricular fibrillation elicited by exercise in a patient with catecholaminergic polymorphic ventricular tachycardia. (b) BiVT and ventricular fibrillation in an RyR2$^+$/RyR2^{R4496C} mouse under conditions that closely resemble those of the CPVT patient. Reproduced by permission from Cerrone M, *et al.*, Bidirectional ventricular tachycardia and fibrillation elicited in a knock-in mouse model carrier of a mutation in the cardiac ryanodine receptor. *Circ Res* 2005; 96:e77–82

release leading to intracellular Ca^{2+} concentration oscillations during diastole. DADs were first demonstrated in Purkinje fibers exposed to toxic concentrations of digitalis and data in the literature strongly suggest that Purkinje fibers are more susceptible to Ca^{2+} overload than ventricular muscle, possibly because of their greater Na$^+$ load. It is well known, for example, that Purkinje fibers become intoxicated by digitalis at a time when ventricular myocardial fibers still show relatively normal action potentials. Hence, the demonstration that CPVT mutations are linked with biVT led to the hypothesis that both digitalis intoxication-induced triggered activity and biVT in CPVT patients may ultimately result from activation of RyR2 and a subsequent DAD inducing SR Ca^{2+} release. Whether such DADs occur primarily in the Purkinje fiber network or in the ventricular muscle was the central focus of a recent investigation aimed at testing the hypothesis that arrhythmias in this mouse model, and by inference in CPVT patients, are triggered by DADs occurring in Purkinje fibers on the right and left branches of the specialized ventricular conducting system. The idea was to use epicardial and endocardial optical mapping, chemical subendocardial ablation with Lugol's solution, and patch clamping in the RyR2/RyR2^{R4496C} knock-in mouse model to investigate the

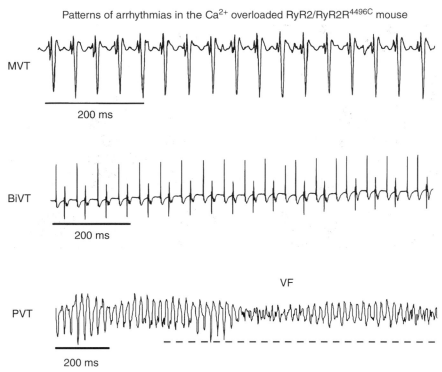

Patterns of arrhythmias in the Ca^{2+} overloaded RyR2/RyR2R^{4496C} mouse

MVT

200 ms

BiVT

200 ms

VF

PVT

200 ms

Figure 10.28 The Ca^{2+}-overloaded or adrenergically stimulated RyR2/RyR2^{R4496C} mouse heart undergoes episodes of monomorphic ventricular tachycardia (MVT), bidirectional ventricular tachycardia (biVT), polymorphic ventricular tachycardia (PVT), and ventricular fibrillation (VF).

arrhythmogenic mechanisms in CPVT. The salient results of that study were as follows. First, the isolated RyR2/RyR2^{R4496C} mouse heart shows no abnormalities of ventricular excitation or propagation during SR in the absence of stimuli leading to Ca^{2+} overload. Second, as illustrated in Figure 10.28, the Ca^{2+}-overloaded or adrenergically stimulated RyR2/RyR2^{R4496C} mouse heart undergoes episodes of monomorphic VT, biVT and PVT. Note that in all cases, epicardial breakthrough patterns are highly focal and strongly suggest that all these arrhythmias may originate from point sources in the His-Purkinje networks of the right and/or left ventricles. Third, endocardial optical mapping of the right ventricle demonstrated that the arrhythmic foci in this model similar to those shown in Figure 10.29 do originate within the specialized conduction system. In the case of monomorphic VT, the arrhythmias are clearly unifocal, whereas in polymorphic VT the arrhythmia is initially multifocal but eventually becomes reentrant upon degeneration into VF. This was further confirmed by the close relation between the onset of the optical signal during arrhythmias and sinus rhythm and the onset of the QRS complex of the ECG. Fourth, as shown in Figure 10.30 in anesthetized RyR2/RyR2^{R4496C} mice, selective chemical ablation of the right ventricular Purkinje network

(a) (b)

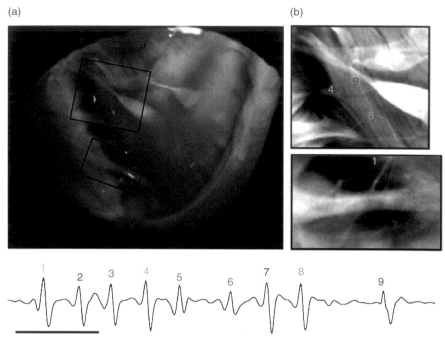

Figure 10.29 Endocardial optical mapping of the right ventricle demonstrated that the arrhythmic foci in the RyR2/RyR2^{R4496C} model originate within the endocardial specialized conduction system. (a) Location of each of the eight consecutive discharges during polymorphic ventricular tachycardia (PVT) superimposed on an image of the right ventricle (RV) endocardium. Each color indicates the location of the corresponding QRS complex in the ECG trace. (b) Magnification of the two boxes shown in panel (a) demonstrates the precise origin of each complex at a Purkinje fiber branch.

changed the biVT into monomorphic VT with wide QRS, demonstrating that in the biVT the focal origin alternates beat-to-beat between Purkinje sources in the right and left ventricles. Finally, single Purkinje cells from RyR2/RyR2^{R4496C} mouse hearts generated DAD-induced TA at lower frequencies than WT. They did so even in the absence of isoproterenol. WT cells did not. In sum, the data strongly suggested that the His-Purkinje system is a major source of focal arrhythmias in CPVT.

From Bidirectional Ventricular Tachycardia to Polymorphic Ventricular Tachycardia and Ventricular Fibrillation

It is likely that the ultimate cause of SCD in the majority of patients suffering from familial CPVT is VF. In Figure 10.27, we showed an example of biVT deteriorating into polymorphic VT and VF in a carrier of the R4497C mutation. The mechanism underlying the transition from tachycardia to VF in isolated, Langendorff-perfused RyR2/RyR2^{R4496C} mouse hearts was documented in optical mapping experiments of the kind shown in Figure 10.31. During coronary perfusion with Tyrode's solution containing 1.8 mmol/L

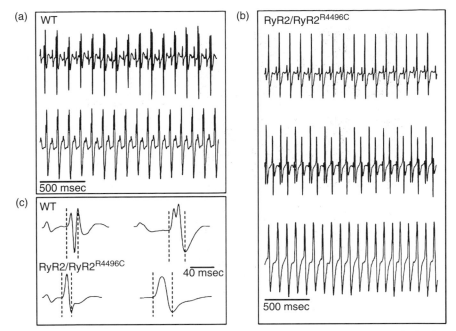

Figure 10.30 Effects of chemical ablation of right ventricle (RV) endocardium in anesthetized wild-type (WT) and RyR2/RyR2^{R4496C} mice. (a) ECG during sinus rhythm (SR) in WT mouse (top) and ECG during SR after Lugol's solution injection (bottom). Note RBB block pattern. (b) ECG during SR in RyR2/RyR2^{R4496C} mouse (top), bidirectional VT (BVT) after administration of 120 mg/kg caffeine and 2 mg/kg epinephrine (middle), and Lugol's solution injection in RV cavity converts BVT to monomorphic VT with RBB block (bottom). (c) Morphology and width of the QRS complex in baseline (left) and after Lugol (right) in WT and RyR2/RyR2^{R4496C} mice.

Ca^{2+} and 1 mmol/L caffeine, the administration of a bolus of epinephrine (1.6 µmol/L) initiated a run of polymorphic VT, which manifested as repetitive multifocal right ventricular epicardial breakthroughs and deteriorated into VF. The top panel on the left shows three 10-millisecond phase maps during one focal discharge. The middle panel shows similar maps obtained during the transition from focal to reentrant activity brought about by a wavebreak formed between the first and second frames. In this episode, the focal activity lasted 1.1 seconds (frequency, 39 Hz) and the rotor lasted 1.7 seconds (frequency, 43 Hz). The maps on the bottom panel demonstrate that VF was maintained by a high-frequency rotor throughout the reminder of the episode (see right panel).

Arrhythmogenic Right Ventricular Cardiomyopathy

Clinical Features
ARVC is an inherited cardiac disease, characterized by progressive myocyte loss and fibro-fatty infiltration primarily to the right ventricular myocardium

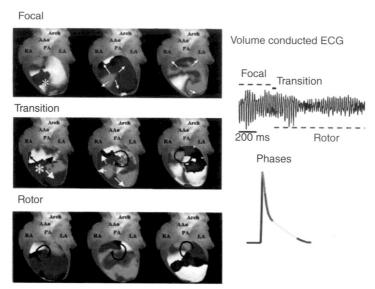

Figure 10.31 Optical mapping experiment demonstrating the mechanisms underlying the transition from tachycardia to ventricular fibrillation (VF) in an isolated, Langendorff-perfused RyR2/RyR2^{R4496C} mouse heart. During coronary perfusion with Tyrode's solution containing 1.8 mmol/L Ca^{2+} and 1 mmol/L caffeine, the administration of a bolus of epinephrine (1.6 µmol/L) initiated a run of polymorphic ventricular tachycardia (VT), which manifested as repetitive multifocal right ventricular epicardial breakthroughs and deteriorated into VF (see text for details).

and the occurrence of ventricular arrhythmias. Overall, it has been reported that 3% to 10% of unexplained cases of SCD at less than 65 years of age are due to ARVC. Typically between the second and fifth decades of life, ARVC patients present with symptoms including palpitations, syncope and symptomatic monomorphic VT with left bundle branch morphology. However, in some patients effort-related SCD may be the first manifestation of the disease. Ventricular arrhythmias can range from frequent isolated premature ventricular beats to sustained VT. Monomorphic VT typical of the disease is thought to be initiated and maintained by reentry. However, the mechanism that leads to the degeneration of VT into VF in these patients is still unknown. Two morphological variants of ARVC have been described: (1) "fatty" ARVC remains confined to the right ventricle and is characterized by substitution of the myocardium with adipose tissue (Figure 10.32), without wall thinning; and (2) "fibro-fatty" ARVC presents as replacement with fibrous tissue and thinning of the ventricular wall, aneurysmal dilatation and inflammation. In this second variant, the left ventricle is most commonly involved in later stages of the disease. The fibro-fatty replacement of the myocardium appears to proceed from the subepicardium to the endocardium. Moreover, in the early stage of the disease, the replacement is generally confined to the inflow tract, the outflow tract, and the apical region of the right ventricle ("triangle of dysplasia").

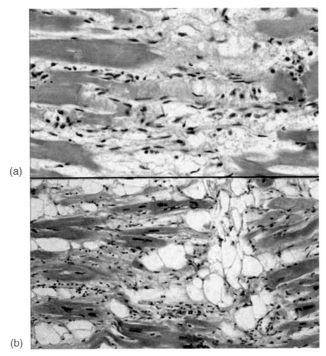

(a)

(b)

Figure 10.32 Typical histologic features of ARVC/D. Ongoing myocyte death (a) with early fibrosis and adipocytes infiltration (b). (Reproduced with permission from Thiene *et al.*, *Orphanet J Rare Dis* 2007;2:1–16.)

Four clinical phases can be distinguished in the severe form of ARVC: (1) "concealed" in which only minor structural changes are present and arrhythmias are absent or non-sustained. In some individuals SCD can be the first clinical sign of ARVC at this stage. (2) "Overt electric disorder" is where right ventricular structural abnormalities are present with the occurrence of sustained VT and/or the risk of cardiac arrest and SCD. (3) "Right ventricular failure" is where the progression of fibro-fatty infiltration in the RV leads to dilatation and right ventricular dysfunction. (4) "Biventricular pump failure" is the latest stage of the disease and the involvement of the left ventricle causes congestive heart failure due to biventricular dysfunction. Although many theories have been advanced, the natural history of disease progression in ARVC is still unclear.

At least three mechanisms have been suggested to contribute to the arrhythmic substrate of ARVC: bouts of myocarditis, fibrous and adipose infiltrates that facilitate macro-reentry, and gap junction remodeling secondary to altered mechanical coupling (see further discussion). It is quite obvious that all those factors interplay in arrhythmogenicity but it is still unknown which factors are the primary trigger of the arrhythmia, which primarily sustain it, or are responsible for its transformation into VF. Understanding the specific contribution of each factor may be important especially in treating ARVC in its early stages.

Arrhythmogenic Right Ventricular Cardiomyopathy is Linked to Mutations in Desmosomal Proteins

The first report of a genetic basis of ARVC occurred in 2002, with the discovery of a missense mutation in the desmoplakin gene in one family with the classic ARVC phenotype. Desmoplakin is a key component of the desmosome (or macula adherens), a highly organized intermediate filament-associated junctional complex that provides tissues with mechanical strength (Figure 10.33). Together with the adherens and gap junctional complexes, the desmosomal complex is part of the intercalated disk (ID) structure at the intercellular interface. Recently, mutations in the plakophilin-2 gene have been identified in ARVC patients and mutations in the plakoglobin gene have been identified in Naxos disease, an ARVC variant with autosomal recessive transmission, woolly hair, and palmoplantar keratoderma in addition to the cardiac phenotype. Thus, causative mutations for ARVC and its variants have been identified in three different components of the desmosome: plakoglobin, desmoplakin, and plakophilin, which suggests a new hypothesis on the pathogenic mechanism underlying ARVC. Altered desmosome function may perturb force transmission between cardiomyocytes triggering myocyte death and subsequent fibro-fatty replacement of the damaged myocardium. The

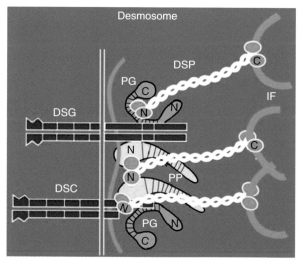

Figure 10.33 Schematic representation of the molecular structure of the desmosome, site of defective proteins in ARVC/D. Desmoplakin is a key component of the desmosome (or macula adherens), a highly organized intermediate filament-associated junctional complex that provides tissues with mechanical strength. PG, plakoglobin; DSP, desmoplakin; PP, plakophilin; DSG, desmoglein; DSC, desmocollin. (Reproduced with permission from Thiene *et al.*, *Orphanet J Rare Dis* 2007;2:1–16.)

heterogeneous distribution of mechanical stress in the ventricle could explain the regional distribution of fibro-fatty replacement, with preference to the thinnest parts of the right ventricular wall. In addition, recent examinations of the distribution of intercalated disk proteins in Naxos disease and Carvajal syndrome, two related disorders, reveal extensive remodeling of the intercalated disk including significant loss of gap junctional plaques. Accordingly, heterogeneous conduction due to alterations in the normal number of gap junctions may also contribute to arrhythmias in ARVC.

Investigating the Molecular Basis of the Arrhythmogenic Right Ventricular Cardiomyopathy Phenotype

The heart relies on specialized structures known as intercalated disks for both mechanical and electrical coupling between its cells. Intercalated disks contain three distinct types of cell-to-cell connection: gap junctions, adherens junctions, and desmosomes. Gap junctions mediate the transfer of ions and small molecules between neighboring cells. Importantly, gap junctions mediate cell-to-cell propagation of the cardiac impulse to ensure synchronous contraction. Each gap junction channel is composed of two hemi-channels, or connexins (Figure 10.34), located within the cytoplasmic membrane of closely apposed cardiomyocytes. Each connexin is formed by an assembly of six connexin subunits, connexin43 (Cx43) being the most important connexin in the mammalian ventricles, including humans. Desmosomes provide mechanical

Gap junctions

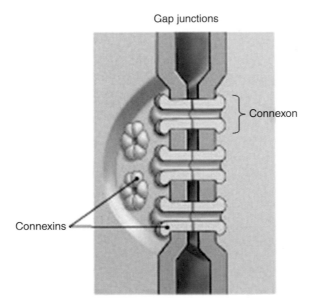

Figure 10.34 Diagrammatic representation of a gap junction plaque and its component proteins. In each plaque, there are multiple gap junctions. Each cell of a pair contributes six connexins to form a connexon and two connexins, one from each cell, form a gap junction.

Adherens junction

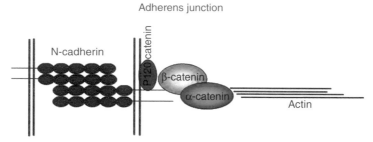

Figure 10.35 Cartoon illustrating the organization of the gap junction. In the human heart, the principal transmembrane protein component of the adherens junction is a Ca^{2+}-dependent glycoprotein known as N-cadherin, which establishes intercellular contact. Attached to the cytoplasmic tail of N-cadherin are β-catenin and plakoglobin (γ-catenin), both of which bind to α-catenin. α-Catenin interacts directly with actin microfilaments within the sarcomere.

attachment between cells. Desmosomes are formed by three separate families of proteins, including the desmosomal cadherins, armadillo proteins, and plakins. These proteins associate with intermediate filaments, including desmin. The major source of force transmission between cardiomyocytes that ensures synchronous contraction are the adherens junctions at the intercalated disk. In the human heart, the principal transmembrane protein component of the adherens junction is a Ca^{2+}-dependent glycoprotein known as N-cadherin, which establishes intercellular contact. As illustrated in Figure 10.35, attached to the cytoplasmic tail of N-cadherin are β-catenin and plakoglobin (γ-catenin), both of which bind to α-catenin. α-Catenin interacts directly with actin micro-filaments within the sarcomere.

Mice deficient in plakoglobin, desmoplakin or plakophilin2 die during embryonic development due to severe myocardial rupture. A conditional desmoplakin knockout mouse develops a severe cardiomyopathy shortly after the deletion of the gene. More relevant from the point of view of clinical cardiology, a number of cases of cardiomyopathy in humans have been linked to mutations in desmosomal proteins. In 2000, Norgett *et al.* provided the first report of a recessive mutation in desmoplakin (truncation of the C-terminal region) that associated with a cardio-cutaneous syndrome, which included a ventricular cardiomyopathy (Carvajal syndrome). In the same year, McKoy *et al.* showed that a deletion in plakoglobin was linked to Naxos disease, an autosomal-recessive cardio-cutaneous syndrome of which ARVC is the cardiac component. Desmoplakin was the first gene linked to an autosomal dominant case of ARVC. More recently, a number of ARVC cases have been linked to mutations in the gene coding for Plakophillin-2. While these mutations have been associated to clinically relevant phenotypes, the consequence of these mutations on the fate of the desmosomal protein, its ability to associate to its partners, or the structural modification to the various components of the intercalated disk (including gap junctions) remains to be determined.

It has been suggested that ARVC may be (at least in most cases) a "disease of the desmosome." Based on the evidence described, it is reasonable to speculate that the arrhythmogenic substrate may be, at least in part, the disruption of the gap junction plaque. In 2004, Dr. Jeffrey Saffitz and his collaborators, then at the University of Washington in St. Louis, reported their observations demonstrating a significant disruption of gap junction integrity in hearts of patients afflicted with Naxos disease (caused by plakoglobin mutation). Further evidence of a link between desmosomes and gap junctions in the heart came recently from the analysis of cardiac tissue obtained from patients with Carvajal syndrome (desmoplakin truncation). Immunofluorescence staining of intercalated disk proteins showed the preservation of N-cadherin and other intercalated disk proteins at the sites of cell-to-cell apposition. However, gap junction plaques were absent. Interestingly, Cx43 was still detectable by Western blot, though the proportion of phosphorylated protein was decreased, consistent with the notion that Cx43 had translocated out of the cell membrane. While much research is needed to determine the molecular and biophysical bases of the disease, these studies showed a fundamental link between desmosomal and gap junction integrity and were the first to postulate its failure as a potential pathophysiologic mechanism.

Summary

We have briefly discussed some important aspects of the clinical manifestations, genetic bases, and cellular mechanisms of the arrhythmias seen in some of the most widely studied heritable arrhythmogenic diseases, including LQTS, Brugada syndrome, SQTS, CPVT, and ARVC. Arguably, the intense amount of scrutiny given to these relatively rare diseases has led to an explosion of new knowledge about the molecular and ionic bases of normal cardiac excitation and propagation. Most important, the identification of the disease loci underlying the currently known inherited arrhythmogenic diseases has greatly contributed to the understanding of the substrate for life-threatening arrhythmias. However, recent work has led to the conclusion that identifying a mutation in a given gene need not establish the diagnosis of a single disease and discovering a mutation in an individual with a known disease is not enough to predict the phenotype of that individual. Therefore, important challenges remain in the understanding of the relationship between genetic defects and their clinical consequences. Arguably, original studies on the functional consequences of specific protein mutations in systems that approximate the physiological environment of these proteins—including expression of mutant proteins in cardiac myocytes, development of transgenic models in animal species, and use of realistic numerical models that simulate the cardiac excitation process in humans—will be useful not only in the characterization of individual mutations, but also in the elucidation of the events underlying the initiation and maintenance of the arrhythmias in question.

Bibliography

The following list of articles, chapters, and monographs is presented to the reader as an additional aid in his or her attempts to gain more in-depth understanding of cardiac electrophysiology. It is not an exhaustive list of references and should be taken as a first step into the vast literature on this subject.

Allessie MA, Bonke FIM, Schopman FJC. Circus movement in rabbit atrial muscle as a mechanism of tachycardia. *Circ Res* 1973; 33:54–62.

Allessie MA, Bonke FIM, Schopman FJC. Circus movement in rabbit atrial muscle as a mechanism of tachycardia. II. The role of nonuniform recovery of excitability in the occurrence of unidirectional block as studied with multiple microelectrodes. *Circ Res* 1976; 39:168–177.

Allessie MA, Bonke FIM, Schopman FJC. Circus movement in rabbit atrial muscle as a mechanism of tachycardia. III. The "leading circle" concept: A new model of circus movement in cardiac tissue without the involvement of an anatomical obstacle. *Circ Res* 1977; 41:9–18.

Allessie MA, Schalij MJ, Kirchhof CJHJ, *et al.* Electrophysiology of spiral waves in two dimensions: The role of anisotropy. *Ann N Y Acad Sci* 1990; 591:247–256.

Allessie MA, Schalij MJ, Kirchhof CJHJ, *et al.* Experimental electrophysiology and arrhythmogenicity: Anisotropy and ventricular tachycardia. *Eur Heart J* 1989; 10:2–8.

Allessie MA, Lammers WJEP, Bonke FIM, Hollen J. Experimental evaluation of Moe's wavelet hypothesis of atrial fibrillation. In: Zipes DP, Jalife J, eds. *Cardiac Electrophysiology and Arrhythmias*. Orlando, FL: Grune & Stratton; 1985.

Antzelevitch C, Bernstein MJ, Feldman H, *et al.* Parasystole, reentry and tachycardia: A canine preparation of cardiac arrhythmias occurring across inexcitable segments of tissue. *Circulation* 1983; 68:1101–1115.

Antzelevitch C, Jalife J, Moe GK. Characteristics of reflection as a mechanism of reentrant arrhythmias and its relationship to parasystole. *Circulation* 1980; 61:182–191.

Antzelevitch C, Jalife J, Moe GK. Electrotonic modulation of pacemaker activity. Further biological and mathematical observations on the behavior of modulated parasystole. *Circulation* 1982; 66:1225–1232.

Anumonwo JMB, Delmar M, Vinet A, *et al.* Phase resetting and entrainment of pacemaker activity in single sinus nodal cells. *Circ Res* 1991; 68:1138–1153.

Anumonwo J, Jalife J. Initiation and modulation of pacemaker activity in cardiac cells. In: Fisch C, Surawicz B, eds. *Cardiac Electrophysiology and Arrhythmias*. New York: Elsevier; 1991:35–50.

Atienza F, Almendral J, Moreno J, Vaidyanathan R, Talkachou A, Kalifa J, Arenal A, Villacastin JP, Torrecilla EG, Sanchez A, Ploutz-Snyder R, Jalife J, Berenfeld O. Activation of inward rectifier potassium channels accelerates atrial fibrillation in humans: Evidence for a reentrant mechanism. *Circulation* 2006; 114:2434–2442.

Barr L, Dewey MM, Berger W. Propagation of action potentials and the structure of the nexus in cardiac muscle. *J Gen Physiol* 1965; 48:797–823.

Barr RC, Plonsey R. Propagation of excitation in idealized anisotropic two dimensional tissue. *Biophys J* 1984; 45:1191–1202.

Basso C, Fox PR, Meurs KM, *et al.* Arrhythmogenic right ventricular cardiomyopathy causing sudden cardiac death in boxer dogs: A new animal model of human disease. *Circulation.* 2004; 109:1180–1185.

Beaumont J, Davidenko N, Davidenko JM, Jalife J. Spiral waves in two-dimensional models of ventricular muscle: Formation of a stationary core. *Biophys J* 1998; 75:1–14.

Benito B, Brugada R, Brugada J, Brugada P. Brugada syndrome. *Prog Cardiovasc Dis* 2008; 51:1–22.

Bennett MVL, Goodenough DM. Gap junctions, electrotonic coupling and intercellular communication. *Neurosci Res Prog Bull* 1978; 16:373–486.

Berenfeld O, Mandapati R, Dixit S, Skanes AC, Chen J, Mansour M, Jalife J. Spatially distributed dominant excitation frequencies reveal hidden organization in atrial fibrillation in the Langendorff-perfused sheep heart. *J Cardiovasc Electrophysiol.* 2000; 11:869–879.

Berenfeld O, Zaitsev AV, Mironov SF, Pertsov AM, Jalife J. Frequency-dependent breakdown of wave propagation into fibrillatory conduction across the pectinate muscle network in the isolated sheep right atrium. *Circ Res.* 2002; 90:1173–1180.

Berenfeld O, Pertsov AM. Dynamics of intramural scroll waves in 3-dimensional continuous myocardium with rotational anisotropy. *J Theor Biol* 1999; 199:383–394.

Berenfeld O. Quantifying activation frequency in atrial fibrillation to establish underlying mechanisms and ablation guidance. *Heart Rhythm* 2007; 4:1225–1234.

Beyer EC, Veenstra RD, Kanter HL, *et al.* Molecular structure and patterns of expression of cardiac gap junction proteins. In: Zipes DP, Jalife J, eds. *Cardiac Electrophysiology. From Cell to Bedside*, 2nd ed. Philadelphia, PA: WB Saunders; 1995:31–38.

Billette J. Atrioventricular nodal activation during periodic premature stimulation of the atrium. *Am J Physiol* 1987; 252:11163–11177.

Bleeker WK, Mackaay AJC, Masson-Pevet M, *et al.* Functional and morphological organization of the rabbit sinus node. *Circ Res* 1980; 46:11–22.

Boineau JP, Cox JL. Slow ventricular activation in acute myocardial infarction. A source of reentrant premature ventricular contractions. *Circulation* 1973; 48:702–713.

Bonke FIM. Electrotonic spread in the sinoatrial node of the rabbit heart. *Pflugers Arch* 1973; 339:17–23.

Botteron GW, Smith JM. Quantitative assessment of the spatial organization of atrial fibrillation in the intact human heart. *Circulation* 1996; 93:513–518.

Brachmann J, Scherlag RJ, Rosenshtraukh LV, *et al.* Bradycardia-dependent triggered activity: Relevance to drug-induced multiform ventricular tachycardia. *Circulation* 1983; 68:846–856.

Brooks CMcC, Lu HH. *The Sinoatrial Pacemaker of the Heart.* Springfield, IL: Charles C Thomas; 1972.

Brown G, Eccles J. The action of a single vagal volley on the rhythm of the heart beat. *J Physiol (London)* 1934; 82:211–241.

Brugada J, Brugada R, Brugada P. Channelopathies: A new category of diseases causing sudden death. *Herz.* 2007; 32:185–191.

Buck J, Buck E. Synchronous fireflies. *Sci Am* 1986; 234:74–85.

Cabo C, Pertsov AM, Baxter WT, *et al.* Wave-front curvature as a cause of slow conduction and block in isolated cardiac muscle. *Circ Res* 1994; 75:1014–1028.

Cabo C, Pertsov AM, Davidenko JM, *et al.* Vortex shedding as a precursor of turbulent cardiac electrical activity in cardiac muscle. *Biophys J* 1996; 70:1105–1111.

Carmeliet E, Vereecke J. Electrogenesis of the action potential and automaticity. *The Cardiovascular System. The Heart.* In: Berne RM, Sperelakis N, Geiger SR, eds. *Handbook of Physiology;* vol I, sect 2. Bethesda, MD: American Physiological Society; 1979.

Catterall WA. Structure and function of voltage-sensitive sodium channels. *Science* 1988a; 242:50–61.

Catterall WA. Molecular pharmacology of voltage-sensitive sodium channels. *ISI Atlas Sci Pharmacol* 1988b; 2:190–195.

Cerrone M, Colombi B, Santoro M, di Barletta MR, Scelsi M, Villani L, Napolitano C, Priori SG. Bidirectional ventricular tachycardia and fibrillation elicited in a knock-in mouse model carrier of a mutation in the cardiac ryanodine receptor. *Circ Res* 2005; 96: e77–82.

Cerrone M, Noujaim SF, Tolkacheva EG, Talkachou A, O'Connell R, Berenfeld O, Anumonwo J, Pandit SV, Vikstrom K, Napolitano C, Priori SG, Jalife J. Arrhythmogenic mechanisms in a mouse model of catecholaminergic polymorphic ventricular tachycardia. *Circ Res* 2007; 101:1039–1048.

Chadda KD, Banka VS, Helfant RH. Rate-dependent ventricular ectopia following coronary occlusion. The concept of an optimal antiarrhythmic heart rate. *Circulation* 1974; 49:654–658.

Chen PS, Wolf PD, Dixon EG, *et al.* Mechanism of ventricular vulnerability to single premature stimuli in open chest dogs. *Circ Res* 1988; 62:1191–1209.

Chen J, Mandapati R, Berenfeld O, Skanes AC, Gray RA, Jalife J. Dynamics of wavelets and their role in atrial fibrillation in the isolated sheep heart. *Cardiovasc Res* 2000; 48:220–232.

Chialvo DR, Gilmour RF, Jalife J. Low dimensional chaos in cardiac tissue. *Nature* 1990a; 343:653–657.

Chialvo DR, Jalife J. Non-linear dynamics of cardiac excitation and impulse propagation. *Nature* 1987; 330:749–752.

Chialvo DR, Michaels DC, Jalife J. Supernormal excitability as a mechanism of chaotic dynamics of activation in cardiac Purkinje fibers. *Circ Res* 1990; 66:525–545.

Clapham DE, Shrier A, DeHaan RL. Junctional resistance and action potential delay between embryonic heart cell aggregates. *J Gen Physiol* 1980; 75:633–654.

Clay JR, Guevara MR, Shrier A. Phase resetting of the rhythmic activity of embryonic heart cell aggregates. *Biophys J* 1984; 45:699–714.

Clerc L. Directional differences of impulse spread in trabecular muscle from mammalian heart. *J Physiol (London)* 1976; 255:335–346.

Coraboeuf E, Deroubaix E, Coulombe A. Acidosis-induced abnormal repolarization and repetitive activity in isolated dog Purkinje fibers. *J Physiol (Paris)* 1980; 76:97–106.

Cranefield P. Action potentials, afterpotentials, and arrhythmias. *Circ Res* 1977; 41:415–423.

Cranefield PF, Klein HO, Hoffman BF. Conduction of the cardiac impulse. I. Delay, block, and one-way block in depressed Purkinje fibers. *Circ Res* 1971; 28:199–219.

Crotti L, Celano G, Dagradi F, Schwartz PJ. Congenital long QT syndrome. *Orphanet J Rare Dis* 2008; 3:18.

Dangman KH, Dresdner KP Jr, Zaim S. Automatic and triggered impulse initiation in canine subepicardial ventricular muscle cells from border zones of 24-hour transmural infarcts. New mechanisms for malignant cardiac arrhythmias? *Circulation* 1988; 78:1020–1029.

Daut J, Maier-Rudolph W, von Beckerath N, *et al.* Hypoxic dilation of coronary arteries is mediated by ATP-sensitive potassium channels. *Science* 1990; 247:1341–1344.

Davidenko JM. Spiral wave activity as a common mechanism for polymorphic and monomorphic ventricular tachycardias. *J Cardiovasc Electrophysiol* 1993; 4:730–746.

Davidenko JM. Spiral waves in the heart: Experimental demonstration of a theory. In: Zipes D, Jalife J, eds. *Cardiac Electrophysiology. From Cell to Bedside.* Philadelphia, PA: WB Saunders; 1994:478–488.

Davidenko JM, Antzelevitch C. The effects of milrinone on conduction, reflection, and automaticity in canine Purkinje fibers. *Circulation* 1984; 69:1026–1035.

Davidenko MJ, Pertsov AM, Salomonsz R, *et al.* Stationary and drifting spiral waves of excitation in isolated cardiac muscle. *Nature* 1991; 355:349–351.

De Bakker JMT, vanCapelle FJL, Janse MJ, *et al.* Reentry as a cause of ventricular tachycardia in patients with chronic ischemic heart disease: Electrophysiologic and anatomic correlations. *Circulation* 1988; 77:589–606.

de la Fuente D, Sasyniuk B, Moe GK. Conductance through a narrow isthmus in isolated canine atrial tissue: A model of the W-P-W syndrome. *Circulation* 1971; 44:803–809.

Delgado C, Steinhaus B, Delmar M, *et al.* Directional differences in excitability and margin of safety for propagation in sheep ventricular epicardial muscle. *Circ Res* 1990; 67:97–110.

Delmar M, Glass L, Michaels DC, *et al.* Ionic bases and analytical solution of the Wenckebach phenomenon in guinea pig ventricular myocytes. *Circ Res* 1989; 65:775–788.

Delmar M, Ibarra J, Davidenko J, *et al.* Dynamics of the background outward current in single guinea pig ventricular myocytes. Ionic mechanisms of hysteresis in cardiac cells. *Circ Res* 1991; 69:1316–1326.

Delmar M. Jalife J. Wenckebach periodicity: Rom deductive electrocardiographic analysis to ionic mechanisms. In: Zipes DP, Jalife J, eds. *Cardiac Electrophysiology. From Cell to Bedside.* Philadelphia, PA: WB Saunders; 1990:128–138.

Delmar M, Jalife J, Michaels DC. Effects of changes in excitability and intercellular coupling on synchronization in the rabbit sino-atrial node. *J Physiol (London)* 1986; 370:127–150.

Delmar M, Michaels DC, Jalife J. The single ventricular myocyte as a model for Wenckebach periodicity. In: Clark WA, Decker RS, Borg TK, eds. *Biology of Isolated Adult Cardiac Myocytes.* New York: Elsevier; 1988:426–429.

Delmar M, Michaels DC, Jalife J. Slow recovery of excitability and the Wenckebach phenomenon in the single guinea pig ventricular myocyte. *Circ Res* 1989; 65:761–774.

Delmar M, Michaels DC, Johnson T, *et al.* Effects of increasing intercellular resistance on transverse and longitudinal propagation in sheep epicardial muscle. *Circ Res* 1987; 60:780–785.

Delmar M, Duffy HS, Soren PL, Taffet SM & Spray DC. Molecular organization and regulation of the cardaic gap junction channel connexin43. In: Zipes DP, Jalife J, ed. *Cardiac Electrophysiology: From Cell to Bedside.* 4th Edition ed. Philadelphia, PA: Saunders; 2004:66–76.

DeMello WC. Passive electrical properties of the atrio-ventricular node. *Pflugers Arch* 1977; 371:135–139.

Di Francesco D. The cardiac hyperpolarizing activated current, I_f. Origins and developments. *Prog Biophys Mol Biol* 1982; 46:163–183.

Di Francesco D. Characterization of single pacemaker channels in cardiac sinoatrial cells. *Nature* 1984; 324:470–473.

Di Francesco D, Tromba C. Muscarinic control of the hyperpolarizationactivated current (I_f) induced by acetylcholine in rabbit sinoatrial node myocytes. *J Physiol (London)* 1986; 371:201–217.

Dillon SM, Allessie MA, Ursell PC, *et al.* Influence of anisotropic tissue structure on reentrant circuit in the epicardial border zone of subacute canine infarcts. *Circ Res* 1988; 63:182.

Dominguez G, Fozzard HA. Influence of extracellular K^+ concentration on cable properties and excitability of sheep cardiac Purkinje fibers. *Circ Res* 1970; 26:565–574.

Downar E, Harris L, Mickleborough LL, *et al.* Endocardial mapping of ventricular tachycardia in the intact human ventricle: Evidence for reentrant mechanisms. *J Am Coll Cardiol* 1988; 11:783–791.

Doyle DA, Morais Cabral J, Pfuetzner RA, Kuo A, Gulbis JM, Cohen SL, Chait BT, MacKinnon R. The structure of the potassium channel: Molecular basis of K+ conduction and selectivity. *Science.* 1998; 280:69–77.

Durrer D, Schoo L, Schuilenburg RM, *et al.* The role of premature beats in the initiation and the termination of supraventricular tachycardia in the Wolff-Parkinson-White syndrome. *Circulation* 1967; 36:461–464.

Ek-Vitorin JF, Calero G, Morley GE, *et al.* pH regulation of connexin43: Molecular analysis of the gating particle. *Biophys J* 1996; 71:1273–1284.

Elharrar V, Surawicz B. Cycle length effect on restitution of action potential duration in dog cardiac fibers. *Am J Physiol* 1983; 244:H782–H792.

El-Sherif N. The figure 8 model of reentrant excitation in the canine post-infarction heart. In: Zipes DP, Jalife J, eds. *Cardiac Electrophysiology and Arrhythmias.* New York: Grune & Stratton; 1985:363–378.

El-Sherif N, Scherlag BJ, Lazzara R, *et al.* Pathophysiology of tachycardia- and bradycardia-dependent block in the canine proximal His-Purkinje system after acute myocardial ischemia. *Am J Cardiol* 1974; 33:529–540.

El-Sherif N, Caref EB, Restivo M. The electrophysiological mechanism of ventricular arrhythmias in the long QT syndrome—Tridimensional mapping of activation and recovery patterns. *Circ Res* 1996; 79:474–492.

Escande D, Coraboeuf E, Planche C. Abnormal pacemaking is modulated by sarcoplasmic reticulum in partially-depolarized myocardial from dilated right atria in humans. *J Mol Cell Cardiol* 1987; 19:231–241.

Farwell D, Gollob MH. Electrical heart disease: Genetic and molecular basis of cardiac arrhythmias in normal structural hearts. *Can J Cardiol* 2007; 23:16A–22A.

Fast VG, Darrow BJ, Saffitz JE, *et al.* Anisotropic activation spread in heart cell monolayers assessed by high-resolution optical mapping. Role of tissue discontinuities. *Circ Res* 1996; 79:115–127.

Fast VG, Kléber AG. Cardiac tissue geometry as a determinant of unidirectional conduction block: Assessment of microscopic excitation spread by optical mapping in patterned cell cultures and in a computer model. *Cardiovasc Res* 1995a; 29:697–707.

Fast VG, Kléber AG. Block of impulse propagation at an abrupt tissue expansion: Evaluation of the critical strand diameter in 2- and 3-dimensional computer models. *Cardiovasc Res* 1995b; 30:449–459.

Fast VG, Kléber AG. Role of wavefront curvature in propagation of cardiac impulse. *Cardiovasc Res* 1997; 33:258–271.

Fast VG, Pertsov AM. Drift of a vortex in the myocardium. *Biophysics* 1990; 35:489–494.

Feinberg WM, Blackshear JL, Laupacis A, Kronmal R, Hart RG. Prevalence, age distribution, and gender of patients with atrial fibrillation. *Arch Intern Med.* 1995; 155:469–473.

Fenoglio JJ, Pham TD, Harken AH, *et al.* Recurrent sustained ventricular tachycardia: Structure and ultrastructure of subendocardial regions in which tachycardia originates. *Circulation* 1983; 68:518–533.

Ferrier GR, Saunders JH, Mendez C. A cellular mechanism for the generation of ventricular arrhythmias by acetylstrophanthidin. *Circ Res* 1973; 32:600–609.

Fozzard HA, Levin DN, Walton M. Control of conduction velocity in cardiac Purkinje fibers. In: Paes de Carvalho A, Hoffman BF, Lieberman M, eds. *Normal and Abnormal Conduction in the Heart.* Mount Kisco, NY: Futura; 1982:105–116.

Francis J, Antzelevitch C. Atrial fibrillation and Brugada syndrome. *J Am Coll Cardiol* 2008; 51:1149–1153.

Frazier DW, Krassowska W, Chen PS, *et al.* Transmural activations and stimulus potentials in three-dimensional anisotropic canine myocardium. *Circ Res* 1988; 63:135–146.

Frazier DW, Wolf PD, Wharton JM, *et al.* Stimulus-induced critical point: Mechanism for the electrical initiation of reentry in normal canine myocardium. *J Clin Invest* 1989; 83:1039–1052.

Friedman DL, Steward JR, Wit AL. Spontaneous and induced cardiac arrhythmias in subendocardial Purkinje fibers surviving extensive myocardial infarction. *Circ Res* 1973; 32:612–626.

Furuse A, Matsuo H, Saigusa M. Effects of intervening beats on ectopic cycle length in a patient with ventricular parasystole. *Jpn Heart J* 1981; 22:201–209.

Gallavardin L. Extrasystolic ventriculaire a paroxysmes tachycardiques prolonges. *Arch Mal Coeur Vaiss* 1922; 15:298–306.

Gallicano GI, Kouklis P, Bauer C, Yin M, Vasioukhin V, Degenstein L, Fuchs E. Desmoplakin is required early in development for assembly of desmosomes and cytoskeletal linkage. *J Cell Biol* 1998; 143:2009–2022.

Garfinkel A, Spano ML, Ditto WL, *et al.* Controlling cardiac chaos. *Science* 1992; 257:1230–1235.

Garrey WE. Auricular fibrillation. *Physiol Rev* 1924; 4:215.

Gellens ME, George AL, Chen L, *et al.* Primary structure and functional expression of the human cardiac tetrodotoxin-insensitive voltage-dependent sodium channel. *Proc Natl Acad Sci USA* 1992; 89:554–558.

Gerisch G. Standienpezifische aggregationsmuster bei dictyostelium discoideum. *Wilhelm Roux Archiv Entwick Org* 1965; 156:127–144.

Gerull B, Heuser A, Wichter T, *et al.* Mutations in the desmosomal protein plakophilin-2 are common in arrhythmogenic right ventricular cardiomyopathy. *Nat Genet* 2004; 36:1162–1164.

Giles W, van Ginneken A, Shibata EF. Ionic currents underlying cardiac pacemaker activity: A summary of voltage-clamp data from single cells. In: Nathan RD, ed. *Cardiac Muscle: The Regulation of Excitation and Contraction.* New York: Academic Press; 1986:1–27.

Giles WR. Shibata EF. Voltage clamp of bull-frog cardiac pacemaker cells: A quantitative analysis of potassium currents. *J Physiol (London)* 1985; 368:265–292.

Gillete PC, Garson A Jr. Electrophysiologic and pharmacologic characteristics of automatic ectopic atrial tachycardia. *Circulation* 1977; 56:571–575.

Gilmour RF Jr, Watanabe M. Dynamics of circus movement reentry across canine Purkinje–muscle junctions. *J Physiol (London)* 1994; 476:473–485.

Goldenberg I, Moss AJ. Long QT syndrome. *J Am Coll Cardiol* 2008; 51:2291–2300.

Goldreyer BN, Gallagher JJ, Damato AN. The electrophysiologic demonstration of atrial ectopic tachycardia in man. *Am Heart J* 1973; 85:205–215.

Goodenough DA. Gap junction dynamics and intercellular communication. *Pharmacol Rev* 1979; 30:383–392.

Gorelova NA, Bures J. Spiral waves of spreading depression in the isolated chicken retina. *Neurobiology* 1983; 14:353–363.

Grossmann KS, Grund C, Huelsken J, *et al.* Requirement of plakophilin 2 for heart morphogenesis and cardiac junction formation. *J Cell Biol* 2004; 167:149–160.

Grant AO, Katzung BG. The effects of quinidine and verapamil on electrically induced automaticity in the ventricular myocardium of guinea pig. *J Pharm Exp Ther* 1976; 196:407–419.

Gray RA, Jalife J, Panfilov A, *et al.* Nonstationary vortexlike reentrant activity as a mechanism of polymorphic ventricular tachycardia in the isolated rabbit heart. *Circulation* 1995a; 91:2454–2469.

Gray RA, Jalife J, Panfilov A, *et al.* Mechanisms of cardiac fibrillation. *Science* 1995b; 270:1222–1225.

Gray RA, Pertsov AM, Jalife J. Incomplete reentry and epicardial breakthrough patterns during atrial fibrillation in the sheep heart. *Circulation* 1996; 94:2649–2661.

Gray RA, Pertsov AM, Jalife J. Spatial and temporal organization during cardiac fibrillation. *Nature* 1998; 392:75–78.

Greenbaum RA, Ho SY, Gibson DG, *et al.* Left ventricular fiber architecture in man. *Br Heart J* 1981; 45:248–263.

Guevara MR, Glass L. Phase locking, period-doubling bifurcations and chaos in a mathematical model of a periodically driven oscillator: A theory for the entrainment of biological oscillators and the generation of cardiac dysrhythmias. *J Math Biol* 1982; 14:1–23.

Guevara MR, Glass L, Shrier A. Phase locking, period-doubling bifurcations, and irregular dynamics in periodically stimulated cardiac cells. *Science* 1981; 214:1350–1353.

Gul'ko FB, Petrov AA. Mechanism of the formation of closed pathways of conduction in excitable media. *Biophysics* 1972; 17:271–281.

Gutstein DE, Morley GE, Tamaddon H, *et al.* Conduction slowing and sudden arrhythmic death in mice with cardiac-restricted inactivation of connexin43. *Circ Res* 2001; 88:333–339.

Gutstein DE, Morley GE, Vaidya D, *et al.* Heterogeneous expression of gap junction channels in the heart leads to conduction defects and ventricular dysfunction. *Circulation.* 2001; 104:1194–1199.

Hagiwara N, Irisawa H, Kameyama M. Contribution of two types of calcium currents to the pacemaker potentials of rabbit sino-atrial nodel cells. *J Physiol (London)* 1998; 395:85–100.

Haïssaguerre M, Jais P, Shah DC, Takahashi A, Hocini M, Quiniou G, Garrigue S, Le Mouroux A, Le Metayer P, Clementy J. Spontaneous initiation of atrial fibrillation by ectopic beats originating in the pulmonary veins. *N Engl J Med* 1998; 339:659–666.

Hamill OP, Marty A, Neher E, *et al.* Improved patch clamp techniques for high resolution current recording from cells and cell-free membrane patches. *Pflugers Arch* 1981; 391:85–100.

Hanck D. Biophysics of sodium channels. In: Zipes D, Jalife J, eds. *Cardiac Electrophysiology. From Cell to Bedside.* 2nd ed. Philadelphia, PA: WB Saunders; 1995:65–74.

Harada A, Sasaki K, Fukushima T, Ikeshita M, Asano T, Yamauchi S, Shoji T. Atrial activation during chronic atrial fibrillation in patients with isolated mitral valve disease. *Ann Thorac Surg* 1996; 61:104–112.

Harris AL. Emerging issues of connexin channels: Biophysics fills the gap. *Q Rev Biophys* 2001; 34:325–472.

Hauswirth O, Noble D, Tsien RW. The mechanism of oscillatory activity at low membrane potentials in cardiac Purkinje fibers. *J Physiol (London)* 1969; 200:255–265.

Henthorn RW, Okumura K, Olshansky B, *et al.* A fourth criterion for transient entrainment: The electrogram equivalent of progressive fusion. *Circulation* 1988; 77:1003–1012.

Hille, B. *Ionic Channels of Excitable Membrane*, 2nd ed. Sunderland, MA: Sinauer Associates; 1992.

His W. Ein fall von Adams-Stokes'scher Krankeit mit ungleichzeitigem schlagen der vorhofe u. Herzkammern (Herzblock). *Dtsch Arch Klin Med* 1899; 64:316–331.

Hodgkin AL. Evidence for electrical transmission in nerve. I. *J Physiol (London)* 1937a; 90:183–210.

Hodgkin AL. Evidence for electrical transmission in nerve. II. *J Physiol (London)* 1937b; 90:211–232.

Hodgkin AL, Huxley AF. A quantitative description of membrane current and its application to conduction and excitation in nerve. *J Physiol (London)* 1952; 117:500–544.

Hoffman BF. Cardiac electrogenesis. In: *Frontiers of Cardiac Electrophysiology.* The Hague, The Netherlands: Martinus Nijhoff; 1983:1–12.

Hoffman BF, Cranefield PF. *Electrophysiology of the Heart.* New York: McGrawHill; 1960.

Hoffman BF, Dangman KH. Are arrhythmias caused by automatic impulse generation? In: Paes de Carvalho A, Hoffman BF, Lieberman M, eds. *Normal and Abnormal Conduction in the Heart.* Mount Kisco, NY: Futura; 1982:429–448.

Hoffman BF, Paes de Carvalho A, DeMello WC. Transmembrane potentials of single fibers of the atrio-ventricular node. *Nature* 1958; 181:66–67.

Hoshi T, Zagotta W, Aldrich R. Biophysical and molecular mechanisms of shaker potassium channel inactivation. *Science* 1990; 250:568–571.

Hoshino K, Anumonwo J, Delmar M, *et al.* Wenckebach periodicity in single atrioventricular nodal cells from the rabbit heart. *Circulation* 1990; 82:2201–2216.

Hulot JS, Jouven X, Empana JP, Frank R, Fontaine G. Natural history and risk stratification of arrhythmogenic right ventricular dysplasia/cardiomyopathy. *Circulation* 2004; 110: 1879–1884.

Hunter PJ, Smail BH. The analysis of cardiac function: A continuum approach. *Prog Biophys Mol Biol* 1988; 52:101–164.

Imanishi S. Calcium-sensitive discharge in canine Purkinje fibers. *Jpn J Physiol* 1971; 2:443–463.

Irisawa H, Hagiwara N. Pacemaker mechanism of mammalian sinoatrial node cells. In: Mazgalev T, Dreifus L, Michelson E, eds. *Electrophysiology of Sinoatrial and Atrioventricular Nodes.* New York: Alan R. Liss; 1988:33–52.

Jack JJB, Noble D, Tsien RW. *Electric Current Flow in Excitable Cells.* London: Oxford University Press; 1983.

Jalife J. The sucrose gap preparation as a model of AV nodal transmission: Are dual pathways necessary for reciprocation and AV nodal echoes? *Pacing Clin Electrophysiol* 1983; 6:1106–1122.

Jalife J. Mutual entrainment and electrical coupling as mechanisms for synchronous firing of rabbit sino-atrial pace-maker cells. *J Physiol (London)* 1984; 356:221–243.

Jalife J. Chaos theory and the study of arrhythmogenesis. I. *ACC Curr J Rev* 1993a; May/June:13–16.

Jalife J. Chaos theory and the study of arrhythmogenesis. II. *ACC Curr J Rev* 1993a; July/August:13–16.

Jalife J, Antzelevitch C, Moe GK. The case for modulated parasystole. *Pacing Clin Electrophysiol* 1982; 5:911–926.

Jalife J, Antzelevitch C, Moe GK. Rate-dependent changes in excitability of depressed cardiac Purkinje fibers as a mechanism of intermittent bundle branch block. *Circulation* 1983; 62:912–922.

Jalife J, Delmar M. Ionic basis of the Wenckebach phenomenon. In: Glass L, Hunter P, McCulloch A, eds. *Theory of Heart*. New York: Springer-Verlag; 1991:359–376.

Jalife J, Gray R. Drifting vortices of electrical waves underlie ventricular fibrillation in the rabbit heart. *Acta Physiol Scand* 1996; 157:123–131.

Jalife J, Hamilton AJ, Lamanna VR, *et al.* Effects of current flow on pacemaker activity of the isolated kitten sino-atrial node. *Am J Physiol* 1980; 238:H307–H316.

Jalife J, Michaels DC. Phase-dependent interactions of cardiac pacemakers as mechanisms of control and synchronization in the heart. In: Zipes DP, Jalife J, eds. *Cardiac Electrophysiology and Arrhythmias*. Orlando, FL: Grune & Stratton; 1985:109–119.

Jalife J, Moe GK. Effect of electrotonic potentials on pacemaker activity of canine Purkinje fibers in relation to parasystole. *Circ Res* 1976; 39:801–808.

Jalife J, Moe GK. A biologic model of parasystole. *Am J Cardiol* 1979; 43:761–722.

Jalife J, Moe GK. Excitation, conduction and reflection of impulses in isolated bovine and canine cardiac Purkinje fibers. *Circ Res* 1981; 49:233–247.

Jalife J, Sicouri S, Delmar M, *et al.* Electrical uncoupling and impulse propagation in isolated sheep Purkinje fibers. *Am J Physiol* 1989; 257:H179–H189.

Jalife J, Slenter VAJ, Salata JJ, *et al.* Dynamic vagal control of pacemaker activity in the mammalian sinoatrial node. *Circ Res* 1983; 52:642–656.

Jalife J, Berenfeld O, Mansour M. Mother rotors and fibrillatory conduction: A mechanism of atrial fibrillation. *Cardiovasc Res* 2002; 54:204–216.

Jalife J, Berenfeld O. Molecular mechanisms and global dynamics of fibrillation: An integrative approach to the underlying basis of vortex-like reentry. *J Theor Biol* 2004; 230:475–487.

James TN. Pulse and impulse in the sinus node. *Henry Ford Hosp Med J* 1967; 15:275–299.

James TN. The sinus node. *Am J Cardiol* 1977; 40:965–986.

James TN, Sherf L, Fine G, *et al.* Comparative ultrastructure of the sinus node in man and dog. *Circulation* 1966; 34:139–163.

Janse MJ, Opthof T. Mechanisms of ischemia-induced arrhythmias. In: Zipes D, Jalife J, eds. *Cardiac Electrophysiology. From Cell to Bedside*. 2nd ed. Philadelphia, PA: Grune & Stratton; 1995:489–496.

January C, Cunningham P, Zhou Z. Pharmacology of L- and T-type calcium channels in the heart. In: Zipes D, Jalife J, eds. *Cardiac Electrophysiology. From Cell to Bedside*. 2nd ed. Philadelphia, PA: Grune & Stratton; 1995:269–277.

Jiang Y, Ruta V, Chen J, Lee A, MacKinnon R. The principle of gating charge movement in a voltage-dependent K+ channel. *Nature* 2003; 423:42–48.

Jiang D, Xiao B, Zhang L, Chen SR. Enhanced basal activity of a cardiac Ca2+ release channel (ryanodine receptor) mutant associated with ventricular tachycardia and sudden death. *Circ Res* 2002; 91:218–225.

Jiang D, Xiao B, Yang D, Wang R, Choi P, Zhang L, Cheng H, Chen SR. RyR2 mutations linked to ventricular tachycardia and sudden death reduce the threshold for store-overload-induced Ca2+ release (SOICR). *Proc Natl Acad Sci U S A* 2004; 101:13062–13067.

Jiang D, Wang R, Xiao B, Kong H, Hunt DJ, Choi P, Zhang L, Chen SR. Enhanced store overload-induced Ca2+ release and channel sensitivity to luminal Ca2+ activation are common defects of RyR2 mutations linked to ventricular tachycardia and sudden death. *Circ Res* 2005; 97:1173–1181.

Johnson N, Danilo P, Wit A, *et al.* Response to pacing of triggered activity occurring in catecholamine-treated canine coronary sinus. *Circulation* 1986; 74:1168–1179.

Jongsma HJ, Masson-Pevet M, Hollander CC, *et al.* Synchronization of the beating frequency of cultured rat heart cells. In: Lieberman M, Sano T, eds. *Development and Physiological Correlates of Cardiac Muscle.* New York: Raven; 1973:185–196.

Josephson ME, Horowitz LN, Farshidi A. Continuous local electrical activity. A mechanism of recurrent ventricular tachycardia. *Circulation* 1978; 57:659–665.

Joyner RW, Westerfeld M, Moore JW. Effects of cellular geometry on current flow during a propagated action potential. *Biophys J* 1980; 31:183–194.

Kalifa J, Jalife J, Zaitsev AV, Bagwe S, Warren M, Moreno J, Berenfeld O, Nattel S. Intra-atrial pressure increases rate and organization of waves emanating from the superior pulmonary veins during atrial fibrillation. *Circulation* 2003; 108:668–671.

Kalifa J, Klos M, Zlochiver S, Mironov S, Tanaka K, Ulahannan N, Yamazaki M, Jalife J, Berenfeld O. Endoscopic fluorescence mapping of the left atrium: A novel experimental approach for high resolution endocardial mapping in the intact heart. *Heart Rhythm* 2007; 4:916–924.

Kass RS, Lederer WJ, Tsien RW, *et al.* Role of calcium ions in transient inward currents and aftercontractions induced by strophantidin in cardiac Purkinje fibers. *J Physiol (London)* 1978; 281:187–208.

Kaplan SR, Gard JJ, Protonotarios N, *et al.* Remodeling of myocyte gap junctions in arrhythmogenic right ventricular cardiomyopathy due to a deletion in plakoglobin (naxos disease). *Heart Rhythm* 2004; 1:3–11.

Kaplan SR, Gard JJ, Carvajal-Huerta L, Ruiz-Cabezas JC, Thiene G, Saffitz JE. Structural and molecular pathology of the heart in carvajal syndrome. *Cardiovasc Pathol* 2004; 13:26–32.

Katz A. *Physiology of the Heart.* 2nd ed. New York: Raven; 1992.

Katz B. *Nerve, Muscle and Synapse.* New York: McGraw-Hill; 1966.

Katzung B, Morgenstern J. Effects of extracellular potassium on ventricular automaticity and evidence for a pacemaker current in mammalian ventricular myocardium. *Circ Res* 1977; 40:105–111.

Kauffman R, Rothberger CJ. Beitrage zur kenntnis der entstehungsweise extra systolischer Allorhythmien IV. *Ges Exp Med* 1920; 11:40–62.

Kay GN, Epstein AE, Plumb VJ. Resetting of ventricular tachycardia: Implications for localizing the area of slow conduction. *J Am Coll Cardiol* 1988; 11:522–529.

Keener JP. On cardiac arrhythmias: AV conduction block. *J Math Biol* 1981; 12:215–225.

Keener JP. An eikonal-curvature equation for action potential propagation in myocardium. *J Math Biol* 1991; 29:629–651.

Keener JP, Panfilov AV. Three-dimensional propagation in the heart: The effects of geometry and fiber orientation on propagation in myocardium. In: Zipes DP, Jalife J, eds. *Cardiac Electrophysiology. From Cell to Bedside.* 2nd ed. Philadelphia, PA: WB Saunders; 1995:335–347.

Keener JP, Tyson JJ. Spiral waves in the Belousov-Zhabotinskii reaction. *Physica D* 1986; 21:307–324.

Kléber AG, Rudy Y. Basic mechanisms of cardiac impulse propagation and associated arrhythmias. *Physiol Rev* 2004; 84(2):431–488.

Kobayashi Y, Kikushima S, Tanno K, *et al.* Sustained left ventricular tachycardia terminated by dipyridamole. Cyclic cAMP-mediated triggered activity as a possible mechanism. *Pacing Clin Electrophysiol* 1994; 17:377–385.

Kodama I, Boyett MR. Regional differences in the electrical activity of the rabbit sinus node. *Pflugers Arch* 1985; 404:214–226.

Krinsky VI. Mathematical models of cardiac arrhythmias (spiral waves). *Pharm Ther B* 1978; 3:539–555.

Laitinen PJ, Brown KM, Piippo K, Swan H, Devaney JM, Brahmbhatt B, Donarum EA, Marino M, Tiso N, Viitasalo M, Toivonen L, Stephan DA, Kontula K. Mutations of the cardiac ryanodine receptor (RyR2) gene in familial polymorphic ventricular tachycardia. *Circulation* 2001; 103:485–490.

Lauer MR, Rusy BF, Davis LD. H+-induced membrane depolarization in canine cardiac Purkinje fibers. *Am J Physiol* 1984; 247:H312–H321.

Lazar S, Dixit S, Marchlinski FE, Callans DJ, Gerstenfeld EP. Presence of left-to-right atrial frequency gradient in paroxysmal but not persistent atrial fibrillation in humans. *Circulation* 2004; 110:3181–3186.

Lechleiter J, Girard S, Peralta E, *et al.* Spiral calcium wave propagation and annihilation in *Xenopus laevis* oocytes. *Science* 1991; 252:123–126.

Lehnart SE, Wehrens XH, Marks AR. Calstabin deficiency, ryanodine receptors, and sudden cardiac death. *Biochem Biophys Res Commun* 2004; 322:1267–1279.

Lerman BB, Stein K, Engelstein EF, *et al.* Mechanism of repetitive monomorphic ventricular tachycardia. *Circulation* 1995; 92:421–429.

Lerman BB, Wesley RRC, DiMarco JP Jr., *et al.* Antiadrenergic effects of adenosine on His-Purkinje automaticity. Evidence for accentuated antagonism. *J Clin Invest* 1988; 82:2127–2136.

Levy MN, Martin PJ, Zieske H, *et al.* Role of positive feedback in the atrioventricular nodal Wenckebach phenomenon. *Circ Res* 1974; 24:697–710.

Lewis T. *The Mechanism and Graphic Registration of the Heart Beat.* London: Shaw and Sons; 1925.

Li M, West JW, Lai Y, Scheuer T, Catterall WA. Functional modulation of brain sodium channels by cAMP-dependent phosphorylation. *Neuron* 1992; 8:1151–1159.

Liu S, Taffet S, Stoner L, *et al.* A structural basis for the unequal sensitivity of the major cardiac and liver gap junctions to intercellular acidification: The carboxyl tail length. *Biophys J* 1993; 64:1422–1433.

Loewenstein WR. Junctional intercellular communication. The cell-to-cell membrane channel. *Physiol Rev* 1981; 61:829–913.

Long SB, Campbell EB, MacKinnon R. Voltage-sensor of Kv1.2: Structural basis of electromechanical coupling. *Science* 2005; 309:903–908.

Luo CH, Rudy Y. A dynamic model of the cardiac ventricular action potential. I. Simulations of ionic currents and concentration changes. *Circ Res* 1994; 74:1071–1096.

Mandapati R, Skanes A, Chen J, Berenfeld O, Jalife J. Stable microreentrant sources as a mechanism of atrial fibrillation in the isolated sheep heart. *Circulation.* 2000; 101:194–199.

Manjunath CK, Page E. Cell biology and protein composition of cardiac gap junctions. *Am J Physiol* 1985; 248:H783–H791.

Mann JE, Spereklakis N. Further development of a model for electrical transmission between myocardial cells not connected by low resistance pathways. *J Electrocardiol* 1979; 12:23–33.

Mansour M, Mandapati R, Berenfeld O, Chen J, Samie FH, Jalife J. Left-to-right gradient of atrial frequencies during acute atrial fibrillation in the isolated sheep heart. *Circulation* 2001; 103:2631–2636.

Masson-Pevet M, Bleeker WM, Cyros D. The plasma membrane of leading pacemaker cells in the rabbit sinus node: A qualitative and quantitative ultrastructural analysis. *Circ Res* 1979; 45:621–629.

Mendez C, Mueller WJ, Urquiaga X. Propagation of impulses across the Purkinje fiber-muscle junctions in the dog heart. *Circ Res* 1970; 26:135–150.

Merideth J, Mendez C, Mueller WJ, *et al.* Electrical excitability of atrioventricular nodal cells. *Circ Res* 1968; 23:69–85.

Michaels DC, Matyas EP, Jalife J. A mathematical model of the effects of acetylcholine pulses on sinoatrial pacemaker activity. *Circ Res* 1984; 55:89–101.

Michaels DC, Matyas EP, Jalife J. Dynamic interactions and mutual synchronization of sino-atrial node pacemaker cells. *Circ Res* 1986; 58:706–720.

Michaels DC, Matyas EP, Jalife J. Mechanisms of sinoatrial pacemaker synchronization: A new hypothesis. *Circ Res* 1987; 61:704–714.

Mines GR. On circulating excitation on heart muscles and their possible relation to tachy-cardia and fibrillation. *Trans R Soc Can* 1914; 4:43–53.

Mironov S, Jalife J, Tolkacheva EG. Role of conduction velocity restitution and short-term memory in the development of action potential duration alternans in isolated rabbit hearts. *Circulation* 2008; 118:17–25.

Moak JP, Rosen MR. Induction and termination of triggered activity by pacing in isolated canine Purkinje fibers. *Circulation* 1984; 69:149–162.

Mobitz W. Uber die unvollstandige storung der erregungsuberleitung zwischen Vorhof and Kammer des Menschlichen Herzens. *Z Ges Exp Med* 1925; 41:180–237.

Moe GK, Childers RW, Merideth J. An appraisal of "supernormal" A-V conduction. *Circulation* 1968; 38:5–28.

Moe GK, Jalife J, Mueller WJ, *et al.* A mathematical model of parasystole and its application to clinical arrhythmias. *Circulation* 1977; 56:968–979.

Moe GK, Abildskov JA. Atrial fibrillation as a self-sustaining arrhythmia independent of focal discharges. *Am Heart J* 1959; 58:59–70.

Moe GK, Rheinboldt WC, Abildskov JA. A computer model of atrial fibrillation. *Am Heart J* 1964; 67:200–220.

Morillo CA, Klein GJ, Jones DL, Guiraudon CM. Chronic rapid atrial pacing: Structural, functional, and electrophysiological characteristics of a new model of sustained atrial fibrillation. *Circulation* 1995; 91:1588–1595.

Morita H, Wu J, Zipes DP. The QT syndromes: Long and short. *Lancet* 2008; 372:750–763.

Muller SC, Plesser T, Hess B. The structure of the core of the spiral wave in the Belousov-Zhabotinsky reagent. *Science* 1985; 230:661–663.

Muñoz V, Grzeda KR, Desplantez T, Pandit SV, Mironov S, Taffet SM, Rohr S, Kléber AG, Jalife J. Adenoviral expression of IKs contributes to wavebreak and fibrillatory conduction in neonatal rat ventricular cardiomyocyte monolayers. *Circ Res* 2007; 101:475–483.

Myerburg RJ, Kessler KM, Interian A Jr., *et al.* Clinical and experimental pathophysiology of sudden cardiac death. In: Zipes DP, Jalife J, eds. *Cardiac Electrophysiology. From Cell to Bedside.* Philadelphia, PA: WB Saunders; 1990:666.

Nakayama T, Kurachi Y, Noma, A, *et al.* Action potentials and membrane currents of single pacemaker cells of the rabbit heart. *Pflugers Arch* 1984; 402:248–257.

Nanthakumar K, Jalife J, Massé S, Downar E, Pop M, Asta J, Ross H, Rao V, Mironov S, Sevaptsidis E, Rogers J, Wright G, Dhopeshwarkar R. Optical mapping of Langendorff-perfused human hearts: Establishing a model for the study of ventricular fibrillation in humans. *Am J Physiol Heart Circ Physiol* 2007; 293:H875–H880.

Napolitano C, Bloise R, Priori SG. Long QT syndrome and short QT syndrome: How to make correct diagnosis and what about eligibility for sports activity. *J Cardiovasc Med (Hagerstown)* 2006; 7:250–256.

Nathan RD. Two electrophysiologically distinct types of cultured pacemaker cells from rabbit sinoatrial node. *Am J Physiol* 1986; 250:H325–H329.

Nattel S. New ideas about atrial fibrillation 50 years on. *Nature* 2002; 415:219–226.

Nattel S, Shiroshita-Takeshita A, Cardin S, Pelletier P. Mechanisms of atrial remodeling and clinical relevance. *Curr Opin Cardiol* 2005; 20:21–25.

Nau GJ, Aldariz AE, Acunzo R, *et al.* Modulation of parasystolic activity by nonparasystolic beats. *Circulation* 1982; 66:462–469.

Nay-Ungvarai A, Pertsov AM, Hess B, *et al.* Lateral instabilities of a wave front in the Ce-catalized Belousov-Zhabotinsky reaction. *Phys D* 1992; 61:205–212.

Nernst W. *Theoretical Chemistry From the Standpoint of Avogadro's Rule and Thermodynamics.* London: McMillan; 1895.

Nielsen PMF, Le Grice IJ, Smaill BH, *et al.* Mathematical model of geometry and fibrous structure of the heart. *Am J Physiol* 1991; 260:H1365–H1378.

Noble D. Ionic basis of rhythmic activity in the heart. In: Zipes D, Jalife J, eds. *Cardiac Electrophysiology and Arrhythmias.* Orlando, FL: Grune & Stratton; 1985:3–11.

Noble D. *The Initiation of the Heartbeat.* New York: Oxford University Press; 1979.

Noma, A. ATP-regulated K^+ channels in cardiac muscle. *Nature* 1983; 305:147–148.

Noma A, Irisawa H. Membrane currents in the rabbit sinoatrial node as studied by the double microelectrode method. *Pflugers Arch* 1976; 364:45–52.

Noujaim SF, Pandit SV, Berenfeld O, Vikstrom K, Cerrone M, Mironov S, Zugermayr M, Lopatin AN, Jalife J. Up-regulation of the inward rectifier K+ current (IK1) in the mouse heart accelerates and stabilizes rotors. *J Physiol* 2007; 578:315–326.

Noujaim SF, Berenfeld O, Kalifa J, Cerrone M, Nanthakumar K, Atienza F, Moreno J, Mironov S, Jalife J. Universal scaling law of electrical turbulence in the mammalian heart. *Proc Natl Acad Sci U S A* 2007; 104:20985–20989.

Olgin JE, Kalman JM, Fitzpatrick AP, *et al.* Role of right atrial endocardial structures as barriers to conduction during human type I atrial flutter. Activation and entrainment guided by intracardiac echocardiography. *Circulation* 1995; 92:1839–1848.

Ono K, Fozzard A, Hanck D. Mechanisms of cAMP-dependent modulation of cardiac sodium channel current kinetics. *Circ Res* 1993; 72:807.

Opthof T, de Jonge B, Mackaay AFC, *et al.* Functional and morphological organization of the guinea-pig sinoatrial node compared with the rabbit sinoatrial node. *J Mol Cell Cardiol* 1985; 17:549–564.

Oral H, Pappone C, Chugh A, Good E, Bogun F, Pelosi F Jr., Bates ER, Lehmann MH, Vicedomini G, Augello G, Agricola E, Sala S, Santinelli V, Morady F. Circumferential pulmonary-vein ablation for chronic atrial fibrillation. *N Engl J Med* 2006; 354:934–941.

Paes de Carvalho A, de Almeida DF. Spread of activity through the atrioventricular node. *Circ Res* 1960; 8:801–809.

Panfilov AV, Keener JP. Reentry in an anatomical model of the heart. *Chaos Solitons Fractals* 1995; 5:681–689.

Patel C, Antzelevitch C. Pharmacological approach to the treatment of long and short QT syndromes. *Pharmacol Ther* 2008; 118:138–151.

Perkel DH, Schulman JH, Bullock TH, *et al.* Pacemaker neurons: Effect of regularly spaced synaptic input. *Science* 1964; 145:61–63.

Pertsov AM, Davidenko JM, Salomonsz R, *et al.* Spiral waves of excitation underlie reentrant activity in isolated cardiac muscle. *Circ Res* 1993; 72:631–650.

Pertsov AM, Ermakova EA. Mechanism of the drift of spiral wave in an inhomogeneous medium. *Biophysics* 1988; 33:338–341.

Pertsov AM, Emarkova EA, Panfilov AV. Rotating spiral waves in modified FitzHugh-Nagumo model. *Physica D* 1984; 14:117.

Pertsov AM, Jalife J. Three-dimensional vortex-like reentry. In: Zipes DP, Jalife J, eds. *Cardiac Electrophysiology. From Cell to Bedside.* 2nd ed. Philadelphia, PA: WB Saunders; 1995:403–410.

Pfaffinger, PJ, Martin JM, Hunter DD, *et al.* GTD-binding proteins couple cardiac muscarinic receptors to a K channel. *Nature* 1985; 317:536–538.

Pinsker HM. Synaptic modulation of endogenous neuronal oscillators. *Fed Proc* 1977; 36:2045–2049.

Pittendrigh C. On the mechanism of the entrainment of a circadian rhythm by light cycles. In: Aschoff J, ed. *Circadian Clocks.* Amsterdam: Elsevier North-Holland; 1965:277–297.

Pollack GII. Cardiac pacemaking: An obligatory role of catecholamines? *Science* 1965; 196:277–297.

Preisig-Muller R, Schlichthorl G, Goerge T, Heinen S, Bruggemann A, Rajan S, Derst C, Veh RW, Daut J. Heteromerization of Kir2.x potassium channels contributes to the phenotype of Andersen's syndrome. *Proc Natl Acad Sci U S A* 2002; 99:7774–7779.

Priori SG, Napolitano C. Cardiac and skeletal muscle disorders caused by mutations in the intracellular Ca2+ release channels. *J Clin Invest* 2005; 115:2033–2038.

Priori SG, Napolitano C, Tiso N, Memmi M, Vignati G, Bloise R, Sorrentino V, Danieli GA. Mutations in the cardiac ryanodine receptor gene (hRyR2) underlie catecholaminergic polymorphic ventricular tachycardia. *Circulation* 2001; 103:196–200.

Priori SG, Pandit SV, Rivolta I, Berenfeld O, Ronchetti E, Dhamoon A, Napolitano C, Anumonwo J, di Barletta MR, Gudapakkam S, Bosi G, Stramba-Badiale M, Jalife J. A novel form of short QT syndrome (SQT3) is caused by a mutation in the KCNJ2 gene. *Circ Res* 2005; 96:800–807.

Randall WC. Sympathetic control of the heart. In: Randall WC, ed. *Neural Regulation of the Heart.* New York: Oxford University Press; 1977:45.

Robinson GA, Butcher RW, Sutherland, EW. Cyclic AMP. New York: Academic Press; 1971.

Roden DM. Clinical practice. Long-QT syndrome. *N Engl J Med* 2008; 358:169–176.

Rogers JM, Huang J, Melnick SB, Ideker RE. Sustained reentry in the left ventricle of fibrillating pig hearts. *Circ Res.* 2003; 92:539–545.

Rohr S, Kucera JP, Fast V, *et al.* Paradoxical improvement of impulse conduction in cardiac tissue by partial cellular uncoupling. *Science* 1997; 275:841–844.

Rosen MR, Anyukhovsky EP. Arrhythmias triggered by afterdepolarizations. In: Fisch C, Surawicz B, eds. *Cardiac Electrophysiology and Arrhythmias.* New York: Elsevier; 1991:67–75.

Rosen MR, Gelband HB, Merker C, *et al.* Mechanism of digitalis toxicity. Effects of ouabain on phase 4 of canine Purkinje fiber transmembrane potentials. *Circulation* 1973; 47:681–689.

Rosenblueth A. Functional refractory period of cardiac tissues. *Am J Physiol* 1958a; 194:171–183.

Rosenblueth A. Mechanism of the Wenckebach-Luciani cycyles. *Am J Physiol* 1958b; 194:491–494.

Rozanski GJ, Jalife J, Moe GK. Determinants of post-repolarization refractoriness in depressed mammalian ventricular muscle. *Circ Res* 1984; 55:486–496.

Rudenko AN, Panfilov AV. Drift and interaction of vortices in two-dimensional heterogeneous active medium. *Stud Biophys* 1983; 98:183–188.

Rushton WAH. Initiation of the propagated disturbance. *Proc Roy Soc B Biol Sci* 1937; 124:210.

Rushton WAH, Klebes AG, Fleischhauer J, Cascio W. Ischemia-induced propagation failure in the heart. In: Zipes DP and Jalife J, eds. *Cardiac Electrophysiology. From Cell to Bedside.* 2nd ed. Philadelphia, PA: WB Saunders; 1995:174–182.

Saffitz JE. Dependence of electrical coupling on mechanical coupling in cardiac myocytes. In: Thiene G, Pessina AC, ed. *Advances in Cardiovascular Medicine.* Padova, Italy: Universita degli Studi di Padova; 2003:15–28.

Sahadevan J, Ryu K, Peltz L, Khrestian CM, Stewart RW, Markowitz AH, Waldo AL. Epicardial mapping of chronic atrial fibrillation in patients: Preliminary observations. *Circulation* 2004; 110:3293–3299.

Sakakibara Y, Wasserstrom JA, Furukawa T, *et al.* Characterization of the sodium current in single human atrial myocytes. *Circ Res* 1992; 71:535–546.

Salama G, Morad M. Merocyanine 540 as an optical probe of transmembrane electrical activity in the heart. *Science* 1976; 191:485–487.

Samie FH, Berenfeld O, Anumonwo J, Mironov SF, Udassi S, Beaumont J, Taffet S, Pertsov AM, Jalife J. Rectification of the background potassium current: A determinant of rotor dynamics in ventricular fibrillation. *Circ Res* 2001; 89:1216–1223.

Sanders P, Berenfeld O, Hocini M, Jais P, Vaidyanathan R, Hsu LF, Garrigue S, Takahashi Y, Rotter M, Sacher F, Scavee C, Ploutz-Snyder R, Jalife J, Haissaguerre M. Spectral analysis identifies sites of high-frequency activity maintaining atrial fibrillation in humans. *Circulation* 2005; 112:789–797.

Sanguinetti M, Jurkiewicz N. Delayed rectifier potassium channels of cardiac muscle. In: Spooner P, Brown A, Catteral A, *et al.* eds. *Ion Channels in the Cardiovascular System.* Armonk, NY: Futura; 1994:121–143.

Sano T, Sawanobori T, Adaniya H. Mechanism of rhythm determination among pacemaker cells of the mammalian sinus node. *Am J Physiol* 1978; 235:H379–H384.

Sano T, Takayama N, Shimamoto T. Directional difference of conduction velocity in cardiac ventricular syncytium studied by microelectrodes. *Circ Res* 1959; 7:262–267.

Sarmast F, Kolli A, Zaitsev A, Parisian K, Dhamoon AS, Guha PK, Warren M, Anumonwo JMB, Taffet SM, Berenfeld O, Jalife J. Cholinergic atrial fibrillation: I-K,I-ACh gradients determine unequal left/right atrial frequencies and rotor dynamics. *Cardiovas Res* 2003; 59:863–873.

Sasyniuk BI, Mendez C. A mechanism for reentry in canine ventricular tissue. *Circ Res* 1971; 28:3–15.

Scheinman MM, Basu D, Hollengerg M. Electrophysiologic demonstration of atrial ectopic tachycarida in man. *Am Heart J* 1973; 85:205–215.

Scherf D. Studies on auricular tachycardia caused by aconitine administration. *Proc Soc Exp Biol Med* 1947; 64:233–239.

Scherlag BJ, El-Sherif N, Hope RR, *et al.* Characterization and localization of ventricular arrhythmias resulting from myocardial ischemia and infarction. *Circ Res* 1974; 35:372–383.

Schimpf R, Borggrefe M, Wolpert C. Clinical and molecular genetics of the short QT syndrome. *Curr Opin Cardiol* 2008; 23:192–198.

Schmitt FO, Erlanger J. Directional differences in the conduction of the impulse through the heart muscle and their possible relation to extrasystolic and fibrillatory contractions. *Am J Physiol* 1928; 87:326–347.

Schuessler RB, Grayson TM, Bromberg BI, *et al.* Cholinergically mediated tachyarrhythmias induced by a single extrastimulus in the isolated canine right atrium. *Circ Res* 1992; 71:1254–1267.

Schuessler RB, Kawamoto T, Hand DE, *et al.* Simultaneous epicardial and endocardial activation sequence mapping in the isolated canine right atrium. *Circulation* 1993; 88:250–263.

Schwartz PJ, Crotti L. Ion channel diseases in children: Manifestations and management. *Curr Opin Cardiol* 2008; 23:184–191.

Schwieler JH, Zlochiver S, Pandit SV, Berenfeld O, Jalife J, Bergfeldt L. Reentry in an accessory atrioventricular pathway as a trigger for atrial fibrillation initiation in manifest

Wolff-Parkinson-White syndrome: A matter of reflection? *Heart Rhythm* 2008; 5:1238–1247.

Segers M. Les phenomenes de synchronisation au niveau du Coeur. *Arch Int Physiol* 1946; 54:87–105.

Sen-Chowdhry S, Syrris P, McKenna WJ. Genetics of right ventricular cardiomyopathy. *J Cardiovasc Electrophysiol* 2005; 16:927–935.

Shibata G. Ionic currents which generate the spontaneous diastolic depolarizations in individual cardiac pacemaker cells. *Proc Natl Acad Sci U S A* 1985; 82:7796–7800.

Shibata J. The effects of barium on the action potential and the membrane current of sheep heart Purkinje fibers. *J Pharmacol Exp Ther* 1973; 183:418–426.

Shrier A, Adjemian RA, Munk AA. Ionic mechanisms of atrioventricular nodal cell excitability. In: Zipes DP, Jalife J, eds. *Cardiac Electrophysiology. From Cell to Bedside.* 2nd ed. Philadelphia, PA: WB Saunders; 1995:164–173.

Shrier A, Dubarski H, Rosengarten M, *et al.* Prediction of complex atrioventricular conduction rhythms in humans with use of the atrioventricular nodal recovery curve. *Circulation* 1987; 76:1196–1205.

Sih HJ, Zipes DP, Berbari EJ, Adams DE, Olgin JE. Differences in organization between acute and chronic atrial fibrillation in dogs. *J Am Coll Cardiol* 2000; 36:924–931.

Skanes AC, Mandapati R, Berenfeld O, Davidenko JM, Jalife J. Spatiotemporal periodicity during atrial fibrillation in the isolated sheep heart. *Circulation* 1998; 98:1236–1248.

Smits JP, Blom MT, Wilde AA, Tan HL. Cardiac sodium channels and inherited electrophysiologic disorders: A pharmacogenetic overview. *Expert Opin Pharmacother* 2008; 9:537–549.

Spach MS, Dolber PC, Heidlage JF. Influence of the passive anisotropic properties on directional differences in propagation following modification of sodium conductance in human atrial muscle: A model of reentry based on anisotropic discontinuous propagation. *Circ Res* 1988; 62:811–832.

Spach MS, Dolber PC, Heidlage JF. Interaction of inhomogeneities of repolarization with anisotropic propagation in dog atria. A mechanism for both preventing and initiating reentry. *Circ Res* 1989; 65:1612–1631.

Spach MS, Kootsey JM. The nature of electrical propagation in cardiac muscle. *Am J Physiol* 1983; 244:H3–H22.

Spach MS, Kootsey JM, Sloan JD. Active modulation of electrical coupling between cardiac cells in the dog: A mechanism for transient and steady state variations in conduction velocity. *Circ Res* 1982a; 51:347–362.

Spach MS, Miller WT III, Dolber PC, *et al.* The functional role of structural complexities in the propagation of depolarization in the atrium of the dog. Cardiac conduction disturbances due to discontinuities of effective axial resistivity. *Circ Res* 1982b; 50:175–191.

Spach MS, Miller WT III, Geselowitz DB, *et al.* The discontinuous pattern of propagation in normal canine cardiac muscle. *Circ Res* 1981; 48:39–54.

Spach MS, Miller WT III, Miller-Jones, E, *et al.* Extracellular potentials related to intracellular action potentials during impulse conduction in anisotropic canine cardiac muscle. *Circ Res* 1979; 45:188–204.

Sperelakis N. Electrical properties of embryonic heart cells. In: De Mello WC, ed. *Electrical Phenomena of the Heart.* New York: Academic Press; 1972:1–61.

Sperelakis N. Propagation mechanisms in heart. *Annu Rev Physiol* 1976; 41:441–457.

Sperelakis N. Origin of the cardiac resting potential. The cardiovascular system. The heart. In: Berne RM, Sperelakis N, Geiger SR, eds. *Handbook of Physiology*, vol I, sect 2. Bethesda, MD: American Physiological Society; 1979.

Sperelakis N. Cable properties and propagation of action potentials. In: Sperelakis N, ed. *Cell Physiology. Source Book.* San Diego, CA: Academic Press; 1994:245–254.

Stockbridge N. Differential conduction at axonal bifurcations. II. Theoretical basis. *J Neurophysiol* 1988; 59:1286–1295.

Stockbridge N, Stockbridge LL. Differential conduction at axonal bifurcations. I. Effect of electrotonic length. *J Neurophysiol* 1988; 59:1277–1285.

Streeter D. Gross morphology and fiber geometry of the heart. The heart. The cardiovascular system. In: Berne RM, ed. *Handbook of Physiology*, vol I, sect 2. Baltimore, MD: American Physiological Society; 1979:61–112.

Sung RJ, Huycke EC, Lai WT, *et al.* Clinical and electrophysiologic mechanisms of exercise-induced ventricular tachyarrhythmias. *Pacing Clin Electrophysiol* 1988; 11:1347–1357.

Sutherland EW Jr., Wosilait WD. Inactivation and activation of liver phosphorylase. *Nature* 1955; 175:169–70.

Syrris P, Ward D, Asimaki A, Sen-Chowdhry S, Ebrahim HY, Evans A, Hitomi N, Norman M, Pantazis A, Shaw AL, Elliott PM, McKenna WJ. Clinical expression of plakophilin-2 mutations in familial arrhythmogenic right ventricular cardiomyopathy. *Circulation* 2006; 113:356–364.

Taccardi B, Macchi E, Lux RL, *et al.* Effect of myocardial fiber direction on epicardial potentials. *Circulation* 1994; 90:3076–3090.

Talajic M, Papadatos D, Villemarie C, *et al.* A unified model of atrioventricular nodal conduction predicts dynamic changes in Wenckebach periodicity. *Circ Res* 1991; 68:1280–1293.

Tanaka K, Zlochiver S, Vikstrom KL, Yamazaki M, Moreno J, Klos M, Zaitsev AV, Vaidyanathan R, Auerbach DS, Landas S, Guiraudon G, Jalife J, Berenfeld O, Kalifa J. Spatial distribution of fibrosis governs fibrillation wave dynamics in the posterior left atrium during heart failure. *Circ Res* 2007; 101:839–847.

Tiso N, Stephan DA, Nava A, Bagattin A, Devaney JM, Stanchi F, Larderet G, Brahmbhatt B, Brown K, Bauce B, Muriago M, Basso C, Thiene G, Danieli GA, Rampazzo A. Identification of mutations in the cardiac ryanodine receptor gene in families affected with arrhythmogenic right ventricular cardiomyopathy type 2 (ARVD2). *Hum Mol Genet* 2001; 10:189–194.

Tiso N, Salamon M, Bagattin A, Danieli GA, Argenton F, Bortolussi M. The binding of the RyR2 calcium channel to its gating protein FKBP12.6 is oppositely affected by ARVD2 and VTSIP mutations. *Biochem Biophys Res Commun* 2002; 299:594–598.

Tourneur Y. Action potential-like responses due to the inward rectifying potassium channel. *J Membr Biol* 1986; 90:115–122.

Tranum-Jensen J. The fine structure of the atrial and atrioventricular (AV) junctional specialized tissues of the rabbit heart. In: Wellens HJJ, Lie KI, Janse MJ, eds. *The Conduction System of the Heart.* Leiden, The Netherlands: Stenfert Kroese BV; 1976:51–81.

Trautwein W, Osterrieder W. Mechanisms of beta adrenergic modulation and cholinergic control of Ca and K currents in the heart. In: Hathan RD, ed. *Cardiac Muscle: The Regulation of Excitation and Contraction.* Orlando, FL: Academic Press; 1986:87–128.

Tsuobi N, Kodama I, Takayama J, *et al.* Anisotropic conduction properties of canine ventricular muscles. *Jpn Circ J* 1985; 49:487–498.

Tyson JJ, Keener JP. Singular perturbation theory of travelling waves in excitable media. Review. *Physica D* 1988; 32:327–361.

Ursell PC, Gardner PI, Albala A, *et al.* Structural and electrophysiological changes in the epicardial border of canine myocardial infarcts during infarct healing. *Circ Res* 1985; 56:436–451.

Vaquero M, Calvo D, Jalife J. Cardiac fibrillation: From ion channels to rotors in the human heart. *Heart Rhythm* 2008; 5:872–879.

Vasalle M. Cardiac pacemaker potentials at different extra- and intracellular K concentration. *Am J Physiol* 1965; 208:770.

Vasalle M. The relationship among cardiac pacemakers. Overdrive suppression. *Circ Res* 1977; 41:47–55.

Vassalle M, Levine MJ, Studkey JH. On the sympathetic control of ventricular automaticity: The effect of stellate ganglion stimulation. *Circ Res* 1968; 23:249.

Veenstra RD, DeHaan RL. Electrotonic interactions between aggregates of chick embryo cardiac pacemaker cells. *Am J Physiol* 1986; 250:H453–H465.

Walsh B, Kass R. Distinct voltage-dependent regulation of a heart delayed IK by protein kinase A and C. *Am J Physiol* 1991; 261:C1081–C1090.

Warren M, Guha PK, Berenfeld O, Zaitsev A, Anumonwo JMB, Dhamoon AS, Bagwe S, Taffet SM, Jalife J. Blockade of the inward rectifying potassium current terminates ventricular fibrillation in the guinea pig heart. *J Cardiovasc Electrophysiol* 2003; 14:621–631.

Wehrens XH, Lehnart SE, Huang F, Vest JA, Reiken SR, Mohler PJ, Sun J, Guatimosim S, Song LS, Rosemblit N, D'Armiento JM, Napolitano C, Memmi M, Priori SG, Lederer WJ, Marks AR. FKBP12.6 deficiency and defective calcium release channel (ryanodine receptor) function linked to exercise-induced sudden cardiac death. *Cell* 2003; 113:829–840.

Wehrens XH, Lehnart SE, Reiken SR, Deng SX, Vest JA, Cervantes D, Coromilas J, Landry DW, Marks AR. Protection from cardiac arrhythmia through ryanodine receptor-stabilizing protein calstabin2. *Science* 2004; 304:292–296.

Weidmann S. Effect of current flow on the membrane potential of cardiac muscle. *J Physiol (London)* 1951; 115:227–236.

Weidmann S. The electrical constants of Purkinje fibers. *J Physiol (London)* 1952; 118:348–360.

Weidmann S. The effect of cardiac membrane potential on the rapid availability of the sodium carrying system. *J Physiol (London)* 1955; 127:213–224.

Weidmann S. The diffusion of radiopotassium across intercalated disks of mammalian cardiac muscle. *J Physiol (London)* 1966; 187:323–342.

Wellens HJJ, Durrer DR, Lie Kl. Observations on mechanisms of ventricular tachycardia in man. *Circulation* 1976; 54:237–244.

Wellens HJJ, Schuilenburg RM, Durrer D. Electrical stimulation of the heart in patients with ventricular tachycardia. *Circulation* 1972; 46:216–226.

Wellner M, Berenfeld O, Jalife J, Pertsov AM. Minimal principle for rotor filaments. *Proc Natl Acad Sci U S A* 2002; 99:8015–8018.

Wenckebach KF. Zur analyse des unregelmassigen pulses. II. Ueber den regelmassig intermittirenden puls. *Z Kin Med* 1899; 37:475–488.

Wiener N, Rosenblueth A. The mathematical formulation of the problem of conduction of impulses in a network of connected excitable elements, specifically in cardiac muscle. *Arch Inst Cardiol Mex* 1946; 16:1.

Wijffels MC, Kirchhof CJ, Dorland R, Allessie MA. Atrial fibrillation begets atrial fibrillation. A study in awake chronically instrumented goats. *Circulation* 1995; 92:1954–1968.

Wilders R, Jongsma HJ, van Ginneken AC. Pacemaker activity of the rabbit sinoatrial node. A comparison of mathematical models. *Biophys J* 1991; 60:1202–1216.

Winfree A. Estimating the ventricular fibrillation threshold. In: Glass L, Hunter P, McCulloch A, eds. *Theory of Heart*. New York: Springer-Verlag; 1991:477–532.

Winfree AT. Spiral waves of chemical activity. *Science* 1972; 175:634–636.

Winfree AT. Scroll-shaped waves in chemical activity in three dimensions. *Science* 1973; 181:937–939.

Winfree AT. *The Geometry of Biological Time.* New York: Springer-Verlag; 1980.

Winfree AT. *When Time Breaks Down.* Princeton, NJ: Princeton University Press; 1987.

Winfree AT. Electrical instability in cardiac muscle: Phase singularities and rotors. *J Theor Biol* 1989; 138:353–405.

Winfree AT. Electrical turbulence in three-dimensional heart muscle. *Science* 1994; 266:1003–1006.

Winfree AT. Theory of spirals. In: Zipes DP, Jalife J, eds. *Cardiac Electrophysiology. From Cell to Bedside.* 2nd ed. Philadelphia, PA: WB Saunders; 1995:379–389.

Winkle RA. The relationship between ventricular ectopic beat arrhythmias. In: Levy M, Vassalle M, eds. *Excitation and Neural Control of the Heart.* Baltimore, MD: American Physiological Society; 1982.

Wit AL, Dillon SM, Coromilas J, *et al.* Anisotropic reentry in the epicardial border zone of myocardial infarcts. *Ann N Y Acad Sci* 1990; 591:86–108.

Wit AL, Hoffman BF, Cranefield PF. Slow conduction and reentry in the ventricular conducting system. I. Return extrasystole in canine Purkinje fibers. *Circ Res* 1972; 30:1–10.

Wit AL, Janse MJ. Relationship of experimental delayed ventricular arrhythmias to clinical arrhythmias. In: Wit AL, Janse MJ, eds. *The Ventricular Arrhythmias of Ischemia and Infarction: Electrophysiological Mechanisms.* Mount Kisco, NY: Futura; 1993:285–291.

Yazawa K, Kameyama M. Mechanisms of receptor-mediated modulation of the delayed outward potassium current in guinea pig ventricular myocytes. *J Physiol* 1990; 421:135–150.

Yanagihara K, Noma A, Irisawa H. Reconstruction of sinoatrial node pacemaker potential based on the voltage clamp experiments. *Jpn J Physiol* 1980; 30:841–857.

Yatani A, Codina J, Imoto Y, *et al.* Direct regulation of mammalian cardiac calcium channels by a G protein. *Science* 1987; 238:1288–1292.

Ye B, Valdivia CR, Ackerman MJ, *et al.* A common human SCN5A polymorphism modifies expression of an arrhythmia causing mutation. *Physiol Genomics* 2003; 12:187–193.

Zimmerman M, Maisonblanche P, Cauchemez B, *et al.* Determinants of the spontaneous ectopic activity in repetitive monomorphic idiopathic ventricular tachycardia. *J Am Coll Cardiol* 1986; 7:1219–1227.

Zipes DP, Bailey JC, Elharrar V, eds. *The Slow Inward Current and Cardiac Arrhythmias.* The Hague, The Netherlands: Martinus Nijhoff; 1980.

Zipes DP, Jalife J. *Cardiac Electrophysiology. From Cell to Bedside.* Philadelphia, PA: WB Elsevier, Inc. 2004.

Zipes DG, Mendez C. (1973) Actions of manganese ions and tetrodotoxin on atrioventricular nodal transmembrane potentials in isolated rabbit hearts. *Circ Res* 1973; 32:447–454.

Zipes DG, Mendez C, Moe GK. Some examples of Wenckebach periodicity in cardiac tissues, with an appraisal of mechanisms. In: Elizari MV, Rosenbaum MB, eds. *Frontiers of Cardiac Electrophysiology.* Boston, MA: Martinus Nijhoff; 1983:357–375.

Zlochiver S, Munoz V, Vikstrom KL, Taffet SM, Berenfeld O, Jalife J. Electrotonic myofibroblast-to-myocyte coupling increases propensity to reentrant arrhythmias in 2-dimensional cardiac monolayers. *Biophys J* 2008; 95:4469–4480.

Zykov VS. *Simulations of Wave Processes in Excitable Media.* Manchester, England: Manchester University Press; 1987.

Index

Page numbers in *italics* indicate figures. Page numbers followed by "t" indicate tables.